Tasks for the Veterinary Assistant

Tasks for the Veterinary Assistant

Fourth Edition

Teresa F. Sonsthagen, BS, LVT

WILEY Blackwell

Registered Office
John Wiley & Sons, Inc., 111 River Street, Hoboken, NJ 07030, USA

Editorial Office
111 River Street, Hoboken, NJ 07030, USA

For details of our global editorial offices, customer services, and more information about Wiley products visit us at www.wiley.com.

Wiley also publishes its books in a variety of electronic formats and by print-on-demand. Some content that appears in standard print versions of this book may not be available in other formats.

Library of Congress Cataloging-in-Publication Data
Names: Sonsthagen, Teresa F., author. | Pattengale, Paula. Tasks for the veterinary assistant.
Title: Tasks for the veterinary assistant / Teresa F. Sonsthagen, BS, LVT.
Description: Fourth edition. | Hoboken, NJ : Wiley-Blackwell, 2020. | Revised edition of: Tasks
    for the veterinary assistant / Paula Pattengale, Teresa Sonsthagen. Third edition. 2014. | Includes bibliographical
    references and index.
Identifiers: LCCN 2019025690 (print) | LCCN 2019025691 (ebook) | ISBN 9781119466826 (paperback) |
    ISBN 9781119466802 (adobe pdf) | ISBN 9781119466833 (epub)
Subjects: LCSH: Veterinary medicine–Handbooks, manuals, etc. | Animal health technicians–Handbooks,
    manuals, etc.
Classification: LCC SF748 .P38 2020 (print) | LCC SF748 (ebook) | DDC 636.089/069–dc23
LC record available at https://lccn.loc.gov/2019025690
LC ebook record available at https://lccn.loc.gov/2019025691

Cover images: © Dmytro Zinkevych/Shutterstock (cat standing), © didesign021/Shutterstock (dog at vet),
© Maria Sbytova/Shutterstock (female vet doctor using stethoscope), © Viktoriia Hnatiuk/Shutterstock
(syringe with injection of medicine)
Cover design by Wiley

Set in 10/12pt New Baskerville by SPi Global, Pondicherry, India

SKY10079471_071224

CONTENTS

Preface   ix

Acknowledgments   xi

About the Companion Website   xiii

1 Professional Conduct and Foundation Skills   1

Determining Your Role in a Veterinary Practice   1
Meeting Employer Expectations – 10 Behaviors to Master   4
Professional Appearance   8
Effective Communication Skills Within the Veterinary Practice   10
    Verbal Communication   10
    Non-verbal Communication   10
    Client Communication   10
    Written Communication   11
Computer Competency   11
Use and Misuse of Social Media   12
Determining Credible Web Sources   12
Anticipation of Workflow   12
Application of Veterinary Ethics   13
Human–Animal Bond   13
Grief Process   14
Foundation Skills – Veterinary Practice Math and Medical Terminology   14
    Basic Math Used in the Veterinary Practice   14
    Estimating   16
    Volume Measurements – Dilutions   16
    Drug Calculation   18
    Medical Terminology   18

2 Laws, Policies, and OSHA Standards Affecting Veterinary Practice   21

Laws and Regulations for Veterinary Practices   21
    Federal Laws   21
    State Laws   23
    Common or Case Law   24
    Local Ordnances   25
Guidelines of Practice from Veterinary Organizations   26
Occupational Safety and Health Administration (OSHA) – Workplace Safety   26
    Labeling   27
    Personal Protection Equipment   27

3 Veterinary Business Protocols   33

Front Office Skills   34
    Telephone Skills   34
    Scheduling Appointments   35
    Handling Non-Client Calls   37
Client Interactions at the Facility   38
    Arrivals   38
    Admitting Patients   39
    Discharging Clients   39
Veterinary Medical Record Keeping Procedures   40
    Computerized Versus Paper Patient Records   40
    Paper Patient Record Assembly   41
    Paper Filing Systems   41
    Chronological Order or SOAP File Format   42
    Transferring Medical Records   42
    Forms, Certificates, and Logs   43
Day's End Protocols   45
Inventory Control   46
    Daily Inventory Control   47
    Ordering Supplies   48
    Receiving Shipments   48
    Handling Shipments and Invoices   48
    Restocking Shelves   48

4 Facility and Equipment Maintenance – Cleaning for Disease Control   51

Basic Cleanliness and Orderliness   52
    Cleaning   54
    Disinfecting   54
Hospital Waste – Non-Hazardous versus Hazardous   55
Cleaning Techniques When Caring for Hospitalized Animals   57
    Order of Cleaning   57
Facility Maintenance   60
    Hospital Laundry   61
Equipment Maintenance   62

5 Anatomy and Physiology   73

"Speaking" Anatomy   73
Body Systems   75
    Skeletal System   75
    Muscular System   78
    Cardiovascular System   78
    Respiratory System   81

Immune System	81
Digestive System	82
Urinary System	84
Reproductive System	85
Nervous System	86
Endocrine System	88
Integumentary System	88
Suggested Reading	89

6 Introduction to Animals   91

Scientific Classification of Animals	91
Phenotypes	92
Introduction to Genetics	94
Breeds of Animals	96
Herding Group	96
Hound Group	96
Non-Sporting Group	97
Sporting Group	97
Terrier Group	99
Working Group	100
Toy Group	101
Cat Breeds	101
Pocket Pets	104
Determining the Sex of Companion Animals	107

7 Feeds and Feeding   111

Essential Nutrients –The Basics	112
Understanding Pet Food Labels	113
Learning to Read Labels	113
List of Ingredients	114
Adequacy Statement	114
Feeding Guidelines	115
Dry Matter Basis	115
Application of Basic Nutrition	115
Calorie Requirements	115
How Much to Feed	116
Prescription Diets	117
Feeding the Hospitalized Patient	117
Water Availability and Consumption	119
Feeding Livestock and Poultry	119
Feeding Other Species	120
References	120
Suggested Reading	120

8 Restraint of Animals   121

Restraint of Companion Animals	122
Patient Defenses	122
Assessing Behavior and Safely Approaching Companion Animals	123
Utilize Fear Free Techniques	129
Safely Moving Patients from One Location to Another	131
General Restraint Techniques for Dogs and Cats	133
Restraint for Examinations, Medications, and Procedures	134
Restraint Equipment	139
Restraint of Pocket Pets	143

Restraint of Pet Birds	143
Restraint of Livestock	144
Assessing Behavior and Safely Approaching Livestock	145
Restraint Techniques for Horses and Livestock	146
Reference	151
Suggested Reading	151

9 Knots and Ropes   153

Knot Tying Terminology	153
Types of Ropes	154
Prevent Fraying	154
Hanking a Rope	156
Types of Knots and Hitches	157
Types of Knots	157
Hitches	162
Suggested Reading	165

10 Management of Hospitalized and Boarding Pets   167

Housing Requirements – Kennel Set-up	168
Water and Food Consumption – Elimination	168
Environmental Considerations	169
Socialization and Exercising Hospitalized Patients	170
Patient Care Based on Reason for Being in the Hospital	170
Boarding	170
Surgical Patients	171
Recumbent Patient Care	171
Constipated Patients – Enemas	172
Contagious Patients	173
Feral and Quarantine Animal Housing	173
Pocket Pets and Birds	174
Treatments and Procedures	174
Medical Records	174
Understanding the Disease Process	174
Treatment Plan Protocols	175
In-hospital Grooming	179
Combing and Brushing	179
Clipping Hair or Fur	179
Identifying Ectoparasites	180
Bathing and Dipping	181
Collection of Fecal and Urine Samples	182
Pain Evaluation and Monitoring	183
Discharging Patients	184
Veterinary Hospice Care	184
Euthanasia and Post Mortem Protocols	185
After the Euthanasia	186
Reference	187
Suggested Reading	187

11 Clinical Techniques   189

Toenail Trimming	190
Clipping Birds' Wings	191
Expressing Anal Glands	192

Administration of Medications   193
    Ear Cleaning and Medicating   194
    Topical Medications   196
    Oral Medications   197
    Ophthalmic Medications   200
Syringes and Needles   201
    Preparing Syringe and Needle for Use   203
    Solution Bottle Preparation   204
    Preparing Vaccines   204
Injections   205
    Subcutaneous Injections   206
    Subcutaneous Fluid Administration   206
    Intramuscular Injections   207
    Intranasal Infusion   208
Monitoring IV Fluid Administration and IV
    Catheter Maintenance   208
Wound Care and Bandaging   210
    Apply a Simple Bandage   211
    Bandage Failure   214
    Bandage Removal   214
Emergency Support   214
    Maintenance of Crash Cart Kit or
        Emergency Station   215
Suggested Reading   215

12   Laboratory Skills   217

Maintenance of Stain Sets   218
Staining Protocol   219
Laboratory Log Book   219
Maintenance of the Common Laboratory
    Equipment in the Veterinary Lab   220
    Binocular Microscope   220
    Centrifuge   221
    Refractometer   222
Sample Collection   222
    Parasitology   223
Blood Collection and Handling   229
    Equipment Set-up   229
    Blood Sample Handling   230
    Blood Chemistry and Electrolyte
        Determinations   234
    Serologic Test Kits   235
    Urine Collection   235
    Microbiology – Sample Collection   238
Necropsy: Preparation and Follow-Up   240
    Preparing Samples for Shipment
        to Reference Laboratory   241
Vaginal Cytology Collection   242

13   Pharmacy Skills   243

Controlled Drugs   244
Reading a Prescription   245
Labeling a Prescription Container   246
Safe Handling of Dispensed Drugs   247
Prescription Packaging   248
Explaining Prescriptions to the Owner   248
Classification of Medications   250
Suggested Reading   250

14   Surgical Room Skills   251

Cleaning and Maintaining the
    Surgery Suite   252
    Gas Anesthesia Machine   255
    Cleaning the Surgical Instruments   256
    Assembling Surgical Packs   257
    Cold Sterilization   269
Surgery Skills and Maintaining an Aseptic
    Environment   270
    Pre-Surgical Phase   270
    Peri-Surgical Phase   274
    Post-Surgical Phase   278
    Post-Surgical Emergencies   279
Client Communication   279
Removing Sutures   279
Reference   281

**15   Dental Skills for the Veterinary
       Assistant   283**

Assistant's Role in Veterinary Dentistry   283
Dental Anatomy   283
Dental Terminology   284
Directional Terms   284
Dental Formulas   285
Age Approximation Based on Dental Eruption   285
Head Type   285
Dental Instruments, Equipment, and Maintenance   285
    Preparation of Dental Instruments   287
    Sharpening Hand Instruments   287
Power Scalers   287
    Selection of the Correct Handpiece Tip   288
Air-Driven Dental Units   288
Dental Prophylaxis   289
Polishing Follows Dental Cleaning   289
Charting the Oral Examination   289
    Triadan Numbering System   289
    Anatomical Numbering System   290
    Charting Symbols   291
Basics of Pocket Pet Dentistry   292
Dental Formula for Pocket Pets   292
    Ferret Dentition   292
    Hedgehog Dentition   292
Intraoral Radiography   293
    Patient Positioning for Dental Radiography   293
    Manual Developing of Dental Radiographs   294
Patient Care and Clean-up   294
Client Education   294
    Daily Dental Care   295
    Dental Patient Discharge Instructions   295
Suggested Reading   295

**16   Diagnostic Imaging and
       Endoscopy   297**

Introduction to Diagnostic Imaging   298
Digital Radiography   298
Advanced Imaging Technologies   298
Quality Assurance   299

Radiation Safety   299
Radiography Abbreviations   301
Radiography Procedure   302
Radiography Log   302
Measuring the Anatomy with Calipers   302
Setting Exposure Factors Using the
  Technique Charts   303
Cassette Selection   304
Film Labeling   304
Taking a Radiograph   304
Developing Radiographic Film   306
Cassette Routine Maintenance   307
Patient Film Filing   307
Darkroom Maintenance   307
    Checking for Light Leaks   308
    Processor Maintenance   308
Diagnostic Ultrasonography   309
    Set-up for Ultrasonography   309

Endoscopy   310
Introduction to Endoscopy   310
Parts of an Endoscope   310
Endoscopy Preparation   311
Endoscopy: Post Procedure   312
    Gas Sterilization   314
    Cold (Liquid) Sterilization   314
End of Procedure Cleaning   315
References   315
Suggested Reading   315

**APPENDIX: Suffixes, Prefixes, and Anatomic
Terms (Roots)**   **317**

Glossary   **323**

Index   **331**

PREFACE

Reference Book and Task Card Box

A usual day in most veterinary practices is often fast paced and demanding. As a new person it is sometimes difficult to find someone that is free to answer a question or clarify an instruction. The amount of information an assistant needs to know can be staggering, and it seems like you have to know it *all* on the first day!

A technique used in many veterinary technology programs is to have the students put together a reference book or a task card box. The idea is to put key activities and information at your fingertips or in a central location for quick reference. The information in the reference book is usually common information or standard operating procedures and the task card box is usually reminders for tasks that need to be performed weekly, monthly, or yearly. This information can be tailored to the practice in which you work or can be used right from this book as a means to study for exams. The information you gather from this textbook should be close to the standards of care maintained at any veterinary clinic in which you find employment and just needs to be modified to the "way they like things."

The reference book and task card box can be made very simply with prehole punched index cards that can be kept bound together with "D-rings" or a binder made for index cards. The index card fits nicely into scrub or lab coat pocket and can be changed out as duties or procedures change. The task card box also utilizes index cards kept in a recipe box with dividers for weekly, monthly, and yearly tasks. However you put your reference book and task card box together, make it yours! Be as creative as you wish; just try to keep in mind that as you grow in your job, you will be given more or at least different tasks, which in turn will require more or different information. So keep it flexible and changeable.

ACKNOWLEDGMENTS

I wish to acknowledge Dr. Paula Pattengale, the originating author of *Tasks for the Veterinary Assistant*, and all the contributors to the third edition. Their work was the foundation of this remodeled edition.

I also wish to acknowledge my family and friends for their encouragement and support while working on this edition. Special thanks go to my husband for helping me find a good internet signal in the middle of the Mojave desert!

ABOUT THE COMPANION WEBSITE

This book is accompanied by a companion website:

www.wiley.com/go/sonsthagen/tasks

The website includes:

- Suggestions for classroom discussions and activities
- Exam questions
- PowerPoint slides
- Auxiliary websites

CHAPTER 1

Professional Conduct and Foundation Skills

LEARNING OBJECTIVES
- Determining your role in a veterinary practice
- Meeting employer expectations, mastering 10 professional behaviors
- Develop a professional appearance
- Utilize effective communication skills – verbal, written, computer, social media, and credible web resources
- Anticipate work flow
- Application of ethics in the veterinary practice
- Understand the human–animal bond
- Understand and recognize the grief process
- Master foundation skills:
  - Veterinary practice math
  - Medical terminology

NAVTA GUIDELINES COVERED IN THIS CHAPTER
I. Office and Hospital Procedures
A. Front desk
   8. Demonstrate elementary computer skills
   9. Utilize basic medical terminology and abbreviations

Determining Your Role in a Veterinary Practice

A veterinary practice may be conducted in a hospital or a clinic. In human medicine there is a distinct difference. Hospitals are where patients are treated and cared for "in-house" or in a facility. A clinic is where patients are seen and sent home to recover or are sent to a hospital for more intensive care. In veterinary practice, the words "hospital" and "clinic" are used interchangeably, as both will admit critical patients into their facility for intensive care. However, some cities have access to a relatively new type of veterinary practice that does nothing but intensive

Tasks for the Veterinary Assistant, Fourth Edition. Teresa F. Sonsthagen.
© 2020 John Wiley & Sons, Inc. Published 2020 by John Wiley & Sons, Inc.
Companion website: www.wiley.com/go/sonsthagen/tasks

and emergency care. Patients are transferred to these facilities for around the clock care, thereby freeing general clinic and hospital practices to focus on general care. What this means is that whatever the type of clinic or hospital, it requires staffing. Let's discuss the staffing required in a veterinary practice.

A veterinary practice consists of many staff members. It takes the specialized skills of each to provide the competent care that pet owners expect for their pets. The veterinary assistant is just one member of the veterinary team. Synchronization of their duties with those of other members of this specialized team requires an awareness of the responsibilities of each. Understanding how the assistant fits into the complex pattern is crucial to successful coordination of patient care and implementation.

Every practice requires at least one veterinarian. This person can either be the owner of the practice or an employee. To become a veterinarian one must complete an undergraduate course at a college or university. It usually takes four years to complete the undergrad requirements, with most receiving a bachelor's degree in the subject of their choice. Then students must be accepted at a college of veterinary medicine which is another four years of education to receive either a Doctor of Veterinary Medicine (DVM) or a Veterinariae Medicinae Doctoris (VMD) depending on the college of veterinary medicine attended. In order to practice veterinary medicine, new graduates must pass a licensing exam for each state in which they wish to practice. Without this they cannot practice in a state even with a degree in hand! Some veterinarians chose to specialize in a specific area of veterinary medicine which involves additional years of study and another round of exams administered by an organization dedicated solely to that field of study. For example, a DVM interested in ophthalmology does everything required by the College of Veterinary Ophthalmologists and passes their exam to become a Diplomat in Veterinary Ophthalmology. But the learning still isn't finished! The state the veterinarian is practicing in, and if specialized the "College," requires several hours of continuing education per year to maintain their license to practice in that state and their diplomat status as a specialist.

The role of a veterinarian in practice is generally one that provides a diagnosis, prognoses, prescribes treatments and medications, and performs surgery on animals. The mission of the American Veterinary Medical Association (AVMA) is to lead the profession by advocating for its members and advancing the science and practice of veterinary medicine to improve animal and human health. It provides a Model Veterinary Practice Act that succinctly spells out the duties performed by a licensed veterinarian. In addition, the veterinarian is held legally responsible for the safety of all employees and all actions of each employee within the practice. The final word on the treatment of a patient is the veterinarian's.

According to the AVMA Model Veterinary Practice Act, technicians cannot diagnose, prognose, prescribe medicine, or perform surgery. Veterinary technicians are educated to perform the same tasks as human nurses, surgery technicians/nurses, anesthetic nurses, laboratory, dental, and radiology technicians on animals in a veterinary practice. In addition, they play an integral part in client education and communication.

There are several ways to become a veterinary technician. One way is to attend an AVMA accredited veterinary technology program. This is a program that has met stringent guidelines for didactic and medical skills training. Most programs offer an Associate degree that can take from two to three years to complete and is offered in community, technical, or private colleges. There are also several bachelor's degree veterinary technologist programs across the USA that are offered in public and private colleges and universities. This may seem like overkill; however, if you change your mind about working in a veterinary practice a bachelor's degree opens the door to jobs within industry, business, research, and government. Another path to becoming a veterinary technician is to enroll in an AVMA accredited online program. You can work at your own pace and utilize a veterinary practice as your training facility. Once a person has graduated from an accredited program most states require the graduate to sit for a credentialing exam, the Veterinary Technician National Exam (VTNE), administered by the American Association of Veterinary State Boards (AAVSB), and is recorded by a state veterinary medical board. A few states offer voluntary credentialing which is recorded by either the state veterinary technician association or the veterinary medical association. There are also some states that don't require any sort of credentialing. The credential designation also depends upon the state. Those states that recognize veterinary technicians that have passed the VTNE grant them the designation of Certified, Registered, or Licensed Veterinary Technicians. This creates much confusion especially as all states that offer credentialing utilize the VTNE offered by the AAVSB. To address this confusion the National Association of Veterinary Technicians in America (NAVTA) has initiated a move to have all states recognize veterinary technicians and technologists as Registered Veterinary Nurses. It is hoped that with this change in terminology the confusion when moving from state to state will disappear and the public will more readily recognize the role that the veterinary nurse plays in a veterinary practice.

NAVTA offers specialty recognition to those technicians that are interested in various areas of practice, usually within veterinary specialty practices. There are currently 16 Academies that offer training and testing for technicians that are interested in obtaining a specialty designation.

Veterinary technicians are often included in state practice acts. The AVMA has included veterinary technicians/technologists in their Model Veterinary Practice Act.

Veterinary assistants are important members of the veterinary practice team. They are often the "right hand person" for the veterinarian and veterinary technician, meaning that they help wherever and whenever help is needed in the day-to-day activities in the practice. "An assistant provides help under the direct supervision of the veterinarians or veterinary technicians. This allows those team members to perform the tasks and responsibilities of their positions as per their education and training" (NAVTA website). An assistant can be helping to restrain a kitten for an ear exam one minute and mopping up an accident in the reception area, answering the telephone, and scheduling an appointment the next. All the jobs done by an assistant are important to the well-being of the animals, clients, and staff in the veterinary practice. An assistant should be willing to jump in and do "whatever it takes" to keep the practice running smoothly. This is the hallmark of a first-rate veterinary assistant.

Assistants are often trained on the job but there is a certification program offered by many high schools, community colleges (some of which also have veterinary technology programs), and online programs. The NAVTA offers an Approved Veterinary Assistant (AVA) certificate after successful graduation from an approved veterinary assistant program and passing the veterinary assistant exam.

Developing an understanding of the flow of activities within a practice and how other staff members accomplish tasks is essential. This knowledge enables the assistant to prepare both material and patient in anticipation of the work to be done, thus creating an efficient sequence of work within the veterinary practice. It is in the preparation and follow-up phases of patient care, as much as the simultaneous help, that makes assistants so valuable to the practice.

Office personnel are those who handle the business side of a veterinary practice. Included in this group are the receptionists. They are the voice and face of the practice. This means they are the first person a client meets, often in stressful situations. The receptionist must be able to multi-task and keep everything in order to keep the practice running smoothly. This includes scheduling appointments and surgeries, explaining and collecting fees, routing calls to the appropriate person in the practice, and making sure client records are kept up to date. Receptionists are often trained on the job and should have at least a high school education.

Office or business managers often assist with reception duties, but their main duties involve the day-to-day business of the practice: taking care of accounts, paying bills and payroll, settling disputes, and often scheduling staff members. They may have a degree in business management or often they are veterinary technicians or technologists that have taken continuing education courses in practice management. These are just a few of the duties covered by the receptionist and office manager.

Cleaning staff are those personnel that are charged with keeping the clinic clean as well as personnel hired to keep the kennels clean. This may be delegated to one or two people or it could be delegated to the veterinary assistant. It is also the responsibility of every person working in the clinic to clean and make sure the patients are comfortable and have the necessities of life. If this is one of your duties take pride in knowing that often the first impression of a clinic is how clean it is and if it smells good. By doing an excellent job in cleaning both the facility and the kennels you are providing an invaluable service to both your employer and the animals you love.

Cross-training often occurs in veterinary practices, which enables each team member to carry out the tasks of other team members or function in a duel role such as technician–office manager. Cross-training allows for greater flexibility in staff scheduling. It guarantees that when a practice is short staffed, employees can effectively help each other complete their work. Dual roles are often needed in small facilities with fewer employees. Veterinary assistants may be asked to cover the receptionist or kennel care duties on occasion.

Information Discovery

Utilizing the internet, find the veterinary practice act for the state in which you live:
- Find out how many hours of continuing education it takes for a veterinarian to maintain her/his license each year.
- Find out what it means to practice veterinary medicine.
- Develop your written communication skills by explaining what a veterinarian is and what they do in veterinary practice, in your own words, as if you were talking to a high school student.

Utilizing the internet, look up, copy and paste the AVMA's model practice act or continue to work with the practice act from your state:
- Find the definition of a veterinary technician and veterinary technologist and what it means to practice veterinary technology.
- Compare the similarities and differences between a veterinarian and a veterinary technician in a veterinary practice.
- How does your state recognize veterinary technicians?
- What is the credential designation and how many hours of continuing education are required to maintain that credential?

Utilizing the internet, find the NAVTA approved veterinary assistant program guidelines:
- Reflect why passage from such a program versus on the job training may be important to job acquisition and mobility.

Meeting Employer Expectations – 10 Behaviors to Master

Employers in all professions demand behaviors that reflect competent knowledge and good attitudes and veterinary medicine is no exception. This section introduces the veterinary assistant to the professional behaviors specific for success within a veterinary practice. Whether you are a veterinary associate or a kennel assistant, all employers have basic expectations of every employee. The following are 10 behaviors to master in order to meet these expectations:

1. Punctuality
2. Presence
3. Flexibility
4. Cooperation
5. Following directions
6. Working independently
7. Honesty
8. Problem solving
9. Loyalty
    - Adherence to the policies and procedures of the workplace
10. Commitment
    - To customer satisfaction and product quality
    - To client–patient confidentiality
    - To learn now and for a lifetime
    - To take, then act upon constructive criticism without anger or defensiveness.

Punctuality, without excuses. Clients are scheduled to arrive at the clinic at specific times to facilitate seeing their pet, determining a course of action, and treating the pet. If the clinic's personnel are late getting to work, it can have catastrophic effects for the rest of the day. If your shift starts at 8 a.m. you should plan on arriving 5–10 minutes early. This allows you to put your personal belongings away, stow your lunch, make sure you have a pen, leash, roll of tape, and scissors in your pocket, and with name tag in place punch in on time. Walking in the door at 8 a.m. means you have arrived late!

Presence, when you are at work you must concentrate on *work*! Whatever is going on in your personal life needs to be checked at the door of the clinic. Your employer may care about you, but still expects you to do the job you are being paid to perform every day for the times you are scheduled to work. Life is hard, but it gets a lot harder if you are dismissed from your job because your personal life is getting in the way of performing your duties.

Both punctuality and presence can be a morale buster in a clinic. The following scenario demonstrates two divergent behaviors regarding punctuality and presence.

Scenario: Punctuality and Presence

Stew walks in the door right at 8 a.m. or is 5–10 minutes late every morning. He always has an excuse, from traffic jams to his dog running off or his alarm not ringing. When he is finally punched in he is often on his cell phone; arguing with his girlfriend or checking his text or email, which also occurs every chance he gets throughout the day. The other staff members often must ask twice for help or nudge him into action because he is on his phone. He complains to anyone that will listen to him about his car, roommate, or girlfriend. He is often moody and tired because he has stayed up too late playing the latest computer game, which he goes into detail about every chance he gets. Meanwhile, Connie arrives at work by 7.50 a.m. every morning, works with a smile, chats when appropriate but is often on the move all the time. If she isn't helping someone directly she is cleaning something. The only time you see her on her phone is during breaks and lunch. She does use her phone as a timer for vital signs and as a calculator as needed, but that is all during working times.

At the end of the shift an invitation is made to gather at a local coffee shop. Stew readily accepts, but Connie declines. When asked why, she states that her mother is in the hospital critically ill and she needs to be with her. No one knew!

Information Check and Reflection

- Describe how Stew's attitude, presence, and punctuality would wear on the morale in the clinic.
- How do you think Connie keeps so focused at work, especially with a critically ill mother?
- What two behaviors is Connie demonstrating?
- Reflect on how you would plan on being at work on time and how can you stay in the present when life is tough outside of work.

Flexibility and *cooperation* are vital in keeping the workflow going throughout the day. The veterinary assistant may be asked to assist with anesthetizing a patient one moment and to gather a patient in the reception area the next. You are the extra pair of hands often desperately needed in the veterinary clinic. Doing all tasks asked of you willingly and competently builds trust in your abilities. This is not only expected, but also appreciated by everyone in the clinic.

The same is true for working with others in a clinic. It is so important to work well with everyone. Cooperation is a valuable behavior, which can be tough sometimes because each person will often have their own style of accomplishing the same tasks. This makes it difficult sometimes, but it is important to go with the flow and provide the best help you can when taking care of patients. Learn how each veterinarian and veterinary technician likes to accomplish tasks and be a step ahead of them when setting up or be thinking about what they may ask you to do.

Scenario: Flexibility and Cooperation

A new veterinarian, Dr. Kindheart, has been hired and it is her first day at the clinic. Stew has been assigned to be her assistant for the day. He meets her in the prep room and as she walks in informs her that their first task is to neuter a cat. Stew presents the cat for her to examine and restrains it for her to anesthetize. When it is sleeping soundly he automatically places the cat into dorsal recumbency and stretches the back legs up towards its head. Dr. Kindheart is stunned because she has never seen this position before. She asks why he is holding the cat this way and Stew says, "Dr. Alright, the clinic owner, always does them this way." Dr. Kindheart asks Stew to place the cat in lateral recumbency and to hold the tail up and out of the way. Stew heaves big sigh and shakes his head, while slowly repositioning the cat. Dr. Kindheart's confidence is shaken, thinking that she may be doing it wrong. Meanwhile Stew is shifting from foot to foot, heaving more sighs or is babbling about some video game he played the night before which further distracts and heightens the nerves of an already jittery vet. The neuter takes twice as long as usual and Dr. Kindheart feels like a failure.

The next day Connie is assigned to Dr. Kindheart. Stew heaves a sigh of relief and says, "Glad I'm with Dr. Alright today. He knows what he's doing!" Then with an evil grin he quips "Good luck with the newbie!" Connie approaches Dr. Kindheart and introduces herself as the veterinary assistant assigned to her for the day. They proceed to the surgery prep area and Connie asks Dr. Kindheart how she would like to proceed. The relieved vet and Connie have a good discussion about how they will accomplish the neuter, and everything goes according to plan.

Information Check and Reflection

- What behavior skills did Connie employ when working with Dr. Kindheart for the first time?
- How well do you think Stew works with the various people in the clinic compared to Connie?
- Who was more flexible in this scenario?
- Reflect on how you would learn to work with other people in a practice.

Following directions and completing the task to its logical conclusion is very important. To illustrate these behaviors read the following scenario about two very busy veterinary assistants, Stew and Connie.

Scenario: Following Directions

The practice is crazy busy this morning with a full schedule. Already the phone is ringing off the hook with clients seeking to get their pets looked at today. The only option for those pets sounding to be very ill is to have the patients dropped off for the vets to look at when they get a chance. Both Stew and Connie are called to the reception area at the same time to take patients back to the kennel area. Stew approaches the client and asks him to put the dog on the leash he is holding out. He then takes the dog and puts it into a kennel, shuts the door and leaves. Connie approaches the other client, with a smile and a hello. She

confirms that this is the patient that is going to stay with them for a while and assures the client that her dog will be just fine while she is away. Connie takes the dog to a kennel, reassures it with a few pats then shuts the door and leaves, only to return in a few minutes with a water dish and sleeping pad to put in the kennel. She gives the dog a few more pats and then carefully closes the door to the kennel, making sure it latches.

Information Check and Reflection

- Who followed instructions?
- Who followed instructions to their logical conclusion?
- Why was it important to place water and a sleeping pad in the kennel?
- Reflect on who you would want to emulate.

Working independently is a skill all employers check references about. Can you be given a task and complete that task without someone checking up on you constantly? Can you be given instructions and carry out those instructions without asking questions about every step? These are just a few examples of what working independently means. It is also utilizing "moments of time" to learn how to answer the phone, check in or check out a patient, or properly clean and set up a kennel without being directed to do so. These actions increase your value to the practice. "Moments of time" are those down times when the practice isn't busy. Make it a point to look for ways to contribute to the practice. Cleaning out a drawer, observing others doing their jobs, or even washing down a wall are all ways to contribute and make yourself a valuable member of the practice.

Reflection

Do you work independently? If so, describe some of the work you do without supervision or being asked to do something. If you don't, think about ways to start working independently.

Benjamin Franklin is credited with saying, "*Honesty is the best policy.*" But what exactly does that mean. We all have told a "white lie" to avoid hurting someone's feelings. To not tell the truth when we have done something wrong or have forgotten to do something that endangers a person, animal, place, or thing is a moral flaw. It seems to be human nature to either be truthful or dishonest. Which one often depends on how one was raised. Telling the truth, having the punishment fit the crime, and facing the consequences is often a means for teaching that honesty is the best policy. Terrible punishment after telling the truth teaches us to lie the next time to avoid the punishment. Getting away with a lie often reinforces lying because we can get away with it, that is until we get caught in a lie. Telling the truth, facing and dealing with the consequences is still better than being branded a liar and losing the trust of your employer and co-workers. To paraphrase Ankita Bhardwaj, from her essay Honesty is the Best Policy: Origin, Meaning, Explanation, Essay, Speech, honesty is the key to a good life, the benefits of telling the truth always come back to you in the long run. Honest people are trusted and respected. Dishonest people may get by for a while but sooner or later their lies will catch up to them and dire consequences usually follow.

Scenario: Honesty

Remember in our last scenario, when Stew put his patient into a kennel and left? Connie reminded him to get a water dish and sleeping pad for his patient, as he was leaning against the counter looking at his phone. He said "Yeah, as soon as I'm done here." Well, he forgot, two hours have passed. Dr. Kindheart has a break in seeing afternoon patients and goes to check the patients that were dropped off. Remember, these are patients that had to be seen today as their conditions were such that they couldn't wait a few days for an appointment. As she enters the kennel room she sees a very sick dog without a water dish and no sleeping pad. She turns to Stew, who is her assigned assistant, saying, "Who put this dog in a kennel without water? How long has he been here without water?" Stew realizes that he forgot to take care of this patient. He must make a quick decision: tell the truth or lie. Here's what runs through his thoughts:

1. *Blame it on Connie. She brought another dog back at the same time and Dr. Kindheart wouldn't know who brought which dog back. No, that won't work, everyone knows Connie is a stickler for details and would never forget to put water in a patient's kennel.*

2. *Say, "I don't know" and leave it at that. No, that won't work either, everyone knows we were both called to the front to pick up a patient, so it was me or Connie.*

3. *Fess up, I forgot to give him water, tell the truth and hope they don't fire me.*

Stew replies, "Oh no! I am so sorry, little guy, I totally got distracted and forgot to put water in for you! I am sorry, Dr. Kindheart, I will never let this happen again. I hope he is going to be alright." For all of Stew's faults he is not a liar. He does care about animals and would never do anything to intentionally hurt one. Dr Kindheart says, "Well, let's check him out and see if it caused any damage." She continues to say that because of workplace policy she will have to report this and let the owners know what happened. Stew understands and vows to pay better attention to patients while he is at work.

Information Check and Reflection

- What consequences do you think Stew will face because of this incident?
- If the dog is OK do you think Dr. Kindheart should keep this between her and Stew or should she report him?
- What if the dog was harmed by not having water? What would you decide then if you were Dr. Kindheart?
- Reflect on what you would do in the same circumstances when faced with telling the truth or lying, by either omission or outright denial. This does not need to be shared with classmates or instructor, it is simply a means to have you consider if honesty is always the best policy.

Problem solving is an invaluable skill. There are two types of problem solving you'll be exposed to in this world. One is the everyday problems that crop up. For example, not being able to find a specific piece of equipment because it wasn't put back in its storage place. If this is a onetime occurrence there isn't much of a problem other than finding it and putting it back. However, what if this keeps happening because it is used often and never put back into its storage spot? You have three choices: resign yourself to always looking for it and putting it back yourself, you could find out who used it last and tell them to put it back, or you could think about asking the team if another one could be purchased or maybe move the item to an easier storage location. Each of these actions is valid – which one can you live with? Or maybe a better question is which one resolves the problem? Being able to come up with a solution to a problem within the practice's guidelines or protocol manual frees up the owner and office manager to deal with issues far more important than those everyday problems that pop up. Of course, if it means changing a protocol or standard of operation (SOP) then running it past your immediate supervisor first is always a must.

Dealing with a personal problem with another employee is the other type of problem solving that is a skill that is highly valued. These personal conflicts crop up even within the most effective teams. Being able to discuss a problem with the person who is causing the issue is your first mode of action. Utilize "I" or "my" statements to start the conversation. For example, "it is my perception," "it hurts my feelings," "could you help me figure out," or "I need help with…" This puts the person you are having this crucial conversation with into a more receptive mood to help. If you approach the person with a combative, "I wanted to speak to you about…," it immediately puts the person on the defensive and usually nothing gets solved.

If you have approached someone about a problem, remember to ask for a follow-up. This helps to confirm that you both will work on the issue at hand.

If the problem continues or you are met with resistance, determine whether you can live with the issue and let it roll or if you need to take it up the chain of command. This is also important to remember: never jump the chain of command. It often backfires and creates an even worse situation. The chain of command is your immediate supervisor. If the issue is with that person and you have already tried to resolve it with them and gotten nowhere, then move up to that person's supervisor. Again, consider the situation carefully. If it is detrimental to the patients, clients, and practice, then by all means take it up the chain of command. Be sure to have a solution in mind, especially if the problem is about your job specifically. If it is a personal issue and no one else seems bothered, then take a deep look at why it bothers you and come to terms with it and move on.

Information Check and Reflection

- What strategies for starting a crucial conversation do you hope will prevent the person you are speaking to from becoming defensive?
- Reflect on an everyday issue that you have resolved or needs to be resolved. What did you or could you do to resolve it?
- Reflect on a crucial conversation you have had to have with a co-worker, friend, parent, or significant other. How did you approach them? How did the conversation turn out? Was it successful in resolving the problem? Were you able to move forward after the conversation?

Loyalty and commitment to your place of work are so important. This encompasses the preceding information as well as the following points. Adherence to the policies and procedures of the workplace shows a commitment to following the guidelines set out by the owners of the practice. They are usually in place to ensure fair and equal treatment of employees, clients, and patients. These policies and procedures usually dictate how employees dress, ask for time off, how benefits are dispersed, how to report when a policy or procedure has been ignored, to name a few. Client policies are also in place so that all are treated in the same way. For example, there may be a no credit extended policy, or if a client is disrespectful and abusive towards the staff they may be fired from being a client. Patient policies include things like how they are cared for and treated when in the practice. For example, every animal is given a water dish, sleeping pad, and a litter box (as needed) when placed in a hospital kennel. You will also see that procedures are often

written down. For example, how is a patient checked in when they arrive at the practice? How are the clients to be addressed when asking to them enter an exam room? Sometimes you will find a practice that doesn't have policies and procedures written out. This can lead to issues amongst the staff members, especially when employees are doing whatever they think is best and it rubs someone else the wrong way. With clearly stated rules, everyone should commit them to memory and act accordingly. This has the benefit of everyone moving in the same direction. This builds trust and loyalty to the practice and to each other.

Scenario: Reporting a Violation of the Policies and Procedures

Remember our scenario where Stew forgot to put water and a sleeping pad into a patient's kennel and Dr. Kindheart had to report him for this oversight? The reason she had to do this is that at their practice the policy and procedure for hospitalizing a patient is quite clear. Stew failed to protect the health and well-being of this patient and the policy states that "Any employee found to have willingly and/or neglectfully caused harm to a patient of the practice will be dismissed without further consideration. Any employee that has witnessed any such incident is required to report this incident in writing to the practice manager. Failure to report is the same as if the witness perpetrated the harm. The practice manager will interview all parties involved and discuss it with the practice owners and a final decision will be made that may range from retraining, probation status or dismissal from the practice." As you can see, Dr. Kindheart really didn't have a choice in reporting Stew.

Stew did have some things going for him. One was that he didn't leave the patient without water and sleeping pad on purpose. It was a crazy busy day and he did get distracted, albeit on his phone! Secondly, the patient didn't suffer any long-term effect, nor did it exacerbate its symptoms, which Dr. Kindheart did include in her report. She also noted that he was very apologetic and had immediately told the truth that it was his fault. The office manager also noted that this was the first time Stew had ever been reported for a violation of the practice's policies and procedures.

Information Check and Reflection

- What decision would you have come up with if you were the office manager and owner of the practice?
- Why did you reach that conclusion?
- If you were the boss how could you build Stew's and other employees' loyalty and commitment to the practice and still follow the policies and procedures?

Take, then act upon *constructive criticism* without anger or defense. It is human nature to become defensive when someone calls us out on a behavior or action that is detrimental to the practice or to ourselves. It seems that we must justify why we are doing something a certain way. When told about our deficiency it is always wise to take a moment and digest the information. Try to see it from their perspective and be honest with yourself. Remember the person giving you the constructive criticism is doing it with your best interests in mind. They are usually also doing it because your action or behavior may be moving you towards being dismissed from your job.

Scenario: Stew's Meeting with the Practice Manager and Owner

"Stew, we have reviewed your actions with the forgotten patient with Dr. Kindheart, other staff members, and yourself. As per our policy you failed to take adequate action to ensure the comfort of the patient while here. Taking into consideration your years of employment and this being your first major incident we have decided to put you on a 3-month probation with the following stipulations. You are not to use your phone during office hours. It must remain in your locker or vehicle, you may use it on your break and lunch period. You will arrive to work on time every day with no excuses. This means that you are here at least 5–10 minutes early to get settled and be presentable for work. Failure to adhere to either of these stipulations during and after the probation period will be grounds for immediate dismissal. In addition, if another incident occurs where a patient is placed in danger or even compromised you will be dismissed immediately with no justification. Do you have any questions?"

Information Check and Reflection

- Put yourself into Stew's situation, was this a fair means of handling his actions?
- Put yourself into the other employees' shoes, do you think they will think this is a fair decision?
- Why do you think the employers decided to give Stew another chance?

Focus on *customer satisfaction* and *product quality*. The veterinary practice is a business and as such it is essential that clients are well taken care of. They bring their pets to the practice because they are getting value for their money. It isn't always about who is the cheapest in town, it is that your entire team cares about the patient and the owner as well.

Information Check and Reflection

- How can team members show they care about patients' and clients' well-being?
- What are some ways that you can show your practice that you care about client satisfaction and offer quality service?

Lifetime learning keeps you sharp, it expands your experiences, and opens the mind to possibilities. It doesn't have to be only in veterinary medicine, it can be in arts, crafts, hobbies, or in a completely different area of study. With the internet there is really no end to what you can learn. Find your passion outside of work. Yes, work should be fulfilling and enjoyable, but it shouldn't consume your entire life. Outside interests give you a break from the daily grind, keep the mind fresh and spirit open to new possibilities.

Information Check and Reflection

- Reflect on your outside interests. If you are not currently pursuing outside interests, what have you always wanted to do with your spare time?
- If you do pursue outside interests, what are they and what do they do for your mental and physical health?

Professional Appearance

"First impressions are lasting impressions." This saying is important in veterinary medicine as in any other business. Clients have no way of knowing the skill of the veterinarian in surgery; they are not present. They do judge the quality of patient care; not only on how well their animal recovers but judgments are based on the appearance of the facility and staff as well. It may seem hard to believe, but it is true.

Personal grooming includes common sense rules with special adaptations for the work and environment involved. All clothing must be washable in hot water and cleaned daily to reduce the risk of disease transmission. It should be of durable, smooth fabric in a simple style. Scrubs are an excellent answer to these criteria (Figure 1.1). Sleeves should be at or above three-quarter length with a V or round neckline that is modest when bending over. Pants should not be tight, as bending and squatting are done throughout the day. Again, modesty is important when considering the style of waistline. Darker colors or prints are often preferable as they do not show stains and soil as do lighter colors. It is an excellent idea to have an extra set of scrubs at the practice to change into if the set you are wearing is soiled with feces, vomit, blood, or urine. All of which can transmit disease as well as becoming odorous. Scrubs also have an abundance of pockets as it is good to stock your pockets with items that are often used throughout the day.

Shoes must be closed toed, slip or skid resistant, and clean. A solid pair of shoes is an excellent investment in foot health. You will be on your feet for your entire shift and when your feet start to ache it takes your mind off

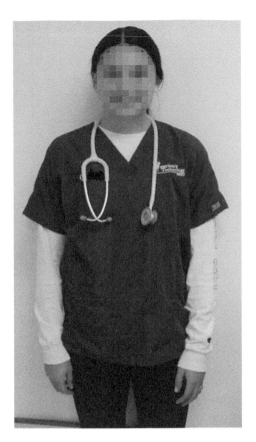

FIGURE 1.1 Clean scrubs ready to work.

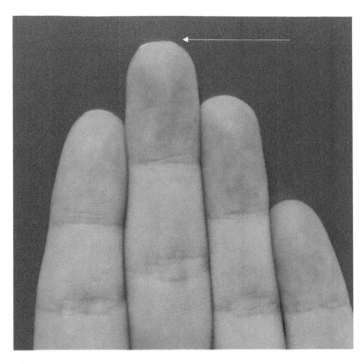

FIGURE 1.2 Fingernail tips.

your work and mistakes can occur. In large animal practices you will be required to wear rubber boots that fit over your shoes. Often, if doing large animal work only, those shoes should have a steel toe. Clean shoes and rubber boots are essential to prevent the transmission of diseases from outside the clinic in and from farm to farm.

Jewelry should be left at home. Loop earrings, rings, and necklaces can become caught on equipment or snag on an animal. An inexpensive wristwatch with a second hand is acceptable to facilitate pulse and respiration readings. The practice may have a policy on facial piercings and tattoos. Check the policy manual or with the office manager before getting any of these things done in an obvious location.

Hair must be kept clean and if long tied back or put up in a bun. Do not allow it to hang free as it will obscure your vision when bending or leaning over. Fingernails should not be longer than just over the top of the tip of the finger and should not be painted (Figure 1.2). Chipped polish or chipped nails makes a person look unkept. If you chew your nails this is a good time to break that habit. Debris and germs can easily get under fingernails and if ingested you can become sick.

If you smoke, drink coffee, or have had food with a strong odor for lunch please be kind and take a breath mint. Chewing gum is usually not appropriate, as the chomping and inadvertent snapping of gum can be interpreted as boredom or non-interest in what you are doing. If you can

smoke on your breaks, make sure to remove your scrub top or to spritz yourself with a deodorizing spray. Non-smokers are often disturbed by the smell of smoke and even if you can't smell it because you are used to it, believe that others can! This also is good advice for perfumes and aftershave lotions. It is important to use them sparingly if at all at work. Many people are affected negatively by scents. Save them for your after hours and weekends.

Men should keep a clean-shaven face but if you have facial hair it should be kept neat. Women, if you wear makeup keep it simple; this is not the time to come glammed up! Bathe regularly and use a perfume-free deodorant. Remember you may be one of the first visual representatives of the clinic so aim for a positive impression!

Help a co-worker. Be the person that notices that there is something in someone's teeth, a zipper isn't quite where it needs to be, or if someone smells bad. Kindly let them know that there is an issue. You can take the sting out of this information by following up your statement with, "I would sure want to know if…"

Information Check and Reflection

- Do you meet the personal appearance expectations?
- What can you do to make sure you are ready for a day at the clinic?
- What items should be stored in your pockets for work?

Effective Communication Skills Within the Veterinary Practice

Verbal Communication

Good manners and common courtesies are always expected in the workplace and in every interaction with clients, team members, and other visitors to the practice. Good manners are nothing more than making social interactions comfortable for everyone involved, which put those with whom you interact at ease. They are like the rules for the road. If everyone follows them, traffic moves smoothly, and everyone is happier. Please, thank you, may I assist and a genuine how are you are all common courtesies that should be used in all interactions. These common courtesies seem to have faded from our society. It is amazing the response they invoke when used, especially in tense situations. They demonstrate that you respect other people and it builds trust and respect for you.

Reflection

Practice common courtesies. Make note of yourself saying thank you, please, may I assist, yes mam, and no sir when addressing classmates, friends, teachers, parents, siblings, clients, and co-workers. Write down their reactions to these courtesies and how they made you feel when using them.

Non-verbal Communication

Humans use body language and facial features to convey feelings and emotions to match or reinforce what they are saying – sometimes! We are very good at verbally saying one thing but non-verbally saying another with our body language. A frown or closed body position will deflate your words, making it seem that you are saying one thing but thinking another. Crossed arms, weight shifted to one foot, and a raised eyebrow gives the appearance of indifference, defensiveness, anger, or aggravation (Figure 1.3a). An open stance with both feet at shoulder width, arms loosely held at your sides, and relaxed facial features or a smile conveys sincerity and interest (Figure 1.3b).

Common courtesies are just one aspect of verbal communication. It also includes using correct grammar. Clients make assumptions about the education and quality of work by the veterinary staff based on their use of language. Listen carefully to the veterinarian's and veterinary technician's manner of speaking to help you expand your vocabulary and grammar.

To check your grammatic ear, read these two sentences out loud:

- I ain't got time to get that mop and bucket to clean up no mess up front!
- I don't have time to get the mop and bucket to clean the mess up in front!

This is an obvious example of improper grammar versus proper grammar. If you are having trouble speaking well, ask someone that does to coach you. This may mean they catch you and correct you on the spot. Be ready to take their advice with good grace and learn from it!

At all times avoid swearing, vulgarities, and the use of slang words as they instantly lower your standing in everyone's estimation. You also want to pay attention to the tone of voice you use. A wise crack or joking tone may be offensive. Baby talk to animals may be OK at home or for a brief time at work, but keep it brief as excessive baby talk can become annoying.

Client Communication

Interacting with clients must integrate all the information shared in the previous section along with the following. All clients should be greeted with a smile, open body language, by their name with an honorific: Mr., Mrs., Ms., Miss, or Dr. Acknowledgment of the pet by name is very important when first meeting a client and patient. It shows respect for the client and care about the pet. The client may ask you to call them by their first name but until that happens use the honorific and last name.

When speaking about the veterinarian to clients always refer to her/him by Dr. Lastname. Veterinarians tend to be more comfortable with Dr. Firstname but that is only acceptable behind the scenes. They worked hard for that title and it should be acknowledged when speaking to clients.

Reflection

Do you speak well? Listen to yourself and others in school, at work, and at home. Document the times that you needed to check your grammar or you caught someone else speaking poorly or well and share it with the class.

(a)   (b)

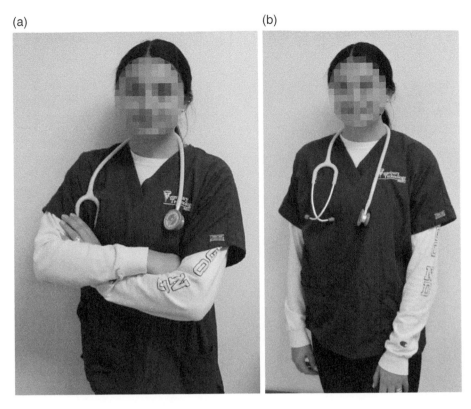

FIGURE 1.3 (a) Closed body language. (b) Open body language.

Written Communication

In veterinary practice the patients' records are legal documents. They are used to record all the treatments, surgeries, medications, and observations carried out by the veterinarian and others in the practice. It is imperative that they are written concisely, completely, and correctly. Therefore, proper grammar and spelling are essential. Making sure you have the correct file is essential. If the practice uses paper files, neat handwriting is essential. More information about what goes into records is covered in Chapter 3.

Computer Competency

The computers used in a veterinary practice will usually have a practice management software package that is very expensive to purchase and maintain but the ease of file management, financial recording, inventory management, and elimination of paper shuffling pays for itself repeatedly.

There are usually several computers networked together, referred to as workstations, which are strategically placed around the clinic. The network allows information placed on one computer to be accessible by all the other computers. For example, the receptionist checks in a patient, taking their chief complaint and indicates that they are ready to be seen. They are escorted

to an exam room where the veterinarian, technician, or assistant calls up the patient's file on that workstation and begins the visit. Once the patient has been examined and a plan is formulated for care, all that information is put into its file at that workstation. A list of charges is completed, and the client is asked to step to the reception desk for their bill. The receptionist calls up that patient's file and sees what fees were applied and asks for payment. There is no waiting for paperwork to be brought to the reception desk or failure to capture all the fees applied to that visit.

Because of the important role these computers have at work they should never be used for personal emails, surfing the internet, or have anything downloaded to them as it could put the entire network in jeopardy from viruses or malware. Each person in a practice is given a password to log into the software and the computer network. This safeguard renders them unavailable to the public. This is to protect client records and practice financial information. It is extremely important to follow the guidelines set out by the practice when utilizing the computers.

Client records are confidential and should never be left open on a workstation, especially between clients. It is to be hoped that the workstations will time out between patients, meaning they have to be logged into to start the next visit. If they don't, the previous client's information is there for anyone to read. This is a violation of client confidentiality and can result in severe consequences for you and the practice. There is more about client confidentiality in the section on application of veterinary ethics later in this chapter.

Determining Credible Web Sources

Credible web sources are sometimes difficult to find. Before utilizing a website for a paper or to increase your knowledge, ask these questions:

- Who has written the information provided on the page?
- What are their credentials, do they possess a degree, or have they studied the topic extensively?
- Do the author(s) have a good reputation?
- Is the information valid, with checkable facts, or is the information provided purely opinion?
- Does more than one source contain the same information?

All these questions should be answered with a yes before utilizing the source as a point of knowledge. Anyone can produce a webpage and make it look and "sound" believable. Many of them are great sites, but there are an equal number of sites that offer poor information if not downright misinformation!

Information Check

- Why is it so important that work computers not be used for personal reasons?
- What could happen if an employee downloads a virus or malware to a business computer?

Use and Misuse of Social Media

For many people social media has become as routine as talking on the telephone. It is amazing how many people can be reached in a short period of time. This works great for events and information the veterinary practice wants to get distributed. There is usually one person in charge of generating social media bursts in the practice. It is important to not post photos of patients or clients on your personal social media. This is an invasion of their privacy and can be grounds for immediate dismissal.

The unfortunate side of social media is a total lack of privacy to this method of communication. Snapchatting, Tweeting, Facebook, and email once posted can never be removed and becomes part of the public domain. It is never appropriate to discuss employee relations, how you feel about your boss or job, patients, or clients. One should never vent about what is going on at work or whom you feel has caused you an injustice. Stories about patients or clients, even if names are not used, is a violation of client privacy.

Social media can also be used to assess your potential fit for a position in a practice. Pictures and stories of wild nights or rants about life's injustices may not paint the picture you would want of your abilities.

Information Challenge

Find a website that talks about a common disease like heartworm. Answer the questions on credible web sources to confirm that it is a reliable site then try finding another site about heartworm and compare them. Do the sites offer the same information? Do both sites meet the criteria? See if you can't find one that offers conflicting information. Compare it to the "reliable" site.

Anticipation of Workflow

One of the most valuable skills is anticipating what comes next. This is an ongoing learning process that may take months to achieve but when you do you will be extremely valuable to the practice. From day one start watching and remembering what needs to be done and when. Learn everyone's routine, know how they coordinate work and use their time. Have everything ready to begin procedures without being asked. The veterinarian and technician should be able to walk into a room and have everything on the counters ready to go to work. Be ready, willing, and able to pitch in and help with whatever is asked of you. Don't wait to be told what to do if there is down time. Restock exam rooms and treatment areas, grab a bucket of soapy water and wash down a wall or completely clean off a counter top, even under the items sitting upon it! This too will increase your value in the practice.

Review the appointment schedule, treatment board, and hospitalized patients throughout the day. Be

Reflection

Examine your social media accounts from a prospective employer's frame of reference:

- What type of person do you appear to be based on pictures and language used?
- Have a classmate or friend check your accounts. Do they come up with the same type of person as your evaluation?
- Would you hire this person to fit into a professional practice?

especially mindful of supplies and equipment necessary to have everything on hand. This also goes for your work duties. Set priories for accomplishing all tasks and work efficiently to stay ahead. Be flexible though, as one never knows how animals will react in a veterinary setting and sometimes things such as schedules can be knocked off track because of an uncooperative patient or a patient that requires extensive care.

Information Exercise

Brainstorm with your classmates on how to develop a strategy for learning and remembering the sequence of various procedures. Start with the very routine procedures like toenail trims, ear cleaning, and vaccinations. Think about what equipment or supplies will be needed. Consider marking down the steps and supplies in a small notebook you can carry in your scrub suit pocket. Utilize this until you are confident that everything is ready to go for those procedures.

Application of Veterinary Ethics

Ethics are defined as the rules or principles that govern right conduct. What is right or correct varies within a culture and society and changes over time. It is to be hoped that you were taught the difference between right and wrong behavior, to be a kind and caring person, and to stand up for what is right or just.

The AVMA and the NAVTA provide codes of ethics on their websites to help make difficult decisions and to provide guidelines for how to behave in a veterinary practice.

Information Exercise

Utilizing the internet, find these key points in both the AVMA's Principles of Veterinary Medical Ethics and the NAVTA's Veterinary Technician Code of Ethics on their respective websites. Then, in your own words, define or describe what each means:
- Establishment of a veterinarian–client–patient relationship
- Confidentiality of medical records
- The principle of doing no harm
- Protection of public health

Reflect how a code of ethics may help you determine a course of action when faced with an ethical dilemma.

Human–Animal Bond

The relationship between a human and an animal can be very complex and often involves a broad range of emotions. Relationships between animals and people have evolved from predominantly the utilitarian model in an agrarian environment to a companionship model in an urban environment. In either instance, the bonds between people and animals is complex, unique, and may change over time and circumstances. It is real, ever-changing in intensity, and induces physical changes in the limbic system of the brain.

Veterinary medicine can improve the human–animal bond. The veterinary staff including the veterinary assistant can either encourage or discourage positive client behaviors towards their animals.

We often associate the human–animal bond with companion animals such as dogs, cats, pocket pets, and birds. However, there is a move towards bringing more livestock and poultry into the urban setting than ever before. Each species of animal plays a part in the client's life ranging from companionship, playmate, surrogate children, and comfort to warmth and food. Regardless of the circumstance, it is our job to understand the different bonds, support the client in decisions, and not pass judgments on the perceived loving or unloving client.

A way to determine how bonded an individual client is to their animal takes some powers of observation. How does the client take care of their animal? How do they interact with their animal? How do they talk about or describe their animal? These are all questions to ask yourself to help interpret how strong the bond is between a client and their animal.

Sometimes there is an aberration in the human–animal bond, ranging from totally absent to an over-reliance on the animal for emotional or physical support. This broad spectrum often causes compassion fatigue in veterinary staff. Clients making decisions because of a lack of knowledge, a lack of caring, or a total dependence on the life of a pet can become very burdensome. By understanding the human–animal bond in its many forms you can interact more effectively with clients, support clients compassionately during times of crisis, and know when to rein back your involvement to prevent burning yourself out.

Reflection

How you can tell if a bond is strong between a client and pet? Use yourself or a friend as an example. Can there be a human–animal bond between a client and his/her livestock?

Grief Process

Dr. Elisabeth Kübler-Ross, in her book *On Death and Dying*, researched and developed the human experience when grieving a loved one who has died. She discovered there are five stages to the grieving process: denial, anger, bargaining, guilt, and acceptance. Further research has shown that humans go through these stages whenever they experience a loss of any magnitude. It was also discovered that we don't necessarily go through the stages in order, there is no timeframe for how long each stage lasts, and that we can get stuck in a stage. It is to be hoped that we do reach acceptance at some point in time. However, a reminder of the loss can trigger a "mini" grief process or a period of experiencing the loss again. It is usually faster than the first process, but it can trigger a period of sadness and grief all over again.

Recognizing the stages of grief can help to explain many behaviors that normally are not part of an individual's behavior. Statements like "I don't believe it" or "There has to be another alternative" are statements often associated with denial. Lashing out or accusing the veterinary staff of "letting a pet die" is an obvious sign of anger. Bargaining could be something like "Do whatever you can to keep him alive until Christmas, then I can let him go." Guilt is demonstrated by statements of blame: "I should have," "I wish I would have," and so on. Acceptance is often demonstrated by being able to speak about the loss without a total and prolonged regression into the previous stages. There may still be tears, but stories, comparisons, and evidence of being able to carry on with their lives are good signs that clients have reached acceptance.

Some people get stuck at a stage during the grief process. They can't move forward until they work through the stage in which they are stuck. Often professional help is required at this point. Otherwise you may see the veterinary staff acting as a sounding board by clients. We of all people understand how it feels to lose a pet or treasured livestock animal. We know about the stages of grief and how to spot trouble if a client isn't moving forward. Have information about professional grief counselors available in your city ready to hand out when the signs appear.

Information Exercise

List the five stages of grief and think about what statement you may hear in a veterinary clinic that may tip you off as to where that client is in the grief process.

Reflection

Reflect on a loss and see if you can pinpoint the stages of grief you went through. Remember it can be about a lost loved one or a lost boyfriend/girlfriend, a lost treasured object.

Foundation Skills – Veterinary Practice Math and Medical Terminology

The veterinary practice is often non-stop action all day long. An employee must be able to adapt to the situations occurring, understand what is said, and to process information quickly and accurately. This chapter covers the basic math used in the practice every day. It touches on the basic medical terminology that is used by veterinarians and technicians when speaking to each other and writing medical records.

Basic Math Used in the Veterinary Practice

Basic math problem solving is an essential function in the daily work of a veterinary assistant. Common occurrences include converting weight in pounds to kilograms and vice versa or milliliters to ounces or diluting a disinfectant to a 10% solution are examples of the math you will be doing all day, every day in a veterinary practice. Estimation skills are another important skill to develop in addition to solving math problems accurately. This is a quick way to check your work as you go. Being able to ask yourself, "Does this amount make sense," and knowing that it does, can keep you moving through the day.

It is to be hoped that you have a good foundation in adding, subtracting, multiplying, and dividing already in place. If you can do these things without a calculator, even better. It is a skill that should be developed because we don't always have a free hand to pull out the phone or calculator on which to figure out a problem. This does take time but is worth the effort as it adds value to you as an employee. A technique to use to polish your math skills is flash cards; this is an old technique but one that does work and can be easily found or made. With this information under control let's move on to the daily math problems you will encounter as a veterinary assistant.

Weight Conversion

This is an important skill to master because medication dosages, solution dilutions, and prescription diets are often prescribed in a per pound or per kilogram format. Let's begin with a comparison of the US system and the metric system for weights.

The US system of weights from smallest to largest are ounces, pounds, and tons. The base unit is the ounce. It takes 16 ounces (oz) to equal 1 pound (lb) and 2000 pounds to equal 1 ton. Anything smaller than 1 ounce is expressed as a decimal point or as a fraction. For example, half of an ounce is either 0.5 oz or as a fraction ½ oz. Once you get to 1/16th of an ounce the name changes to a dram and at 1/7000th of a pound it is called a grain. These are tiny, tiny measurements and are usually used for weighing the ingredients in capsules or powders which a veterinary assistant doesn't need to worry too much about. However, you will need to know how to convert fractions of a pound into ounces. As we said before, 16 ounces equals 1 pound. For example, when you get a weight on a cat that is 8 lb 7 oz, the 7 oz needs to be converted into "pounds" and is expressed as a decimal point. This is necessary to work out drug dosages accurately.

Here is the way the equation would be written: 7 ounces / 16 ounces/lb = 0.____ lb. The ounces cancel each other out 7 / 16 /lb = _0.____ lb, leaving you only a portion of the pound. The 0.__ indicates that you have less than 1 and so your answer is behind the decimal point. Divide 7 by 16 and you get 0.4375 lb. Now place that portion of a pound behind your 8 lb and your animal's weight is 8.4375 lb. Most clinics will have you drop the last two digits and use 8.43 lb, or some may ask you to round that last digit up if is it is above a 6, so you would end up with 8.44 lb. As you can see, this could be a mathematical nightmare for those of us that are a bit challenged by math, but always keep this in mind whenever you are working with a portion of a pound you will *always* divide by 16 oz/lb and you will *always* end up with that portion of a pound as a decimal point that is placed behind your full pound(s).

The metric system is a decimal system based on units of 10. The base unit of measurement is the gram and is designated as 1. You may have pocket pets and birds that weigh 1–9 grams. But what happens when you reach 10 grams? Now for some, the confusion starts. The metric system uses prefixes to indicate what multiplication factor of 10 is being applied to the gram.

For example, let's use a common measurement in veterinary medicine the kilogram. The prefix *kilo* stands for 1000. So, a *kilo*gram is 1 gram × 10^3 or 1000 grams. However, this would be very lengthy to write out, so 1000 grams is expressed as 1 kilogram or 1 kg. Let's explore the math. If you take 1 gram and multiply it by 10 three times you get 1000 (10 × 10 × 10). Or another way of doing it is to place three zeros (10^3) behind the 1-0-0-0 ending up with 1000. The zeros behind the one represents tens (10), hundreds (100), thousands (1000), all the way up to millions (1,000,000), simple right!? A great example of this is our money, we have $1, $10, $100, and $1000 bills all based on the base unit of $1. In US slang, 1000 dollars is often referred to as $1K so in metric terms 1 *kilo*!

What do we do if we have something that weighs less than a gram? We insert a decimal behind the 1 and place zeros behind the decimal. Let's say we have something that weighs 1000 times less than a gram. The prefix milli stands for *minus* 1000 or 10^{-3}. The zeros behind the decimal represents tenths (1/10), hundredths (1/100), and thousandths (1/1000), in that order. If a milligram is 1000th of a gram we would write it as 1 milligram or 1 mg, which is the abbreviation for milligram.

The gram, kilogram, and milligram are three weights often utilized in veterinary medicine to weigh animals, medications, and powders. Understanding this and learning the other prefixes to indicate greater or lesser weights is very important.

Information Exercise

Utilize the internet to fill in this chart:

Name	Number	Prefix	Power of 10	Abbreviation
million				
thousand				
hundred				
tens				
Base unit – gram	1	No prefix	0	g
tenth				
hundredth				
thousandth				
millionth				

Today's scales can often be switched from pounds (US system) to kilograms (metric system). The scale may be one the animal sits upon, giving you a number in either pounds or kilograms, and if tiny like a bird or pocket pet in grams. Often the scales are in pounds, especially in US clinics. Being able to convert pounds to kilograms accurately and vice versa is a skill used constantly in a practice. One trick to remember is that an animal *always* weighs *less* in the metric system; they really don't weigh less, but the number for the weight is smaller.

The most common conversion factor to remember is *1 kilogram (kg) equals 2.2 pounds (lb)*. For example, if you have an animal that weighs 10 lb it will weigh 4.45 kg. How did we arrive at this number? The equation is written like this: 10 lb / 2.2 lb/kg = ___ kg. The pounds cancel each other out: 10 / 2.2 /kg, leaving you with 10/2.2 kg. Divide 10 by 2.2 and you get 4.45, so the answer is 4.45 kg.

If you must convert the other way, kilograms to pounds, you multiply by 2.2 lb/kg. For example, if an animal weighs 5 kg the equation would be written 5 kg × 2.2 lb/kg =___ lb. In this instance the kilograms cancel each other out, 5 × 2.2 ___ lb, and the answer is 11 lb.

This all works easily with whole numbers. What happens when you have an animal that weighs 4 lb 6 oz? Remember how to find the decimal point for a portion of a pound? Here are the equations.

Convert ounces into pounds: 6 oz / 16 oz/lb =___ lb, ounces cancel each other out, 6 / 16 /lb, leaving you with 6/16 = 0.___ lb, the answer is 0.37 lb and if your clinic likes you to round up the working answer is 4.4 lb. Remember we set the portion of a pound behind the decimal which is placed behind the full pounds. Now let's plug the 4.4 lb into the equation to convert pounds to kilograms: 4.4 lb / 2.2 lb/kg = ___ kg. The pounds cancel each other out 4.4 /2.2 /kg so you are just left with kilograms. That gives you 4.4/2.2 = 2 kg.

At the start of this section we briefly mentioned building your estimating skills. This takes some practice, but it is a good way to help check that your work is in range. For example, if you simply divide a number by 2 you are going to be close when converting pounds into kilograms. Here are are some examples.

Estimating kilograms from pounds, if we drop the 0.2 from the equation and divide 6 lb by 2 it equals 3 lb. That is your estimate number and our real answer should be close to 3. Remember it will be a bit less because of the 0.2 decimal.

Answer using the conversion of 1 lb = 2.2 kg: 6 lb / 2.2 lb/kg = 2.72 kg, and if your clinic rounds up the answer is 3 kg!

Estimating

Estimating portions of a pound into a decimal point. Visualize a 1-lb cookie and remember that 1 lb is equal to 16 oz. Now start dividing that cookie into portions. Half of a 16-oz cookie would be 8 oz, 16/2 = 8 and to change that to a decimal we would divide 8 by 16 and we would get 0.5 lb or ½ lb if expressed as a fraction. When estimating for 7 or 9 ounces the number should be something close to 0.5 lb. Let's work the problem and see how close we get. At 7 oz, we can estimate to be just a little under 0.5 lb because 7 is less than 8. We plug the 7 oz into our formula: 7 oz / 16 oz/lb = 0.4375 lb. If we round up, we would use 0.44 lb.

Volume Measurements – Dilutions

Another common occurrence in the veterinary practice is diluting solutions. These are often purchased as a concentrated solution or powder which saves on shipping costs. The veterinary assistant must be able to dilute the concentrate properly to achieve the optimum strength in which to do the job. Too concentrated and a dilution may cause damage and is wasteful. A solution that is too weak will not work as indicated. All products will have the instructions written on the label. Being able to read, understand, and dilute the solution is an important skill. The instructions are often written using the US or the metric system of measurements.

The most common US system of measuring volumes uses teaspoons, tablespoons, fluid ounces, cups, pints, quarts, and gallons for solutions and teaspoons, tablespoons, ounces, cups, pounds, tons for powders. The metric system uses the liter as its base unit for liquid

TABLE 1.1

Comparison of US to Metric Volumes

US liquid measurements	Metric liquid measurements
teaspoon (tsp or t) 3 = 1 tbsp	5 mL
tablespoon (TB, Tbl, tbsp, or T) 2 = 1 fl oz	15 mL
fluid ounce (fl oz)	30 mL
8 oz per 1 cup (C or c) – dry and liquid	250 mL
2 cups per 1 pint (pt)	500 mL
2 pints per 1 quart (qt)	1000 mL or 1 liter*
4 quarts per 1 gallon (gal)	4 liters

* 1 liter is slightly more volume than a quart.

volumes and we have already covered what it uses for powders. Table 1.1 shows a comparison of US to metric volumes.

Often, instructions to dilute a liquid concentrate are given as either ounces per quart or gallon in the US system or milliliters per liter. Here is an example of each:

- 1 oz of solution to 1 gallon of water
- 15 mL of solution to 2 liters of water
- 200 mL to 4 liters of water.

Information Exercise

- Utilizing the measuring devices in Figure 1.4, describe how you would fulfill the diluting instructions given.

A second method of diluting is by using ratios. They are often expressed as a number:number, or as a

decimal point, percentage, or fraction. For example, the instructions for diluting a window cleaner is 1:30. This means that you take 1 part of the concentrate and add it to 30 parts of water. This can be any unit of measurement: cups, milliliters, or liters:

- 1 cup of window cleaner to 30 cups of water
- 1 mL of window cleaner to 30 mL of water.

However, there are also instructions like this: 1:30 per gallon. This indicates that to make 1 gallon of window cleaner you must figure out how many ounces to add to 1 gallon. To figure this out we must remember that 1 gallon is equal to 128 oz. We would take the ratio number 30 and divide it into 128: 128/30 = 4.27 oz. The next issue arises because we don't have a measuring device that we can accurately measure out 0.27 oz. But we work in a veterinary clinic that has graduated cylinders and syringes! These use milliliters and we know that 1 fl oz is equal to 30 mL. Here is the equation: 4.27 oz × 30 mL/oz. The ounces cancel each other, 4.27 oz × 30 mL/oz so we would be left with mL and the answer is 128.1 mL. We have the choice of using the graduated cylinder or 12-mL syringe, refer to Figure 1.4. Which measuring device would it make the most sense to use? Both! You could accurately measure up to 120 mL with the graduated cylinder but would need to add the 8 mL using the syringe. The 0.1 mL would be dropped as it would be such a tiny amount it would not affect the dilution significantly.

Information Exercise

Utilizing Figure 1.4, select the correct implement to mix the following dilutions:
- 1:16 dilution per gallon
- 4 oz to 1 quart
- 120 mL per gallon

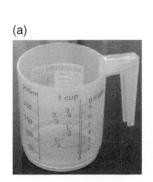

(a)

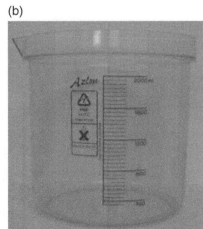

(b)

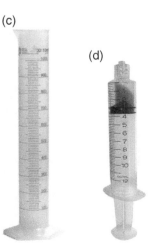

(c)

(d)

FIGURE 1.4 Measuring devices: (a) measuring cup – 250 mL; (b) large beaker – 2000 mL; (c) graduated cylinder – 1000 mL; (d) syringe – 12 mL.

Finally, you may see instructions for diluting a concentrate written as a percentage. This is a three-step formula:

_____(%)×(_____ total amount desired / 100 mL)
= _____ mL of concentrate.

The final amount of solution needed is based on the total amount needed minus the milliliters of solution:

_____ mL (total amount of water required) − _____
mL of concentrate = _____ mL of water.

You have to subtract the starting volume from the final volume to get the amount of water required for the dilution. For example, you need to refill a quart spray bottle with a 3% dilution of bleach with water. We know that a quart is about 1000 mL. Plug the numbers into the formula:

$3 \times (1000 / 100 \, \text{mL}) = 30 \, \text{mL}.$

1000 mL (desired volume) − 30 mL (concentrate)
= 970 mL of water.

30 mL of bleach is added to 970 mL of water
= 1000 mL of 3% diluted bleach solution.

Drug Calculation

Another mathematical problem used consistently in veterinary medicine is that to calculate drug dosages. These calculations are usually handled by veterinarians and veterinary technicians; however, there may come a time when you are asked to figure one out and being able to adds value to you as an employee. Veterinarians prescribe medications based on their knowledge of pharmacology and diseases or conditions that these medications are specifically manufactured to treat. The amount to give an individual is usually based on weight in either pounds (lb) or kilograms (kg). Each medication is formulated to be therapeutic at a certain dosage. The medication is manufactured at a certain concentration, which is found on the label. This information is utilized to figure out how much medication an animal should receive for it to heal the disease or condition the patient is currently suffering from. The formula is expressed as:

Weight (W) × dose (D) / concentration (C)
= number of tablets, capsules, or milliliters required.

For example, a non-steroidal anti-inflammatory drug (NSAID) is a routinely used medication for the treatment of pain in dogs. The dosage is 2 mg/lb of body weight (BW) per day, the patient is a 25-lb dog, and the medication comes in 75 mg tablet concentrations. Plug the information into the formula:

25 lb (W) × 2 mg / lb / 75 mg / tablet.

The pounds cancel each other out:

25 lb (W) × 2 mg /lb. / 75 mg / tablet − 25 × 2 / 75 mg / tablet = 50 / 75 mg / tablet = 0.666 of a tablet.

As tablets cannot be broken into 0.66 portions, your only option in this case is to round down or up. With this medication the clinic will opt to round down to 0.5 or ½ of a tablet. If the answer was in the 0.8 or higher range it would be rounded up. Decisions on when to round up or round down will be those bits of information that you learn when you are working in the practice.

What happens if the dosage of the medication is in mg/kg? The first thing we must do is convert the weight of the patient from pounds to kilograms. Remember how to do that? Then proceed with the drug calculation. Here is an example.

Patient weighs 16 lb 13 oz. Your drug dosage is 4 mg/kg, the concentration of the medication is 20 mg/mL.

Weight conversion − first ounces into pounds : 13 oz / 16 oz / lb − oz cancels out − 13 oz / 16 oz = 0.81 lb

16.81 lb are then converted to kilograms : 16.81 lb / 2.2 lb / kg = lb cancel out 16.81 lb / 2.2 lb / kg = 7.64 kg

Drug calculation formula : 7.64 kg (W) × 4 mg / kg / 20 mg / mL − kg and mg cancel out 7.64 kg (W) × 4 mg / kg / 20 mg / mL = 7.64 × 4 / 20 = 1.528 mL.

We can drop the last two digits and deliver 1.5 mL.

Information Exercise

Solve the following drug calculations. Read each carefully!
- A patient weighs 42 lb 5 oz, and needs an injection of medicine, the dose is 0.04 mg/lb, the concentration is 0.54 mg/mL.
- A patient weighs 6 lb 11 oz and needs an oral antibiotic, the dose is 25 mg/kg and the tablets are 50 mg. They have score marks for breaking them in quarters.

Medical Terminology

The base languages of medical terminology are either Latin or Greek, with some exceptions. Therefore, learning medical terminology is very much like learning a new language. Recognizing and memorizing definitions of frequently occurring word parts is essential to deciphering a word's meaning. The word parts are key to understanding medical terminology. Most words will use one or all the following: a prefix (beginning of a word), root (often the middle part of a word), and suffix (ending of a word). Not all medical terms will have all three parts but are often made up of at least two parts.

Information Exercise

Utilize the Appendix, the Glossary, or the internet to find medical terminology sources on prefixes, root words, suffixes, and combining vowels to determine the meaning of the following terms:

Medical term	Prefix	Root	Suffix	Combining vowel
Tachycardia				
Pneumothorax				
Urinary cystitis				
Otitis				
Hemorrhage				

- Prefixes are often used to indicate intensity, numbers, colors, sizes, position, and time.
- Root words are often related to body systems and/or convey the meaning of the medical term. Root words can be utilized as prefixes and suffixes.
- Suffixes are used to modify the root to indicate a procedure, condition, disease, or part of speech.
- Combining or connected vowels are o, i, e, and a. They are used to build more comprehensive words to describe a condition, disease, or action.

Here are some examples:

- **Intracardial** – [intra] prefix for within, [cardial] root word for heart. Note the absence of a combining vowel because the prefix ended with a vowel.
- **Conjunctivitis** – [conjunctiv] root word for conjunctiva or the white part of the eye, [itis] is the suffix that means inflammation.
- **Hysterectomy** – [hyster] root word meaning uterus, there is no combining vowel because the

suffix starts with one, [ectomy] means surgical removal.
- **Encephalomyelitis** – [encephal] is the root word for brain or inside the skull, [o] is the combing vowel, [myel] is the root word for spinal cord or marrow, [itis] is the suffix for inflammation. Note that there is not a combining vowel between myel and itis, because itis starts with a vowel a combing vowel is not necessary. This also holds true for root words that end with a vowel.

Multiple abbreviations are used by veterinarians to shorten the time it takes to write orders, prescriptions, and instructions for the veterinary technician to carry out for a patient and to educate the client. As a veterinary assistant you may be asked to interpret these orders, prescriptions, and instructions. The ones you may be exposed to the most are those that have something to do with consumption of food and/or medications. Table 1.2 shows some examples.

The abbreviations in Table 1.3 are used for giving medications or treatments to certain areas of the body. These are just a few of the many abbreviations you will see used daily in a veterinary practice. These

TABLE 1.2

Examples of Abbreviations

Abbreviation	Meaning	Abbreviation	Meaning
ad lib	as much as desired	q	every
bw or BW	body weight	h	hour
qd	daily or once a day, every day	q2h	every 2 hours – number is interchangeable
bid	twice a day	NPO	nothing by mouth
tid	three times a day	x	duration of RX
qid	four times a day	PRN	as needed
RX	prescription	TX	prescribed treatment

TABLE 1.3

Abbreviations Used For Giving Medications or Treatments to Certain Areas of the Body

Abbreviation	Meaning
SQ, SubQ	subcutaneous – injection given under the skin
IM	intramuscular – injection given into the muscle
IN	intranasal – liquid squirted into a nostril
IV	intravenous – injection or catheter placed into a vein
PO, po	per os – by mouth or orally
PR, pr	per rectum – rectal medications
as, AS	left ear
as, AD	right ear
au, AU	each or both ears
os, OS	left eye
od, OD	right eye
ou, OU	each or both eyes

abbreviations will crop up in the rest of this textbook. It is suggested that you keep a small notebook in your pocket and when you see an abbreviation or acronym that you don't know the mean of, write it down and look it up.

Information Exercise

One of the best ways to learn these root words, suffixes and prefixes, and abbreviations is to write them on flash cards to test yourself and practice using them every day in a sentence.

Chapter Reflection

Think about all of the information in this chapter. What was the easiest to learn? What was the hardest? What will you need to practice the most?

CHAPTER 2

Laws, Policies, and OSHA Standards Affecting Veterinary Practice

LEARNING OBJECTIVES
- Discover where laws come from and what impact they have on veterinary practices
- Determine how veterinary practice acts protect the public and animals
- Apply OSHA standards to work safely in a veterinary practice

NAVTA GUIDELINES COVERED IN THIS CHAPTER
V. Small Animal Nursing (Large Animal Nursing – Optional)
A. Safety concerns
    2. Utilize personnel safety measures
    7. Be familiar with OSHA standards

Laws and Regulations for Veterinary Practices

Veterinary medicine and the practice of veterinary medicine are regulated by several federal, state, and local laws. They represent the minimum standard to which a veterinarian must comply when practicing veterinary medicine. Ignorance of the law is not an excuse and does not constitute a defense in violation of any law. There are different levels of laws that are set by various entities in government. Let's take a look at where these laws originate and what they do to protect the veterinarian, the animals, and the public. Table 2.1 shows the number of agencies that have a direct impact on veterinary medicine whether by law or by voluntarily following guidelines.

Federal Laws

Federal laws are those made by the US government. They override all state and local laws. These laws tend to be broader in scope and more general in statement, allowing states to decide how to implement policies and penalties. Several federal agencies have been tasked with watching over the different aspects of veterinary medicine and animals and how they impact on public health.

Tasks for the Veterinary Assistant, Fourth Edition. Teresa F. Sonsthagen.
© 2020 John Wiley & Sons, Inc. Published 2020 by John Wiley & Sons, Inc.
Companion website: www.wiley.com/go/sonsthagen/tasks

TABLE 2.1

Agencies and Their Responsibilities

Agency	Acronym	Department	Responsibility
Food and Drug Administration	FDA		Safety of food and pharmaceuticals for animals and humans
		Center for Veterinary Medicine (CVM)	Importation of animal foods, medicines and veterinary equipment
		Food Animal Residue Avoidance Databank (FARAD)	A risk management program to standardize drug withholding times in food animals
US Department of Agriculture	USDA	Animal and Plant Health Inspection Service (APHIS)	Protecting agricultural health, implementing Animal Welfare Act, overseeing Institutional Animal Care and Use Committee (IACUC) actions
National Institutes of Health	NIH	Office of Laboratory Animal Welfare (OLAW)	Sets policies, regulations, and guidance that protect animals used in research, training, and testing
Drug Enforcement Agency	DEA		Licensing and oversight of the use of controlled drugs in veterinary practices
Occupational Safety and Health Administration	OSHA		Sets standards and oversees workplace safety
US Equal Employment Opportunity Commission	EEOC	Civil Rights Act, Equal Pay Act, Americans with Disabilities Act	Enforces laws regarding discrimination and sexual harassment
Environmental Protection Agency	EPA		Guidelines for use and disposal of pesticides and other hazardous materials
State Veterinary Medical Boards	VMB		Administers veterinary licensing exams, veterinary technician exams, upholds practice act, convenes hearings on misconduct and metes out punishments
Association of American Veterinary State Boards	AAVSB	Non-profit	National database for practice acts, foreign veterinary medical student testing, administers the Veterinary Technician National Exam, etc.
American Veterinary Medical Association	AVMA	Non-profit	Sets standards of practice, lobbying for veterinary medicine and animal welfare, continuing education, etc.
American Animal Hospital Association	AAHA	For-profit	Sets high standards of practice and inspects facilities of members
National Association of Veterinary Technicians in America	NAVTA	Non-profit	Networking, continuing education, advocacy for technicians, certification of assistants

The US Food and Drug Administration (FDA) Center for Veterinary Medicine (CVM) regulates animal and veterinary products imported into the USA. This includes all animal food and feed, animal drugs, medicated feed, and veterinary devices. CVM ensures that all imported products are properly labeled for marketing in the USA. All imported human and animal foods must meet the same safety standards as foods produced in the USA. New imported animal drugs are reviewed for safety and effectiveness before they can be marketed in the USA. Any drug used in medicated animal feed must be approved for use in that specific animal feed. Imported veterinary devices must be labeled "for veterinary use only" and radiation-emitting devices are verified and registered according to the radiologic health regulations.

The US Department of Agriculture (USDA) has a role in federal policies and procedures for animal safety. In 1966, the first Animal Welfare Act (AWA) was established, which has been revised and updated numerous times since then. It created a regulatory network with the following areas of main concern:

- Limitations/regulations on how animals are sourced to be sold for research purposes; this is to eliminate the use of stolen animals.
- Issuing of permits to buy and sell animals, and/or the registration of dealers of animals, exhibitors, and research facilities. Research facilities can only purchase animals from licensed dealers.
- Set regulations on animal environmental conditions for housing in and transportation to research and teaching facilities.

- Requires the establishment of an Institutional Animal Care and Use Committee (IACUC) in every research and teaching facility that uses animals. This committee is made up of researchers and/or professors that review all written research and teaching protocols that utilize animals within that facility. They are tasked with making sure the protocols are within the guidelines set by the USDA/AWA and that the animals are cared for as specified in the protocol.
- Inspections by the USDA's Animal and Plant Health Inspection Service (APHIS) are on an annual basis. All licensed facilities (research, exhibition, and sanctuaries) and protocols involving animals are inspected to check if they are complying with the rules.
- Set regulations for transporting animals across state and national borders.
- Prosecute and penalize any person that knowingly sponsors or exhibits an animal in any animal fighting venture.

The USDA oversees the Food Animal Residue Avoidance Databank (FARAD), a risk management program to standardize drug withholding times in food animals. Withholding times minimize drug residue in meat and milk. It is the time necessary for animals to metabolize all traces of these medications before they can be slaughtered, or the milk sold for consumption. The farad.org website contains a full list per species of drugs and their withholding times.

The Drug Enforcement Administration (DEA) is part of the US Department of Justice. Their influence in veterinary medicine is the regulation of controlled drugs such as anesthetics, pain medications, and euthanasia solutions. These drugs have a high incidence of addiction thereby requiring a veterinarian to obtain a DEA license in order to use them. Accurate records of their storage and use in a veterinary practice is required. Surprise inspections can occur and if there are discrepancies legal action and loss of the license to practice veterinary medicine could occur. For more information about these drugs see Chapter 13 on Pharmacy Skills.

Learning Exercise

- Which government agency inspects research and teaching facilities?
- Which US agency is responsible for making sure imported food, drugs, and devices are safe?
- Who is responsible for reviewing research and teaching protocols within a facility?
- Which state agency regulates drugs that have a high incidence of addition?
- Which group is responsible for enforcing drug withholding times?

State Laws

Practice Act Rules and Regulations

As discussed in Chapter 1, veterinary medicine is specifically regulated by a practice act. Each individual state legislates their practice act to fit within the state's laws and culture. The practice act is not changed easily or often as it takes an act of the state's legislative, judicial, and executive branches to be changed. The American Veterinary Medical Association (AVMA) and the American Association of Veterinary State Boards (AAVSB) have model practice acts that can be utilized to update or revamp state practice acts. AAVSB has a current database of each state's practice act and assists with state jurisprudence, veterinary medical exams, and administers the Veterinary Technician National Exam (VTNE).

In addition to the practice act, there are rules and regulations determined by a veterinary state board, whose members are appointed by the governor of the state. These are not legislated and can be adjusted to facilitate the legislated practice act. This board is also responsible for administering veterinary licenses, and in some states veterinary technician credentials by providing an examination for each. They also enforce the practice act and hand out judgments and penalties for violations.

The main purpose of a practice act is to protect the consumer and public health from incompetent and fraudulent veterinary actions. The practice act dictates what the practice of veterinary medicine is, who can call themselves a veterinarian and act as such in a veterinary practice, as well as various state laws and rules of conduct as they pertain to animals and the public. Violation of these laws represent the practice of veterinary medicine without a license, which is prosecutable. Because each state has their own laws and culture, most require a veterinarian to pass their state licensing exam. This means a veterinarian licensed in one state cannot practice veterinary medicine in another state. Some states do have reciprocity, but most do not. Veterinary technicians can have their VTNE scores transferred to another state and, if accepted, is credentialed in that state. Veterinary assistants with a National Association of Veterinary Technicians in America (NAVTA) certificate can work in any state.

The practice act can also provide guidelines as to what veterinary staff may do within a practice. This is usually delineated by levels of supervision such as direct/immediate supervision or indirect/remote supervision. In most states it is up to the veterinarian to determine the competence of the staff members before delegating a task. The veterinarian is directly responsible for the actions of the staff and if a mistake is made it is the veterinarian who will be held responsible including legal ramifications and loss of license.

The last major topic of discussion about practice acts is the establishment of the veterinarian–client–patient relationship. It stipulates that in order to treat an animal the veterinarian must have first-hand knowledge of the animal, have met the owner personally, and be available for follow-up care. Without this a veterinarian may not provide medications or treatment options by law.

Each state has laws that govern the shipment of livestock and companion animals across state lines. This requires that an animal is inspected by and if necessary vaccinated for communicable diseases by a veterinarian. A health certificate is filled out for each companion animal and livestock health certificates can be for 10–20 animals per certificate. In most states this certificate is good for at least 30 days.

Learning Exercise

Utilize the internet to find your state's practice act. In your own words answer these questions:
- What is the definition of "practice veterinary medicine?"
- What does the practice of veterinary medicine include?
- Are there specific levels of supervision for veterinary technicians or specific tasks they can perform in your practice act?
- What does the practice act in your state say about veterinarian–client–patient relationships?
- How many days does a health certificate last in your state?

Common or Case Law

Decisions made by judges over the years have created legal precedence which is used by other lawyers to bring, defend, or not accept future cases in court. Of interest in veterinary practice are laws related to business practices and those that govern the relationships between people and property. In a litigious society, veterinarians protect themselves from lawsuits by practicing good medicine, delegating staff appropriately, and making sure safety is a number one priority. Even with the best of intentions things happen that can lead to a lawsuit being brought against the veterinarian. It is because of this that veterinarians carry liability insurance to cover the cost of legal fees and fines. Here are some examples of past legal cases in which a veterinarian was sued.

A client slips and falls on a wet floor, doesn't matter who or what caused it, if it happens in a business there is legal precedence of suing for bodily injury. Another common case is if an owner is injured by an animal, even their own, while in the veterinary facility they can sue for bodily injury.

Animals are considered as property in the same way as a house or car. Owners have rights when property is stolen, damaged, or destroyed by accident, neglect, or on purpose. A malpractice suit may be brought against a veterinarian because of a perceived substandard of practice, whether willful, because of negligence, ignorance, and/or disregard of the client's wishes. If the actions the veterinarian took led to a decrease in value of, injury to, or death of a companion or livestock animal, the owner has a right to file a malpractice suit. This could result in two outcomes: a malpractice suit in a civil court which could result in a high settlement and/or the loss of the veterinarian's license to practice from the veterinary medical board if found guilty.

Another instance of legal proceedings stem from staff members accidently or mistakenly harming or killing an animal. The veterinarian is legally responsible for the actions taken by all staff members employed by the practice. This is true even if the staff member acted without the knowledge of the veterinarian or overstepped the boundaries set by practice law or policies set by the practice. The consequences for the veterinarian are the same as described in the previous paragraph. The consequences for the employee will depend entirely on the actions taken by the employee. Was it an accident, a mistake, or a willful disregard of rules, policy, and procedure? The employee may find themselves being sued or losing their job.

What can a veterinarian and his/her staff do to protect themselves from liability or malpractice? Adherence to policies and procedures is one way of minimizing the risk. For example:

- Placing wet floor warning signs out and cleaning up accidents quickly in the reception area reduces the chances of someone falling (Figure 2.1). Check outside for potential hazards, like ice or a water hose for the grass on the sidewalk, and fix immediately.
- Multiple suits have been filed because an animal escaped from the clinic or staff member. Make sure doors and windows are latched securely, double leashing works especially well with large dogs that pull excessively. Assisting clients out to their cars with large bags of food and or other take home items rather than having them juggle a dog on a leash or a cat in a carrier plus the items will also reduce the chance of escape.
- Properly identifying animals that are housed in the facility. Utilize the patient files to confirm what treatments or procedures are to be carried out, double check the description of the animal against the one in the kennel or pen. Several previous lawsuits were due to treating the wrong "black lab" or the castrating the "lighter" (owner meant weight) of the two colts – the vet thought it was the lighter colored of the two.

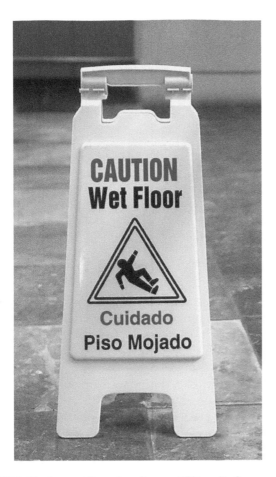

FIGURE 2.1 Caution wet floor sign. Source: Wikimedia Commons. Used under CC BY 2.0, https://creativecommons.org/licenses/by/2.0/deed.cn.

- Utilizing release forms for consent to treat, perform surgery/anesthetic risks, treatment estimates, and euthanasia are also used to prevent misunderstandings or assumptions. These forms are considered contracts and document the expectations of both parties involved. Attach these forms and mark all treatments, observations, and conversations with the owner in the patient's file.
- Never permit the owners to restrain their own animals. They may not know how to keep themselves or the veterinarian from being bitten. Previous cases of owners holding their own animals have resulted in bite wounds that have resulted in loss of limb function and facial nerve damage. If it was the veterinarian who was bitten it may mean shutting down the clinic.
- As an assistant, never provide information to anyone on any subject on which are you are not knowledgeable. Never render a treatment to a patient without orders from a veterinarian; never offer clients advice about their animal's condition, disease, or behavior without orders from a veterinarian. Remember, only the veterinarian can diagnose, prognose, prescribe, and perform surgery in a practice. You should never talk to

clients about the treatments, health concerns, or prognosis of their animal, unless expressly granted permission by the veterinarian. Refer the client to another staff member or back to the veterinarian for answers to their questions.

> ## Learning Reflection
>
> After reading about the many instances in veterinary practice that result in a law suit and/or loss of a license, reflect your feelings about such actions. Are they ever justifiable? Is it fair that the veterinarian is responsible for the actions of her/his employees? How easy would it be for someone to act as a veterinarian, whether knowingly or unknowingly, and what could the consequences be for following that action?

Local Ordnances

As a business the veterinary practice is required to adhere to local ordnances that regulate several aspects. For example, the size and location of signs for the business, zoning laws for where in the city such a business can be, and the requirement of a business license.

Local ordnances also affect the pet owner and who may depend on the veterinary practice staff to inform them correctly of what laws they need to know about. One such ordnance requires dogs and cats to be licensed. Some will limit the number of each species housed in one home, as well as what species or breed of animal may be kept within city limits. Many localities have leash laws requiring dogs and cats to be on a leash when outdoors or secured in a fenced yard. Nuisance laws usually govern noise, soiling, and destruction of private property by companion animals. Barking dogs, failure to clean up feces, and dogs or cats that chase or harm other animals and people can result in a citation. Bites are of major concern and so most localities have ordnances for rabies vaccinations. Some localities differ in only requiring dogs to be vaccinated, some require both dogs and cats, and even others dogs, cats, and ferrets. Most states and/or localities mandate that wolf, wolf–dog hybrids, coyote, coyote–dog hybrids, racoons, and skunks are never vaccinated for rabies. Many states will also allow livestock to be vaccinated; however, they do not require the certificate. Many cities will quarantine vaccinated animals that have bitten someone for up to 10 days at the expense of the owner, and usually in a veterinary facility. Unvaccinated animals are often euthanized immediately for the animal to be tested for rabies. These rules can be found in the state's century code or the local ordnance for details.

This section is only an overview of the many laws and ordnances veterinary practices must observe. Knowledge of these laws is the responsibility of the veterinarian and the practice manager. The polices and procedures of the individual practice should incorporate these laws and regulations. It is the responsibility of the veterinary staff to learn about and adhere to these polices and procedures.

Learning Discovery

- What is the state or local ordnance for vaccinating animals against rabies?
- Which animals are, and which are not to be vaccinated?
- What age is the first vaccination to be given to dogs and cats if mandated?
- Are there ownership limitations on species or breeds in your city?
- How are dogs and/or cat licensed in your city?

Guidelines of Practice from Veterinary Organizations

Federal, state, and local laws represent the required standards to protect the public and animals, the veterinary profession itself makes additional recommendations. The AVMA and the American Animal Hospital Association (AAHA) are organizations that offer enhanced practice recommendations.

The AVMA is a non-profit organization that provides policies and guidelines to the profession, continuing education, accredits colleges of veterinary medicine and programs of education for veterinary technicians. They also lobby on a national level for animal welfare, disease control, and the profession of veterinary medicine.

The AAHA is a for-profit organization that sets a higher practice standard for veterinary hospitals than the usual standards. An AAHA accredited practice has met and adheres to the organization's membership requirements and high standards. Member hospitals are subject to periodic inspections to ensure compliance to these standards. The standards themselves are wide ranging, setting criteria for facilities, pharmacy, anesthesia, surgery, housekeeping, and other areas of practice.

NAVTA is a non-profit organization for veterinary technicians. Their mission is advancing veterinary nursing and technology. They do so by offering continuing education, networking with state associations, membership benefits, advocating the profession to veterinarians and the public, education guidelines, and certification of veterinary assistants.

Exploration Learning

Utilize the internet to find the websites and mission statements for the AVMA, AAHA, and NAVTA. In your own words compare these three organizations' missions for its members. Which one has the biggest impact on your career as a veterinary assistant?

Occupational Safety and Health Administration (OSHA) – Workplace Safety

OSHA is a federal agency that governs workplace safety, enforces laws designed to minimize hazards in the workplace, and metes out fines to those facilities that fail to follow safety guidelines.

Each worksite must have a written plan complying with the laws with a designated person as the plan's administrator, the Hazard Communication Coordinator (HCC), who oversees the implementation of the rules. This person is responsible for training new and existing employees in the safety rules followed in that facility. The AVMA recommends that new employees sign a notification verifying this training. The HCC is also responsible for posting OSHA signage throughout the practice providing information on risks of the job, how to minimize them, what to do in an emergency, and to whom and when to report accidents on the job.

The HCC is also responsible for providing training on and enforcing the use of personal protective equipment (PPE). Goggles, face masks, gloves, rubber boots, and waterproof aprons are the basic safety equipment found in the veterinary facility. All these items must be worn when encountering hazardous chemical and infectious waste materials. For more about these items see the section on Personal Protection Equipment later in the chapter.

The HCC is also responsible for keeping the Material Safety Data Sheets (MSDS) up to date. The MSDS are a source of information about the hazards of each product, including how to handle and store it properly, as well as what to do in case of accidental exposure. They are usually kept in a binder in a central location for ease of access. They are used in case someone is exposed to a chemical that can cause damage.

The HCC is the person to report to if an illness or injury develops on the job or an action or event that might affect job safety. It is especially important for women to notify the HCC as soon as they become pregnant or suspect they are pregnant. There are many hazards associated with birth defects or which can potentially cause miscarriage in a veterinary practice and certain actions must be taken to protect both mother and child.

There are other procedures and policies that cover prevention of bites and other animal-related injuries, accidental needlestick injuries, rabies pre-exposure vaccinations, and other environmental controls that effect health and well-being of the employees. Each practice differs in how they handle such occurrences. Remember to ask for this information if it is not in the policy and procedure manual.

Labeling

Another guideline from OSHA is the use of secondary product labels. Many products used in the veterinary practice come as a concentrate, in gallon bottles, or large bottles of pills and solutions. This is referred to as the source bottle and it comes from the manufacturer with a primary label. A secondary label is required when putting a portion of the source bottle into another container. For example, veterinary practices use gallons of isopropyl alcohol on a weekly basis. To have it readily available it must be divided into spray or smaller bottles and then dispersed around the clinic (Figure 2.2). Each of these bottles must have a secondary label attached to identify what is in the bottle so it isn't used inappropriately.

The secondary labels have adhesive on the back and some have a clear plastic shield cover that is used to protect the label once it is written. The colored squares on the label represent flammability, reactivity, health hazards, and special hazards. Each square should be marked as to the level of flammability, reactivity, health hazards, and special hazards. Each blank line should be filled in with chemical/strength, manufacturer, and date it was set up. All this information is found on the MSDS. Table 2.2 explains how each square is marked on the OSHA secondary labels and what each color represents.

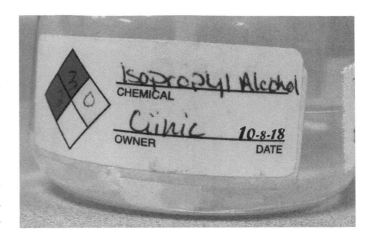

FIGURE 2.2 OSHA secondary label.

Personal Protection Equipment

Veterinary medicine is a hazardous occupation, with dangers including bite wounds, scratches, and kicks, exposure to zoonotic diseases and parasites, noxious chemicals, and radiation, and also hurting yourself by the constant lifting and restraining of heavy animals. The employer is responsible for ensuring a safe working environment, by implementing universal precautions. It is the employee's responsibility to behave in ways that enhance personal safety as well as conform to all OSHA regulations.

There are over 200 zoonotic diseases transmissible from animals to humans, with many of them life-threatening. As there is no way of knowing what disease an animal may be harboring, assume that every encounter with a patient poses the threat of a zoonotic infection. Part of the policies and procedures manual in the practice will have an Infection Control Plan that implements universal precautions. It will have instructions on how to prevent transmission of diseases and what PPE is required for protecting the employees from becoming infected.

Universal precautions are measures taken whenever there is the possible transmission of infection from a patient or the patient's body fluids to the handlers, the possibility of exposure to agents that can cause diseases, or conditions that can become fatal to the handler. These precautions were adapted to veterinary medicine from human medicine and they deal with the potential for cross-infection: person–person, animal–person, person—animal, and animal–animal. These precautions should always be kept in mind when dealing with bodily fluids and or infected patients. PPE and prudent behavior will minimize the risk of cross-infection.

The following is a list of PPE that should be available throughout the practice facility.

Gloves

Exam gloves are usually made of latex. If the handler is allergic to latex, a nitrile glove made from synthetic rubber is a good alternative. Exam gloves must be worn

Learning Discovery

- What is the role of the HCC in a practice?
- Which organization is concerned with keeping employees safe at work?
- Utilizing the internet find a MSDS for 70% isopropyl alcohol:
  - Where should this product be stored in a hospital?
  - How should it be labeled if put into a secondary container?
- What do the red, blue, yellow, and white symbols mean on a secondary container label?
- Utilize the internet to find an MSDS for Rescue disinfectant spray. Fill in the secondary label in Figure 2.3 utilizing the MSDS.

TABLE 2.2		
Explanation of the OSHA Secondary Label		
Color	Hazard	Score
Red	Flammability	0 – Will not burn 1 – Ignites above 200°F 2 – Ignites below 200°F 3 – Ignites below 100°F 4 – Ignites below 73°F
Yellow	Reactivity	0 – Stable 1 – Normally stable 2 – Unstable 3 – Explosive 4 – May detonate
Blue	Health hazards	0 – No hazard 1 – Slight hazard 2 – Dangerous 3 – Extreme danger 4 – Deadly
White	Special hazards	W – Water reactive Trefoil – Radioactive Cor – Corrosive ACD – Acid ALK – Alkali

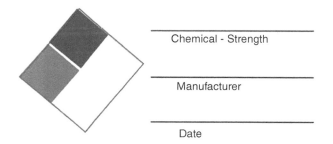

FIGURE 2.3 Empty secondary label.

to protect the hands from exposure or absorption of chemicals and toxic agents as well as infectious materials.

Gloves can develop microscopic holes while being worn, allowing microorganisms or chemical agents to contact the skin. There is also the potential for disease-causing organisms to contact the skin during the de-gloving process despite the most careful efforts to avoid it. After taking the gloves off a thorough washing of the hands and forearms, with a good disinfectant soap, is recommended. After washing hands, dry them thoroughly and apply hand cream to prevent chapping and cracks. Intact skin is the best barrier to the entry of disease into the body; therefore hand care is important for disease prevention. If the used gloves are hazardous to humans, they should be disposed of in a biohazard container or a trash bin that is lined with a biohazard bag.

Gloves are changed whenever handling a new patient, when cleaning or handling bodily fluids, and while working in the laboratory. This prevents transmission of diseases between patients and from patient waste to personnel. Gloves are also changed between dirty and clean tasks on the same patient. If a co-worker or client is injured and bleeding, gloves must be put on before attempting to help and while cleaning up.

Try a couple of sizes to see which fits best; they should fit well without much excess length on the fingers and stay in place, but not so tight that you lose circulation in your fingers! Dirty gloves should be removed in a very careful manner to avoid contaminating your skin. Start by removing the glove from your dominant hand by pinching the outer surface of the glove about 2 inches below the cuff (Figure 2.4a). Pull the glove outward and downward, turning the glove inside out as you pull that hand free of the glove (Figure 2.4b). Gather the removed glove into the palm of the still gloved hand (Figure 2.4c). Slide your fingers under the cuff of the glove on the non-dominant hand and pinch the material. Then pull the glove down and off, turning it inside out with the first glove enclosed inside the glove (Figure 2.4d). Dispose of the gloves properly; don't leave them lying around as they can contaminate the area.

Thorough handwashing follows, this entails moistening hands with water, applying soap, and rubbing the hands together for a minimum of 20 seconds, including wrists, between the fingers, and under the fingernails. Rinse well and leave the water running while you get a paper towel to shut the water off. Discard that paper towel and get another to dry your hands, after which

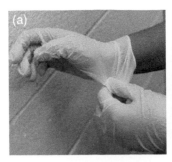 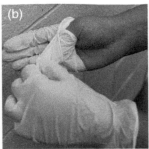 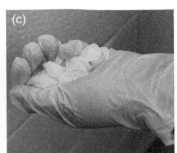 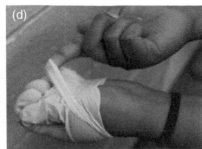

FIGURE 2.4 De-gloving.

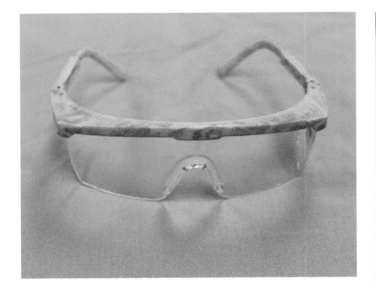

FIGURE 2.5 Safety goggles.

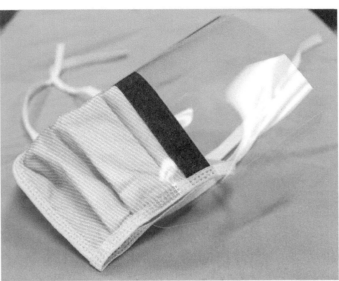

FIGURE 2.6 Face mask and shield.

apply a good hand cream. Twenty seconds is the minimum amount of contact time required for the soap to do its job. Singing the happy birthday song or saying the Pledge of Allegiance twice is about 20 seconds.

Goggles

Safety glasses or goggles are to be worn at any time there is a potential for splashing or spraying of infectious or toxic materials. This includes mixing concentrated chemicals, working with body fluids, or other items that may sting your eyes distracting you from the patient. Goggles should fit so that you can look down without them falling off. If you wear glasses, goggles should be fitted such that they fit well over the glasses and don't make your nose or ears sore. There are a couple of types of goggles that are easily found at building supply stores or uniform shops (Figure 2.5). Never assume that because you wear glasses you don't have to wear safety goggles. Splashes can come from any angle and many people have had to make trips to the emergency room because of this error. Investing in a good pair that is comfortable to wear is worth the expense because your eyesight is priceless.

Masks

Face masks and face shields are used to protect the mouth and nose or the entire face from absorbing or inhaling infectious or toxic materials through the mucus membranes and face (Figure 2.6). Examples of this are the spray from a dental prophylaxis handpiece or dipping a patient with a fungicide. The spray from the dental prophylaxis handpiece is full of bacteria and the fungicide can be toxic if ingested.

Outer Coverings

Waterproof aprons, gowns, or coveralls are used to protect scrubs from becoming soiled or contaminated with infectious or toxic materials. For example, dipping a patient with a fungicide, fecal material when working with cattle, parasites from skin or fecal material, and the spatter of water while cleaning kennels. Some of these microorganisms can live on clothing for a long period of time and have the potential for making you or your pets sick because you brought them home on your clothes.

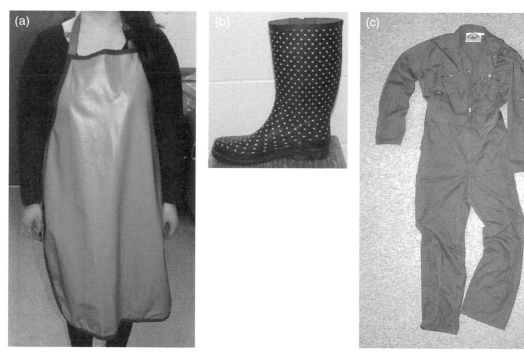

FIGURE 2.7 (a) Apron, (b) rubber boots, and (c) coveralls. Source: Wikimedia Commons. Used under CC BY-SA 3.0, https://creativecommons.org/licenses/by-sa/3.0/deed.en.

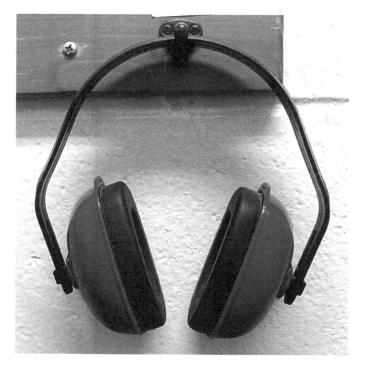

FIGURE 2.8 Ear protectors.

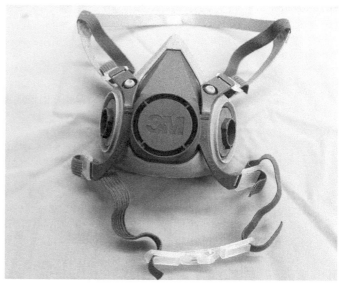

FIGURE 2.9 Respirator.

Footwear

Shoes suitable for a veterinary practice should be supportive and closed toed to protect the foot from spills. Rubber boots are important when working in wet, dirty, or contaminated environments like a farmyard or dirty kennel (Figure 2.7). Shoe covers are used to cover street shoes if going into the surgery suite and isolation ward. It is important to not to drag contaminates into the surgery suite and contaminates out of an isolation ward.

Ear Protection

Ear muffs or buds are important to prevent hearing loss (Figure 2.8). It may not seem as if a veterinary practice is very noisy; however, placing several dogs into a large empty room and when barking starts, the noise level can quickly rise above the acceptable level of safety. Ear muffs or ear buds are appropriate ear protection.

Respirators

Respirators are used when dealing with toxic chemicals that are aerosols or become vapor when exposed to room air or oxygen (Figure 2.9). There are specific respirators to use and the filters should be changed as per the manufacturer's recommendations. An example of when to use a respirator is when filling anesthesia machines with liquid gas.

These are the common PPE found in veterinary practices. The following chapters include more PPE for specific procedures and indicate when to use the PPE discussed in this chapter.

Learning Reflection

Think of working in a veterinary clinic and consider what tasks you will be doing. Now start to envision the PPE that you will need to use for some of these tasks. Write a scenario using PPE and completing a task often asked of a veterinary assistant.

CHAPTER 3

Veterinary Business Protocols

LEARNING OBJECTIVES
- Patient intake/discharge for examination room
- Assist with writing in medical record properly
- Handle front office procedures with skill and confidence
- Keep careful patient records and logs
- Assist with inventory control

NAVTA GUIDELINES COVERED IN THIS CHAPTER

I. Office and Hospital Procedures

A. Front desk
1. Greet clients
2. Demonstrate proper appointment scheduling and make appointments
3. Prepare appropriate forms and certificates for signature
4. Admit patient
5. Discharge patient
6. Perform basic filing and retrieving of medical records
7. Perform basic veterinary medical record keeping procedures
10. Perform basic invoicing, billing, and payment on account procedures

B. Telephone
1. Answer and direct phone call
2. Recognize and respond appropriately to veterinary medical emergencies by notifying the appropriate hospital personnel
3. Request records and information from other veterinary facilities

C. Maintain basic cleanliness and orderliness of a veterinary facility
1. Inventory supplies
2. Restock shelves
3. Perform basic filing and retrieving of medical records, radiographs, lab reports, and so on.

Tasks for the Veterinary Assistant, Fourth Edition. Teresa F. Sonsthagen.
© 2020 John Wiley & Sons, Inc. Published 2020 by John Wiley & Sons, Inc.
Companion website: www.wiley.com/go/sonsthagen/tasks

Front Office Skills

In Chapter 1 we discussed the role each staff member has in the veterinary practice. We said that the receptionist is the person that handles the front desk and is the front line of customer service. A good receptionist is caring, able to multi-task, remains calm, helpful, and is always extremely friendly. A veterinary assistant may be asked to fill in for an absent or overwhelmed receptionist and so this section provides information on what duties are required to run an efficient and welcoming front desk.

If asked to cover the front desk, make sure your appearance is professional. Clean scrubs, change if necessary, hair combed, name tag in place, and a smile planted on your face is a must before stepping foot behind the front desk. This is important because first impressions must be great! The client is often anxious, especially if a new client, when visiting the clinic. Your professionalism will help them relax and build their confidence and trust in the staff. Although being professional is important all the time, it is especially important when acting as a receptionist.

Reflection

Why is appearance so important not only when working as the receptionist, but also when working in all aspects of the job?

Telephone Skills

The telephone is the main means of communicating with clients. It should be answered within three rings with a smile on your face and in your voice. The greeting must contain the name of the hospital, your name, and a question. For example, *"Valley Veterinary Hospital, this is Teresa, how many I help you?"* This should be done in a moderate tone and pace. A hurried or gruff greeting implies that you are bothered by their call. This can amplify or induce anxiety in the client and isn't a very good first impression for new clients. No matter what is going on in the reception area, the phone *must* be answered as if you were waiting for their call and the caller is your best friend.

Discovery Exercise

Practice answering the phone with a smile in your voice and on your face. Then try it with a frown. Can you hear the difference?

TIP BOX 3.1

Always have a functional pen, notepad, and computer open to the appointment screen or the appointment book available when answering the phone.

After the greeting always wait for a reply to your question. It is very off-putting when the phone is answered and the question is "Can I put you on hold?" with an immediate click of the hold button! What if the call is an emergency?! The few seconds it takes to listen is well worth the time as it shows that you care about them and are happy they called.

Once you hear what the client needs, if you have the time to take care of them do so. If you have to redirect their call or put them on hold because you are in the middle of helping someone ask them if it is alright to put them on hold and again wait for an answer. Redirecting means the call is for someone in the practice. You will need to see if that person is available or you will need to take a message.

Most people will accept being placed on hold, but not for very long! It is recommended that you get back to them within a minute, even if it is to ask to them to hold for a bit longer. The endless hold is very frustrating and often anger provoking. At this point you have two options: (i) ask someone else to pick up the call and take care of the customer; or (ii) ask the caller if it would be OK to call them back as soon as you are able. Some clinics have this as a phone service. The call rings in and after several rings it goes to voicemail that offers several options. The client can hang on and wait until someone is available, leave a call back number and the reason for their call, or press a number to indicate this is an emergency and immediate assistance is required. The phone will make a tone to indicate there is someone waiting and another tone to indicate an emergency. If the client opts for a call back do so as soon as possible.

Reflection

Talk about how you like being put on hold, especially if you are anxious or upset. Now translate that into a client that has a very sick pet. How will they feel if placed on hold without a chance to say a word?

Now let's turn our attention toward the reason for the client's call. It could be almost anything and you should be ready for every kind of request! Let us start with the most common reason and that is a request for an appointment.

Scheduling Appointments

Appointments are utilized for several reasons. The first is to keep a practice running smoothly, it lets the staff know what to expect for the day's work and they can plan accordingly. Scheduling depends on the number of veterinarians on staff and who is scheduled to work. If there is just one doctor, time is set aside to examine and treat the hospitalized patients and perform surgeries in the morning. The afternoon is then open for appointments with time set aside at the end of the day to treat hospitalized patients. If there is more than one doctor, the duties may be divided between them such as one sees appointments all day and the other performs surgeries, treats the hospitalized patients, perhaps sees clients in the afternoon, or does triage for dropped off pets and emergencies. That is one example of the many ways the work can be divided and how scheduling varies from one practice to another.

There are two methods for recording appointments: computerized and paper records. Most clinics will utilize a management software program or app with an appointment screen that is connected to the patient's file, so it is quite easy to enter the information for an appointment. It is important to check that phone numbers are correct and enter why the patient is coming to the clinic. If the clinic is still utilizing a paper appointment book, you will need to make the entry in pencil, in case of cancellation. Important information to include is: the correct spelling of the owner's name, phone numbers, name of the pet, and the reason they are visiting. If the client is new to the practice indicate this on the schedule. If utilizing a computer, some clinics will have you start a client file with client information and pet name to begin. If utilizing paper files, it helps the receptionist to know to have a new file shell ready.

It takes a bit of knowledge to schedule appointments and to work clients in if necessary. You want the clinic to be busy but not so busy that every day is a struggle and mayhem is the norm! The following are some guidelines to follow when scheduling an appointment.

1. Know the amount of time veterinarians like to spend with their clients. Most clinics will schedule a 15–20 minute block of time for every appointment. A paper and computer schedule book will have times blocked at these intervals with a column for each veterinarian seeing clients that day.
2. Routine procedures fit into 15-minute time slots very nicely. These appointments should be dispersed throughout the day, with more intense appointments scheduled in between (Table 3.1).
3. Unknown, non-life-threatening sickness or injuries could take up more time so scheduling them between the routine appointments gives the veterinarians and technicians time for running tests or taking radiographs before the next routine visit arrives. Another type of appointment that may take more time is for a new client. Extra time spent is often a good way to build loyalty and trust with a new client, so you may be directed to use a double time slot for new clients.
4. Working clients into the schedule is also a trick to learn. We can't always predict when an animal will present with an illness or injury and if it is non-life-threatening we don't want it to become worse by waiting one or two days. For example, if Monday and Tuesday are filling up with routine appointments, start offering Wednesday or Thursday for those appointments. They can wait for a few days without any harm done, so spread them throughout the week. This allows some flexibility in getting sick animals in the day the client calls. Of course, you don't want to have tons of open slots so fill appointments in as clients call but be aware some types of illnesses and injuries shouldn't wait (Table 3.1).
5. If the appointment book is filled and another client calls with an urgent care concern you may have to offer the client the option of dropping the pet off at the clinic. The veterinarian can examine the pet when there is time. Make sure to let the client know that this option will incur a kenneling fee, but if it is something that can't wait that may be their only

TABLE 3.1

Scheduling Appointments Per Concerns

Routine procedures	Urgent care	Emergency
Vaccinations	Vomiting, diarrhea	Choking, collapse, dyspnea
Toenail trims	Worsening of condition	Poisoning, seizure, snakebite
Anal glands	Blood in urine or feces	Paralysis, bleeding, dystocia
Suture removal	"Ain't doing right" (ADR)	Hit by car (HBC), traumatic injuries
Recheck for disease	Constipation, sore eye	Falling from balcony
Health Certificate Exam	Hives, skin irritations	Bloat, straining to urinate or defecate
	Frostbite, ear infection	

option. A third option is to let the client come in and wait to be worked in, but they must understand that it could be a substantial wait because clients with appointments will be seen first.

6. Emergencies trump all other appointments. Life-threatening injuries or sudden onset diseases or conditions must be seen right away. It is to be hoped that the client has time to call ahead to alert you that they are coming and inform you of the concern. Ask them an estimated time of arrival so that you can alert staff to the impending emergency and approximate time of arrival. Then if there are clients in the reception area let them know what has occurred and offer them the choice of rebooking their appointment, that their appointment may be interrupted when the emergency comes in, or they can wait to be seen after the emergency is stabilized. If this impacts the rest of the day it is best to call clients and reschedule those routine appointments or alert them that they may have a wait and give them their options.

Table 3.1 gives you an idea of what are routine procedures, what conditions should be seen as soon as possible, and what are considered emergencies.

Reflection

Can you think of other reasons a client would bring their pet to the clinic? If so jot down your ideas and share them with the class.

Now that we have that information in place let's offer up appointment times. Once the client indicates what they need done you will look at the appointment book and pick a day or two days depending on the reason for the visit.

Scenario: Telephone

Good morning, Valley Veterinary Hospital, this is Teresa, how may I help you? Hello Mrs. Smith! You need to get Jack in for his vaccinations? Let me look to see what I have open. It looks like there are openings on Tuesday or Thursday. Will either of those days work for you? (Or you can say, did you have a day in mind for the appointment?) Once they have selected a day, offer them two times and wait for their response. *On Tuesday I have a 2p.m. or a 3:15p.m.* Or you can say, do you prefer morning or afternoon if that is an option. If they select morning, then offer them one or two times if available. Mark the appointment book or make the entry in the scheduling screen on the computer. Confirm who it is for, the time of the appointment, and a phone number where they can be reached. *OK, Mrs. Smith, I have you and Jack scheduled for 3:15p.m. on Tuesday, August 8. Is your phone number still 555-822-1234?*

Some clients will ask to see a specific doctor and will wait to see her/him. If it is a routine or non-life-threatening visit it is fine to accommodate them and schedule for that doctor. However, if it is something that shouldn't wait try to convince them to have whomever is available to examine their animal.

Walk-in clients are those that bring their pets in without an appointment. This was more of an issue in the past, but it still happens on occasion. Again, treating these clients well is important but so are your clients that made appointments! If it is a non-life-threatening concern, you can offer them three choices:

1. They can wait and be worked in between clients, but clients with appointments will be seen before them.
2. They could come back if there is an available space later in the day.
3. They can leave their pet at the hospital, again incurring a kennel fee.

It is to be hoped that they will be reasonable and take one of the offered choices. Sometimes, however, people can become a bit combative and if they become angry or abusive you may have to ask them to leave.

There are of course other calls that come into the clinic. Clients will call with questions about their pet's health concerns, but almost always the pet will have to been seen by a veterinarian because diseases and conditions cannot be diagnosed over the phone. Plus, there would not be a veterinary–client–patient relationship established, especially if the client hasn't been to your hospital before. Sometimes, if there is a relationship established and the condition is a reoccurring one, the veterinarian will consent to prescribe medications without seeing the patient. This is up to the veterinarian and you must always ask before promising anything to the client.

Calls also come in asking about the cost of services. This is an opportunity for you to show the value of coming to your hospital. The following scenario demonstrates how.

Good afternoon, Valley Veterinary Hospital, Teresa speaking, how may I help you? Client: I just got a new puppy and I'm calling around to see how much it will cost to get her first vaccinations. *Congratulations! Can I have your name please?* This is Marsha Smith. *I'm so glad you called us, Ms. Smith, we love talking about new puppies! How old is your puppy and what is her name?* She is 8 weeks old and her name is Lottie. *Marvelous, I love the name Lottie! You are calling at the right time. She will require a combination distemper, hepatitis, parainfluenza, and parvovirus injection now with a follow-up booster in 2 weeks. Our puppy visits include a thorough physical exam by a veterinarian, an internal/external parasite check, and nutritional information by our credentialed veterinary technician. The first puppy visit is $120.00 and that includes everything I just mentioned. It will take about 30 minutes as we want to be thorough and make sure your puppy is healthy. Do you have any questions about the visit?*

Wow, $120 seems a bit high, exclaims Ms. Smith! *I know it sounds high, but remember this includes a thorough physical exam by our veterinarian, a parasite check, and nutrition information as well as the vaccination. You will learn so much during your visit. Can I schedule you and Lottie an appointment?* Well, you are the first clinic I've called so I think I want to call a few more before I decide. *I totally understand, Ms. Smith. I forgot to mention that we have a new puppy packet that includes coupons for food and toys, as well as a coupon for puppy kindergarten where your puppy will be socialized to other dogs and people. Can I schedule you and Lottie today?* I would like to see what other clinics offer, but thank you for the information, Ms. Smith replies. *It has been my pleasure talking with you and I hope you will give us a call back. Have a great day!*

Marsha calls the next closest clinic, and this is how the conversation goes. She is a savvy shopper and now knows what questions to ask, thanks to Teresa at Valley Veterinary Hospital.

Hello, Dimond Veterinary Clinic, Kathy, what do you need? Hi, I have just gotten a new puppy and she needs her first vaccinations and I'm wondering how much that will cost. *The first vaccinations are $100, when would you like to come in?* Does that include an examination, Ms. Smith asks? *Of course, the vet will look your puppy over before giving the shot.* Does it include a parasite check, Ms. Smith asks? *Oh, if you want that it will be $15 for a fecal check.* Do you recommend that, Ms. Smith asks? *Yes, we would have you bring in a stool sample at the time of your visit.* Ms. Smith continues, the first clinic I called said something about external parasites, is that a concern? *We can do an ear swab for ear mites and look for fleas if you are concerned about that.* Is there an extra charge for that, Ms. Smith asks? *Let's see, yes, an ear swab is $15 and a flea check is another $10.* Oh! Ms. Smith exclaims, How long does the visit take? *We book a 15-minute slot for new clients.* Ms. Smith asks, do you offer a puppy packet? *Sorry we don't currently.* Can I book you an appointment? in a rather perturbed manner. No thank you, I have a few more clinics to call. Thank you for your time. *OK, goodbye.*

When a new client makes an appointment, get their address, phone numbers, and an email address to start the medical record. The address can be also used to send them a welcome to the clinic card or email. This is a simple marketing tool that can build loyalty to the practice and acts as a paper reminder of the upcoming visit. The card or email can include a map showing the location of the clinic and perhaps a coupon for a percentage off the purchase of an item.

In general, all the appointments scheduled for the next day are called as a reminder of the upcoming appointment. If appointments are scheduled for Monday, a call is made on the Friday before.

Learning Discovery and Reflection

- Of the two receptionists, who did a better job marketing the practice to Ms. Smith?
- How was value for the money demonstrated?
- How did Teresa try to convince Marsha to book an appointment?
- What were the differences in courteousness between the receptionists?
- Why is there a perception of better care by how the receptionists treated Ms. Smith?

Handling Non-Client Calls

There are times when callers will ask for a specific person. Because you are a place of business it is perfectly alright to ask the caller what it is regarding. Depending on the answer, you will need to determine if it should go through to the person right away or if you can take a message. Messages are usually taken for personal calls and the staff member can call back on their break. Unless the call is an emergency, in which case you would want to alert the staff member right way. Calls for staff members that are asking about test results or patient well-being are directed to the most appropriate staff member if available. The receptionist can check to see their availability and if OK send the call to the staff member. If utilizing a management software program, patient status is often available, so you may be able to answer those questions immediately.

It is important to not interrupt staff members in appointments, treatments, or surgeries to take a phone call that can wait. Again, if it is an emergency then it is OK to interrupt. If the staff member is busy, a message is taken: write down who called, with correct spelling of name, call back number, reason for call, the time, and date. Initial the message and make sure it gets to the staff member. If utilizing paper records and the message is about a patient, pull the file and include it with the message slip. All conversations with clients must be recorded in the patient's file. Include the date, time of call, and a summary of the conversation. This is a vital part of keeping accurate client records. We cover what information is included in client records a bit later in this chapter.

Reflection

Why shouldn't you interrupt staff members at work to take a personal call? Think about how it would appear if clients saw and/or heard you talking on your cell phone while working.

Client Interactions at the Facility

Before the first client arrives a scan of the reception area is done. Pick up any trash, restock the refreshment center if available, straighten up magazines, removing outdated ones or ones that are tattered. Check on toys, coloring books, or other items to keep children occupied and make sure there are no animal messes. Check for dust on any of the surfaces and straighten any pictures that have gone astray. Take a good sniff and if necessary spray a deodorizing spray, taking care not to use heavily perfumed sprays as that can affect some clients. Check for tears, tattered or broken furniture, remove any broken piece and make a note for the practice owner if something should be replaced.

Reflection

Why would a neat and clean reception area be important to a client and practice?

Arrivals

Acknowledge every client and patient immediately upon arrival. It is a pretty good chance that the person walking through the door with a pet is the person that is scheduled to be there. Saying hello and addressing either the person or the pet by name in a warm manner helps to start the visit out right. For example,

Good morning! Is this Bongo? Or, *Hello, are you Mrs. Smith and Lottie?* with a smile on your face and in a warm tone!

If by chance you are helping someone at the reception desk as a person walks in or you are on the phone, make eye contact with them, smile, and nod or wave. This lets them know you have seen them, and it gives them permission to have a seat. As soon as possible confirm who they are and check them in on the schedule. Never leave them hanging; this is anxiety producing and not very welcoming.

We don't know what kind of client is going to walk through the door. They come in all shapes, sizes, genders, and races. It should make no difference as all clients must be treated with respect, listened to, and helped if humanly possible. They are the most important person in the world to that clinic and if not treated well they will leave to find another practice.

Clients also come in different moods. Most are those wonderful clients that care deeply about the health and well-being of their pet. The kind that never complain about the cost of the visit and are a joy to have as clients. But even that client could be having a bad day, as they may be juggling kid's activities, having car trouble, and now dealing with a sick pet. That can put even the nicest person in a grumpy mood! Some clients come to the clinic stressed out because they are concerned that the cost of this visit will take them over budget for the week. The client could be a disabled person that relies on their service dog to live on their own. He may be worried that this could be the end of his independence in addition to losing a valued friend. Or it could be a person whose pet is their only companion or family and who is worried about their only friend.

The warm greeting and care will relax most and they appreciate the fact that you are there to help their pet. However, some are too upset, too demanding, or downright nasty and nothing you do will make them calm down or be nice! If you should have to deal with the last group there are some techniques to use to de-escalate the situation if they should get loud or angry. This is also a good technique for emergencies or with clients that are dealing with a euthanasia.

1. Remain calm, greet them, and move them to an empty exam room. Upset, angry, or unhappy people should not be allowed to upset the other clients in the reception area (Figure 3.1).
2. Always maintain your normal tone of voice. It is hard to yell at someone that doesn't yell back!
3. If the person is angry *listen* to what they have to say, without interruption. Then say, "What I hear you saying is…" and reflect to them what you heard. Ask them what they would like to see done to rectify the situation. *Wait* for an answer! This makes the client think and take a breath. Most will see that they are being unreasonable or if they ask for something unreasonable, offer a compromise. Some are never satisfied and if they continue to yell at you or start to swear, ask them to stop swearing at you and, if it continues, step out of the room and get the office manager or owner of the clinic. Let them know what is happening and let them take it from there. They will be the ones to either bring about an amicable conclusion or they can "fire" the client and ask them to leave and not come back.

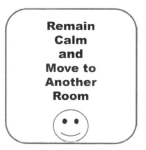

FIGURE 3.1 Remain calm.

4. If it is an emergency alert the staff that they have arrived.
5. If it is for an euthanasia, provide the euthanasia release form and take care of payment in the room.

> ### Reflection
> Envision dealing with an upset, angry, or stressed client. What can you do to de-escalate the situation and provide good customer service? Then reflect on how you can deal with this kind of occurrence on a daily basis and what can you do to decompress.

Admitting Patients

Once you have acknowledged the client and established who they are, you will have to access their pet's record. On the computer type in the client's last name in the Client ID box; this will pull up their record and if they have more than one pet you will need to click on the pet that is visiting that day. Paper files should be pulled already; if not, locate the record in the filing cabinet. Then ask a few questions to make sure the data on the record is current. You should ask:

- Do you still live at _____ address?
- Are your phone numbers _____ for cell and _____ for work?
- Patient today is _____ and is being seen for _____. Is there anything else you need?

Ask the client to have a seat and indicate on the computer that they are ready to be seen. If using a paper file, place it in the designated spot to alert staff that the client is ready to be seen.

If the patient is new to the clinic you will have a bit more information to fill in. Some clinics like to have the client arrive early to fill out a paper form with the required data for a new patient. These same forms would be utilized for computerized or paper records. The forms would include the following:

1. Client information: full name of owner(s), address, phone numbers, emergency contact person if the owner isn't available.
2. Signalment – pet information:
   - Name – confirm spelling
   - Breed – always ask, never assume a breed
   - Species – canine, feline, lagomorphs, rodent, equine, bovine, ovine, caprine, swine
   - Sex: M = male, F = female, N/M = neutered male, S/F = spayed female, date _____

- Description: color of hair, length, markings – i.e., blaze, white paws, white tip on tail
- Date of birth (DOB) – an approximate date is satisfactory
- Previous health issues, medications, and diet – there should be one section for each pet in the household even if just one is present at this appointment.

3. Consent forms: these are often consent to treat, acceptance of financial responsibility, and who can ask for medical information about the pet (usually a spouse, significant other, or part owner). The client is asked to read these forms and then signs on a touch pad at the desk. The receptionist should confirm that the client understands the consent form by asking them specific questions or asking if they have any questions about the consent forms. More about consent forms later in this chapter.

All of the forms are returned to the receptionist, who then puts the information into the database or assembles them into the paper record. It is vital that this information is correct as input mistakes will make it very hard to find a record if a name is misspelled! Once the new client is in the database indicate they are ready to be seen.

> ### Reflection
> Why is all of the information necessary? What difference does it make if we know what color a cat is or whether it is the owner bringing an animal to the clinic?

Discharging Clients

After the veterinarian has seen the patient and client they are given a card or laminated form to take to the reception desk. This insures that they stop and pay before leaving. All medications or supplies should be waiting for them at the desk. The receptionist should greet the client and ask if they are all set to check out. If medications are being sent home, ask them if they understand all the instructions. Be ready to go over the instructions or ask a technician to come up and go over them again with the client. Ask them if they need any food or supplements if that is offered through your clinic. Look at the patient notes to determine if a recheck visit needs to be made and offer up the same options as discussed when answering the phone. Enter the appointment in the schedule and then determine the amount owed for visit. Review each item on the visit list before announcing the total. This explains the value of each service. After the review ask the client if they would like to pay with check, cash, or card.

You should know how to operate the card reader before making the attempt. Some card companies are very protective of the card holder and if a failed attempt is made they may block a second or third attempt. Always print a receipt for the client and staple it to the printed visit list before handing it over to them.

Thank the client for their visit, and express that you hope they will visit again and wish them a good day.

If you have a client that objects to the cost of the day's visit or becomes angry, remember to escort them to another room and work through the issues in private. Never get into an argument in the reception area. It will make other clients uncomfortable and anxious about their bills.

Reflection

Think about how you feel when faced with a huge bill. Now translate that feeling to a client with a sick pet and now a large fee. Without apologising, how could you go about showing the client what they got for their visit and help them understand why it cost so much to help their pet get better?

Veterinary Medical Record Keeping Procedures

Regardless of which type of record a clinic utilizes – paper or computer – it is important to know that these records are considered legal documents. It is the only means of proof that an animal was examined by a veterinarian, immunizations given, tests run, radiographs taken, surgeries performed, and medication prescribed for that patient. Records must be written in a clear, concise, and comprehensive manner, with no spelling errors or mistakes. Ink must be used to write in paper records. If a mistake is made, a single line is drawn through the entry, with the person's initials and date. Never use correction fluid to cover the entry as it may be construed as covering up a mistake. If a mistake is made on the computer, an entry must be made that it was a mistake, and the correct information is added below. Depending on the mistake, one person in the clinic may be designated and know how to remove an entry if caught immediately. Once it has been saved on the hard drive it cannot be erased.

Veterinary assistants do not often enter observations during an appointment. This is the job of the veterinarian.

Only in unusual circumstances might an assistant enter observations before the veterinarian's observation. This is usually in the form of a "warning" notation or behavior of a potentially dangerous or unpredictable patient. Other times, notation of a particularly effective restraint is recorded. These are recorded in red ink.

The veterinary technician and assistants may enter observations, treatments, and test results in the medical records during patient hospitalization. The two circumstances should not be confused.

Reflection

What other reasons would medical records be required in a veterinary practice?

Computerized Versus Paper Patient Records

Computerized records are a major part of the management software utilized by clinics. The individual client records are easy to find; you just type the last name in the client ID box and the record appears. Each record has specific areas for all of the information required in a record so a person doesn't have to read through pages of past history. It generates a visit list which doubles as a bill, a receipt for services, and rabies certificate if needed. A photo of the pet can be easily attached to the file for identification purposes. Best of all, every staff member has access to the file at all times. The different management software programs are fairly intuitive and don't take long to learn. Once you have learnt one program it is fairly easy to move to another.

Paper files are still used in clinics because management software is expensive, even though they are fairly time consuming in assembling, utilizing, and filing. Not everyone has access to them at a given time and they often get misplaced. If the clinic you work at uses paper files there are several steps that you should be familiar with to be a good fill-in receptionist. Each clinic will have their own type of filing system which we will address, but first there are a few standard steps that can be applied to all.

Reflection

For the two methods of keeping patient records, compare and contrast their pros and cons.

Paper Patient Record Assembly

It is prudent to have blank medical records prepared in advance of new client appointments. Even if utilizing management software you will need their information to fill in the database. This accomplishes two things: avoiding a failure to include all pertinent information and making the client wait while the forms are found and put together on a clipboard. The clipboard is given to all new patients to fill out and return. The first form contains the database information already covered in the admitting patient section. The second page will be the consent forms which are discussed after this section. Once everything is completed and returned, place the information into the management software program or if using paper records assemble the sheets into the file shell.

There is usually a specific order in which the clinic likes to have their client records organized in the file shell. It is a good idea for you to learn that order and if in doubt look at other files or ask before assembling or adding more sheets.

The file shell is usually a manila folder which is often divided into sections. The top section is the client database form followed by a page that lists the master problems, medications, immunizations, and lab or test results. A colored divider may used between sections to separate the consent forms from the history sheets.

For established clients, the file is pulled from the filing cabinet and the database information is reviewed to make sure it is correct, corrections are made if necessary, and the reason for the visit is marked on the planning section. Always check to make sure there is room for this visit's notes to be entered into the file. If in doubt add another sheet in the proper order as dictated by the clinic's procedure.

Once the file has been checked over, it can be placed in a designated area indicating that the client has arrived and is ready to be seen.

Reflection

What possible advantage would organizing all paper records in exactly the same way give the practice?

Paper Filing Systems

The retrieval of paper records is a bit more involved than the computerized version. There are many filing systems available and they all involve alphabetizing the client list by last name, first name, and middle initial in some shape or form. One method is to use colored tabs to represent the letters of the alphabet. The first three letters of the last name are placed on the file edge, then the client's full name is written along side the tabs (Figure 3.2). The file is placed in the file cabinet in alphabetical order. Remember, if you have several Smiths, Jones, or Andersons, alphabetize using the first name, and if more than one John use the middle initial. This is often where things go wrong, and files get misfiled because someone doesn't know their alphabet!

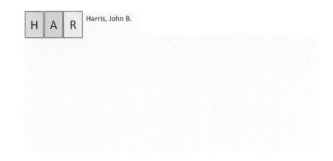

FIGURE 3.2 Color-coded file: alphabetical.

A second method is to assign the client a number; this can be generated by the next number in line. The file folder is marked with tabs that are a different color for each number from 0 to 9. Most systems will start with 100, as three tabs are easier to see a color pattern than two or fewer. The client's name is written on the tab either alongside or under the numbers (Figure 3.3).

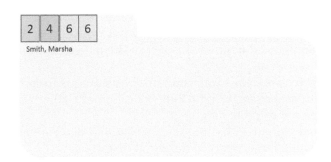

FIGURE 3.3 Color-coded file: numerical.

Both schemes make it easy to find files. If a client has more than one animal, each should have its own file folder. In this case, the name of the pet is placed behind or under the client's name, so you don't have to open every one to find the right pet.

These color-coding systems are touted as foolproof for not losing a file. However, it still takes time to find one if they are alphabetized incorrectly, especially if you are dealing with common last names like Smith, Jones, or Anderson and first names of Bob, Tom, Mary, or Beth. An issue with the numbering system is that clients often do not remember their client number. This is covered by utilizing a client list that is cross-indexed, alphabetized last name, and first name with the client number. So, you can see paper files take a great deal of effort to assemble and file, so they can be retrieved again when needed.

Chronological Order or SOAP File Format

Some paper files will have colored tabs between the different sections of the record. Most will put the client/patient data as the top page followed by the master problem list, medication list, and immunizations page. Then there are two choices for the part of the file that contains the doctor's notes about each visit and any other information about the animal; this is called the history. One type of history page is like a piece of notepaper. The history is written in chronologic order as the veterinarian thinks about the patient and all that needs to be done for the patient. It also includes medications that were prescribed and any other notes as she/he thinks of them. This page is also used by the receptionist if the client called and a question was answered. Other staff members may also write on this page whenever something was done to or for the animal if hospitalized. When the page is full, another is placed on top. The second type of history page is a bit more divided and will be in what is called the SOAP format. This is a page which has specific areas in which to write about the visit, phone call, or other contact with the client/patient. Each letter of SOAP stands for:

- **Subjective information** – client observations, the "chief complaint," patient history as reported by the client and the physical aspect of the patient at the time of visit.
- **Objective data** – veterinarian's observations from the physical exam, weight, and vital signs – in other words the measurable data.
- **Assessment** – what the veterinarian has determined is wrong, tentative, or differential diagnosis.
- **Plans** – where treatment protocols, medications, diagnostic tests, procedures, or surgeries are written, think of them as the "order" for the veterinary technician and assistant to follow for the patient. Daily progress notes are listed here for hospitalized patients with entries concerning nursing care, eating, drinking, and mentation. Follow-up appointments and prescribed drug therapies for the discharged patient are written here too.

There is usually one page per visit and they are kept in the file in chronologic order with the most recent visit on top. This type of record works well when there is more than one doctor on staff. Different doctors can look in specific areas to find quickly what is going on

with the animal and what has been done up to this time. The chronologic history is more time consuming because there is no set order in which it is written so a veterinarian will have to read the entire entry to be able to follow the history of the animal.

Ancillary information can also be included on a paper file. It can indicate at a glance is if the animal is a biter. A red star or tab on the front cover or a red tab placed on the opposite corner from the letter or number tabs can be an indication of this danger. There are also allergy stickers that can be placed on the folder to alert the staff. Other ancillary information for paper history sheets could be in the form of stickers that have an outline of the body or mouth. The mouth ones are used to indicate issues with each tooth. The body sticker can indicate where an animal has sores, lesions, bumps, or lumps on their body, with location and the size noted. Both are filled in as the examination is carried out on the animal. This facilitates recheck visits to determine if the animal is recovering or getting worse.

If using a paper record it is important to make sure that all lab reports, radiographs, and other tests are marked in the file as they are completed. Otherwise, those things can get lost and there would be no indication as to whether or not they had been carried out. This is unacceptable for two reasons. First, it could mean repeating tests that may be painful and costly. Second, if the owner feels there has been a mistake made, sloppy records could cast doubt on the quality of medicine a veterinarian practices and be grounds for a lawsuit, which could cost the clinic money and possibly the veterinarian's license.

When pulling a paper file from the filing cabinet an *out-guide* is put in its place. This is usually larger than the regular folder and is made of thicker cardboard. Some will have a space for the date the file was pulled upon it, otherwise it is just used as a place marker to facilitate replacement.

Reflection

Compare and contrast the two ways to mark files: the color-coded numerical system versus the color-coding alphabetizing last name system.

Transferring Medical Records

People move or decide to switch practices, or a client is referred to a specialty practice and they require the previous medical records. In all instances, a confidentiality waiver must be signed by the client before a copy or summary of the record is sent to a new veterinarian, specialty practice, or even given to the client. The original record remains at the clinic. Medical records are confidential legal documents and a confidentiality waiver ensures that the request for records is made with the owner's knowledge and consent. A copy of the waiver is placed in the paper file or scanned and entered into the patient's file. A notation of when the waiver was signed and when the record was shared is also made in the patient's file. The file is either printed or copied, mailed or emailed to the appropriate person or place.

Reflection

Discuss the reason why medical records belong to the practice but the information belongs to the client.

Forms, Certificates, and Logs

Consent Forms

Consent forms are basic contracts that provide evidence of services requested or agreed upon between the client and veterinarian. They do not protect against malpractice but do provide proof of services rendered. Most forms will have:

1. Hospital name, address, phone numbers
2. Veterinarian's name – maybe a line if more than one doctor is on staff
3. Client's name, address, phone numbers
4. Patient's signalment
5. Statement that the signee is the owner of the animal and is authorized to execute the consent form – initials required
6. Authorization for the specific service being provided – initials required
7. Statement about the risks, complications, and irrevocability associated with procedures and that the client understands the statement – initials required
8. Signature and date line for the client to complete.

The form is kept in the medical record; in paper records it is usually the last page and in the computer it is scanned and saved to the client's file. A copy of the signed consent form is copied and given to the owner.

Some examples of consent forms include: surgery/anesthesia, boarding, euthanasia, and estimates. The AVMA and AAHA have examples of consent forms that can be used if the veterinarian is a member of either organization.

A word about euthanasia forms. These forms must include a statement that verifies that the animal has not bitten anyone in the last 10 days. If the animal has it will need to be tested for rabies or quarantined for 10 days before the euthanasia is performed. This is to protect someone from possibly needing to go through rabies prophylaxis. It is also important to check the files on the patient to make sure the person requesting the euthanasia is the owner. Instances of vindictive euthanasia of a pet have occurred.

Reflection

Discuss how consent forms could protect the clinic from lawsuits.

Certificates

The rabies certificate and health certificate are examples of certificates commonly used in veterinary practice. Rabies certificates are proof that a rabies vaccine has been given by a veterinarian, the only person that can legally administer a rabies vaccination. They are vital if the animal should bite someone. Without it the animal can be legally confiscated and either quarantined for 10 days at the owner's expense or euthanized immediately to be tested for rabies. It is also important if the vaccinated animal is exposed to rabies, such as by being bitten by a skunk, raccoon, or bat. The animal is usually given another vaccination and/or quarantined to watch for symptoms.

The certificate can be filled out by staff members, but the veterinarian must be the person to sign it to make it valid. The certificate must include the manufacturer, type of vaccine, lot and serial number, and expiration date. It will also include the animal's signalment and the owner's address and phone numbers, as well as the clinic's information. The computer will have a printable certificate that will fill in all this information automatically once the vaccine is put into the visit list. The certificate is saved under the animal's name. Paper certificates are in books with triplet copies and need to be filled in by hand, using a pen. One copy is given to the owner, one is put in the patient's file, and the other may be sent to animal control authorities or saved if requested.

A rabies tag with a number, year, and name of the clinic is also included with the certificate. The tag is to be affixed to the patient's collar and serves to indicate when and where the rabies vaccine was given. The number is filled in on the certificate to assist in finding the certificate to prove vaccination status. It is for this reason that rabies tags are dispensed in numerical order.

Health certificates are utilized by federal and state employees to prevent the spread of disease across national and state borders. They are also used to prevent the spread of disease from county to county or region to region at shows and exhibitions like county or state fairs. This is accomplished by examining, vaccinating, and testing animals for disease before the animal is transported. Veterinarians must be accredited by the USDA and the accreditation must be displayed along with the veterinarian's license to practice, along with a business license. Health certificates can be obtained through the state's Department of Agriculture and there are two types: one for companion animals and one for livestock. Both have multiple copies; one is given to the owner, one is sent to the state's Department of Agriculture and/or USDA, one for the patient's files, and one kept in the book for reference.

There can be differing state or country requirements for animal transportation. The staff can call the USDA's toll-free 24-hour service on 800-545-8732 for state requirements. You can also find this information at https://www.aphis.usda.gov/aphis/home/, search animal transportation or importation guidelines.

All certificates require:

1. Owner's name, address, and phone number
2. Animal's signalment including ear tags and/or tattoos, and physical markings
3. Purchaser or consignee name, address, and phone number – if being sold
4. Vaccinations – name, lot or serial number, manufacturer, vaccine type, date of vaccination
5. Small animals – statement saying it has not bitten anyone in the last 10 days
6. Disease status – testing to confirm status, date, and location of testing
7. Veterinarian's signature and date certificate was issued.

Falsifying a health certificate is illegal and can be punished by fines, loss of license, and/or jail time. An animal should be evaluated for a health certificate within 10 days of travel.

Facility Logs

The veterinary practice is required to keep log books for surgeries, controlled drugs, radiographs, laboratory tests, equipment maintenance, and inventory. Table 3.2 indicates what each log is and what information each captures. The following chapters go into more detail for each log.

Reflection

Discuss how the rabies certificate and the health certificate can help prevent the spread of diseases.

TABLE 3.2

Facility Logs

Log	Purpose	Content
Surgical log	Secondary to the patient's file, confirms an animal's surgery and backs up the use of anesthetics. Can also be used if there is a break in sterility issues	Owner's and patient's names, surgeon's name, technician's initials, type of surgery, date
Controlled drug log	Keeps a running total of DEA Controlled Drugs used for surgeries and other procedures	One section per controlled drug, running total of amounts used per day and amounts ordered and entered upon arrival, may also include lot numbers and expiration date information
Radiography log	Secondary to the patient's file, used to document employee's exposure to radiation	Owner's and patient's names, views taken, technician's initials, date
Laboratory log	Secondary to the patient's file, used to quickly document tests run and results	Owner's and patient's names, test(s) run, results, date, and technician's initials
Inventory log	Documents the entire inventory in the practice. Can be used to develop minimum and maximum order points	Quantity, item, size/container, strength/concentration, #/box, storage area, who it is ordered from, minimum/maximum order points, cost
Equipment maintenance	Record of maintenance done on each piece of equipment	Type of maintenance done, who did it and when

Accounts Receivable

Some practices will allow clients to charge for services rendered. This is not a common practice in small animal clinics, but it is done in large animal practices. Large animal veterinarians will fill out a charge form once the visit is completed. Some will give the client a copy before leaving the farm, but most will utilize the management software to generate a bill. Once generated it can be sent via email or by post to the client for payment. The client may have the option of logging into the payment feature and paying online or they will send a check to pay their bill. A payment entry will be made in the management software that requires the amount and check number for it to clear the bill.

Reflection

Why do you think large animal clients can pay after a bill is sent but small animal clients are asked to pay before leaving the clinic.

Day's End Protocols

At day's end there are several things that should be taken care of before leaving for the night. These are tasks that ensure the following day runs smoothly, markets the practice, takes care of the day's receipts and follow-up calls, and ensures that the facility is secured.

Reminder calls   Although these can be done throughout the day when there is a "moment in time" to do so, often there are a few that need to be finished up. Calling to remind clients of their upcoming appointment for the next day ensures that you won't have folks forgetting and big gaps in your schedule.

Sympathy cards   If there were any euthanasias during the day, a sympathy card should be generated, signed by all the employees and put in the mail. This may be the only acknowledgement of a deceased pet a client receives and is greatly appreciated.

Welcome to the practice or thank for the referral cards   These cards are great little marketing tools that show your appreciation for the client giving you their business and for the client that referred business to the clinic. Some practices will offer a little discount on a food item or 5% off a service as a referral thank you, it isn't totally necessary but is a nice gesture.

Reminder cards   These are used to remind clients that their pet's yearly vaccinations are due. They are usually sent out a week before the due date. They can be paper cards that were filled out a year ago by the client as a wrap up to their visit or they can be a generated email utilizing the management software.

Day's receipts   Two team members complete the tally of the receipts and prepares the bank deposit. This increases the accuracy and honesty of the staff members. This is often on a rotational basis, with perhaps the office manager always being one of the members. The bank deposit slip is a listing of the day's receipts that includes cash, checks, and card slip totals. The deposit slip is dated and signed by both staff members. Everything is placed into a bank deposit bag and either placed in a safe or taken to the bank by the practice manager or owner of the clinic.

Follow-up calls   Often the technician or the veterinarian will call the day's surgery patients that have been discharged or the patients from the day before that were sick to see how they are doing and answer any questions the client may have. However, if they are dealing with some emergency or difficult case you may asked to do this. You will need to pull up the file, call the best contact number, and simply ask how the patient is doing. If you can answer the questions with confidence do so, if not let the client know that the technician or the veterinarian will call them back later in the evening, ask them if the number you used is a good number to use, mark a call back slip, and make sure the appropriate staff sees it before you go home. Always mark the patient file with the date, summary of the call, and your initials.

Other tasks to complete before leaving the facility include:

1. Backup the computer data – this may be an automatic setting but checking to make sure it is doing it is important
2. Close and lock all doors and windows
3. Turn off all but the safety lights that are left on throughout the night
4. Turn on the answering machine
5. Adjust the thermostat for the front part of the building to an energy saving temperature; the animal wards should remain at a comfortable temperature
6. Pull client records – if using paper files – for the next day
7. Check exam rooms, bathrooms, and reception area. Are they empty? Are they clean?
8. Set alarms if everyone has left the building. If not alert the remaining staff that you are leaving and ask them to turn on the alarm when they leave.

Reflections

- Why is it important that different people are involved in taking care of the money at the end of the day?
- Why should one person be in charge of making sure the doors are locked and everyone has left the building?

Inventory Control

The largest non-wage expense for a veterinary clinic is inventory. Inventory is everything inside a clinic that isn't a wall! It is the goods required to medicate, run tests, take radiographs, perform procedures, and to feed and care for hospitalized patients. It is the equipment required for procedures, like surgery tables, otoscopes, and instruments. It is cleaning and office supplies, reception area furniture, chairs, desks, and computers. This is a huge outlay of money and the only way to pay for it is to have clients! The reason to have inventory is to take care of patients. The more clients you have, the more inventory must be on hand and in good working condition. Inventory control is a fine balance between having enough on hand to meet needs and having too much on hand that it becomes outdated before it can be used and the products tie up cash flow that could have been invested.

Management software includes an inventory section. This has automated the process to the point where in a few clicks the office manager, inventory manager, or owner can determine where the inventory is as far as amounts on premises, dollars tied up in inventory, what items are ordered numerous times per year, month, or week, and what items are sitting on a shelf taking up valuable space. Therefore, one or two people are designated to control the inventory. Any more than that and mistakes occur, cost the clinic money, or cost an animal its life.

The key to having this work well is making sure *all* the products ordered are entered correctly. It is equally important that when products are used or opened, each tablet or milliliter dispensed, every roll of tape and syringe used is deducted from the inventory. Some clinics will allow staff to remove items from the inventory, such as when they take a roll of tape or open a bag of food it is marked in the inventory. Others will have you indicate this on a whiteboard or notebook and the inventory control person takes it off the inventory. The computer will also deduct inventory as it is dispensed to clients. For example, if the veterinarian prescribes a bottle of amoxicillin, the computer will deduct it from inventory once the visit list is generated.

Most clinics will carry out a physical inventory once a year of the "disposable" goods. This entails counting everything that is used to treat, test, or perform procedures upon patients. This accounting is compared with the previous year's and can tell the practice owner if the inventory control is making money, paying for itself, or losing money. You may be asked to help do inventory and will usually be given a form that either has the product list with the size, strength, number/container, already marked on the page or you fill in the lines as you come across the products.

Most clinics have inventory gathered into areas within the facility. There may be a storage room for food, bandage materials, syringes, needles, source bottles for cleaners or alcohol, and so on. The medications are usually kept in a pharmacy area, laboratory supplies in the lab, radiography supplies in the radiography room, surgical supplies in the surgery room, and so on. The trick is to learn where everything is kept so that a thorough count can be executed.

Note how the columns in Table 3.3 include:

- Quantity – this is the number of items on hand. There are several ways to mark this depending on the item: 1 could stand for 1 bottle, 1 box, or 5 tablets, so always quantify the quantity. It will depend on how you mark size/container or #/box columns.
- Item is the name of the product, some will also ask for the manufacturer.
- Strength/concentration is marked as mg/capsule or tablet, %, mg/mL, and so on.
- Size/container – this is gallons, quarts, mL, 500 tabs/bottle, g, and so on.

TABLE 3.3

Inventory Pages

Quantity	Item	Size/Container	Strength/Concentration	#/Box
6 btls	Isopropyl alcohol	Gallon	70%	4/box
½ btl	Carprofen	250/bottle	75 mg/tablet	
2 bxs	Artificial tears ointment	25 g/tube		12/box
8.5 bxs	Syringes	3 mL slip tip		100/box

TABLE 3.4

Inventory Abbreviations

Bottle	btl	Gram	gm
Box or boxes	bx or bxs	Kilogram	kg
Tablet	tab	Ointment	oint
Capsule	cap	Percentage	%

- #/Box is used when you have things like syringes: they come 100/box; or gallons of alcohol, they come 4/box.

Look at the last entry in Table 3.3; the quantity of syringes is marked as 8.5 bxs, syringes, 3 mL slip tip, 100/box. The inventory manager now knows there are 850 syringes on hand. When marking the inventory record make sure to mark all items in a similar manner. For example, the next item might be 6 mL syringes and there is ½ box left, you mark 25 in the quantity column and 50/box in the #/box column. Does that mean you have 1250, 6 mL syringes? If you are going to mark the actual number, mark it as 25 syringes, do not fill in the 50/box column! It is OK to leave some areas on the inventory sheet blank if it will cause confusion.

Another area of difficulty is what to count and what not to count. We always count the opened bottle of carprofen, there are 125 tablets in there, but we usually don't count the opened tube of lubricant or that roll of tape that is three-fourths gone in the exam rooms. If the clinic wants these items counted, a good way to go about this is to look in every exam room and treatment area that would have an open container of lube, keep a running tally, and mark it in the inventory on the lube line in the closest approximation of full tubes. For example, exam room 1 has ½ tube of lube, exam room 2 has an almost full tube, the treatment area has ¼ tube, and the surgery has a ¾ full tube. That equals out to 2.5 tubes, find the line on the inventory sheet, and add 2.5 tubes to the total count.

It is appropriate to abbreviate while marking the inventory sheets, Table 3.4 lists a few of the commonly used abbreviations.

Reflection

What surprised you about the amount of work involved in inventory control? Is this something that you would enjoy helping with or something you would do only if paid a great deal of money? Why?

Carprofen | 75 mg/cap | 250/btl | mini ½ btl | max 1 btl

FIGURE 3.4 Inventory reorder tag.

Daily Inventory Control

Everyone on staff interacts with the inventory every day. There may be one or two people in charge of the entire inventory, but if you have a "moment in time" perhaps you could offer to help, or you may even be asked to help with the steps required to maintain inventory.

A good inventory manager develops a sense of what is used, how rapidly it is used, and how quickly it can be replaced. Good records and a keen awareness of the clinic's activity all come into play when ordering supplies. There are several manual methods of knowing when to order a product, this is called an order point. Order points can also be set in the management software if in use.

Here is an example, carprofen is a non-steroidal anti-inflammatory drug used for pain in dogs. The 75 mg tablet is dispensed on almost a daily basis. The trick is to determine what the order point or minimum amount is so that you don't have too many or not enough. This is where order tags or inventory markers come into play. These can be small or large tags that are placed upon the item using tape, rubber bands, paper clips, and so on. When the item reaches the order point, the tag is removed and placed in a box or envelope for the inventory manager. This tag will have all the same information upon it that the inventory sheet has, plus an order point or minimum and a maximum reorder number. Again, using carprofen, the reorder tag would look like Figure 3.4.

The order point or the minimum amount available would be ½ bottle and 1 bottle or maximum amount will be ordered. The inventory manager knows that by the time the new bottle arrives the bottle on the shelf will be at ¼ or less, so she orders 1 bottle. This knowledge comes from experience and a keen awareness of the activity in the practice.

The management software can generate a reorder list if reorder points were placed into the database at the start and if everyone input items they took out that are not paid for directly by the client. For example, lube and rolls of tape are items utilized in the clinic but not sold very often to clients directly. This means that if a reorder point is 1 box of tape or a ½ box of lube, they are not manually deducted each time one is taken from the inventory room or the clinic will find themselves out of tape and lube because the reorder point was never reached according to the computer.

Another simpler method of letting the inventory manager know a product is either gone or getting low is to write the item on a whiteboard or clipboard. This works well if everyone actually does it. Everyone must be committed to making sure products are written down before they are used up. However, during a crazy busy day, someone grabs the last roll of gauze, instead of writing it down right away she rushes off because an animal is bleeding! No one knows that was the last roll until the next patient needs it. If a product is out then the treatment of an animal may have to wait one or two days and that could be critical in some instances.

Reflection

Compare and contrast the two techniques of inventory control – the reorder point tags versus writing items needed on a whiteboard.

Ordering Supplies

Supplies are ordered from businesses that specialize in veterinary medicine products. The most common is a distributor that sells several brand name products in addition to their "house" brand. Some companies will only sell direct to veterinarians; their brand name products are ordered through their company's website. Both will have online ordering platforms that require an account set-up prior to ordering which will require a payment method, name, and license number of the veterinarian and a user ID and password. The inventory manager usually handles the orders by gathering all the inventory tags or information from the whiteboard. A smart inventory manager will take a quick spin through the storage areas and see if there are items that are close to the ordering point and grab those tags as well. If possible, ordering once a week is preferable. This often ensures that an order will ship for free because a certain dollar amount gains free shipping. Also, it takes the inventory control person out of caring for patients only once a week!

Reflection

In everyday life we deal with goods that either are name brands or "house" or generic brands. Have you ever compared the two? For example, most grocery stores will carry a name brand spaghetti sauce, but alongside of it will be their store brand. What could be the differences between these two products and what could they mean to you as a client?

Receiving Shipments

Orders are usually delivered in one to two days by the distributors. Most have warehouses strategically located to service an area that facilitates a one-day turnaround. When boxes are delivered they should be inspected for damage before being signed for. If visibly damaged you can refuse them, and the driver will have to take them for shipment back to the distributor. Otherwise, sign for the delivery and alert the inventory manager that the boxes have arrived.

Handling Shipments and Invoices

To unpack the boxes, they should be opened carefully with a box cutter so as not to cut the products inside. Set all the items out in piles and then compare the number of items ordered with the number of items that were shipped using the invoice. The invoice is either packed inside the box or in a plastic envelope on the outside of the box. For example, if 5 boxes of 3 mL syringes were ordered, there should be 5 boxes in the shipping box and 5 boxes should be shown on the invoice. Mark a check alongside that item and continue to check the invoice against the actual items to ensure everything that was ordered was shipped. Invoices have the price of the items on them and those will have to be adjusted to reflect the mark-up the clinic assigns to pay for the costs of ordering, stocking, storing, and selling the item. This is usually 50–100% of the purchase price. If the item is sold outright to clients a price is marked on the item. Invoices are considered bills and once every item in the box is checked against the invoice it goes to the office manager for payment.

If utilizing the management software, the number of items is placed in the appropriate spots in the database, and the invoice is used to check the price of the object. If the price needs to be adjusted, it is updated at this point as well.

Restocking Shelves

The inventory tags need to be placed on the appropriate reorder point item and then are ready to be put away. Check the packaging for storing instructions. There will be instructions for temperature tolerance and whether to store in a dark or dry place or in the refrigerator. If a cart is available, use it to facilitate moving the items to their storage areas. Group items for the refrigerator, storage room, or pharmacy, and so on, on the cart. This will reduce the number of trips needed to get things put away. Place all the new items behind any items that are still on the shelf. This is called stock rotation or "first in, first out." This is especially important if there is an expiration date on the product. Most medications and some cleaning products will have these printed on the box or bottle. It is important that the products with the shortest expiration date are used first so they are not wasted if the date is past before they are used up. This is wasteful and costs the clinic money. Make sure the inventory tags are on the appropriate order point item so that more can be ordered when it reaches the right number. This may mean taking an inventory tag off and putting it on the new item. For example, remember the carprofen on our inventory list? There was a ½ bottle left and that was the reorder point, so when the new bottle comes in the tag is removed from the ½ full bottle and placed on the new bottle. Straighten the other items on the shelf if bumped during the rotation process.

Once everything is put away, break the cardboard boxes down into flats and place into the recycle bin. Some items come with an ice pack. These are good to keep for shipping lab samples to diagnostic labs and if your practice treats livestock you can use them to keep vaccines cool. Otherwise, if the clinic has multiple packs then go ahead and toss them. If there are quite a few and the clinic doesn't mind, they are great for keeping lunches cool as well!

Reflection

Discuss what you learned about inventory management. What surprised you, and what made you stop and think about how you would do inventory control.

Chapter Reflection

Think about what you learned in this chapter. Now that you know a bit about how to run a front desk, pay attention to how other businesses run their client or customer service. Did they follow any of the guidelines discussed in this chapter? Were they building client/customer loyalty or were they "just there for the paycheck?"

CHAPTER 4

Facility and Equipment Maintenance – Cleaning for Disease Control

LEARNING OBJECTIVES

- Maintain basic cleanliness and orderliness of the veterinary facility
- Identify and deal with hazardous and non-hazardous waste
- Utilize proper cleaning techniques when caring for hospitalized animals in all wards
- Discuss the methods by which diseases are spread
- Prevent nosocomial infections and the spread of disease with the use of disinfectants or antiseptics and proper cleaning and waste management
- Restock supplies throughout the facility to ensure quality care
- Maintain the various pieces of equipment utilized in the veterinary practice

NAVTA ESSENTIAL SKILLS COVERED IN THIS CHAPTER

I. Office and Hospital Procedures
C. Maintain basic cleanliness and orderliness of a veterinary facility
    4. Demonstrate knowledge of basic sanitation and disinfection techniques of animal kennels and bedding, examination rooms, hospital facilities, and surgical suites
V. Small Animal Nursing (Large Animal Nursing – Optional)
A. Safety concerns
    2. Utilize patient and personnel safety measures
    4. Describe isolation procedures
    5. Describe hazardous waste disposal

Tasks for the Veterinary Assistant, Fourth Edition. Teresa F. Sonsthagen.
© 2020 John Wiley & Sons, Inc. Published 2020 by John Wiley & Sons, Inc.
Companion website: www.wiley.com/go/sonsthagen/tasks

6. Describe basic sanitation as associated with animal handling and clinical care:
   a. clean and disinfect cages and kennels (stalls optional)

B. Animal care
   1. Provide routine record-keeping, and observation of hospitalized patients (i.e., stress importance of notations made when cleaning and feeding)
   11. Provide care and maintenance of nursing equipment (i.e., otoscope, ophthalmoscope, thermometer, etc.)

Basic Cleanliness and Orderliness

Veterinary assistants play a vital part in the prevention of nosocomial infections. These are infections acquired at a clinic or hospital. Animals become infected in one of two ways:

1. Direct transmission from animal to animal by way of contact with body fluids or secretions such as blood, urine, feces, saliva, or tears. Ingestion or absorption are the most common means of acquiring an infection. Bites, playing, living in dirty conditions, rubbing against each other, or lying together are all examples of direct transmission.

2. Indirect transmission of disease to an animal can occurs in several ways:
   • Coming into contact with contaminated inanimate objects termed **fomites**. Fomites can be virtually anything; exam tables, clothing, hands, shoes, grooming tools, phones, and doorknobs are examples. An example of a fomite transmission would be a grooming tool used on an animal with ringworm (fungus – not always apparent – can be highly infectious) and then used on another, or a bandage scissor used to remove an extremely infected bandage is then used to cut bandage material for another patient.
   • Airborne disease is considered as indirect transmission. Infectious organisms are transmitted by coughing, sneezing, or hissing. The organisms in the saliva are suspended as droplets or absorbed by the dust in the air, then inhaled or absorbed through the mucous membranes or breaks in the skin.
   • Vector-borne diseases are transmitted indirectly by an intermediate host, often insects or rodents. The organisms are transmitted through bites or are ingested by the animal.

Reflection

Think about how diseases can be transmitted in everyday life between humans. What daily activities do you participate in that could directly or indirectly cause you to become sick?

Organisms that cause disease are called **pathogens**. They are **microscopic** in nature and are referred to as **microbes**, although not all microbes are pathogens. Pathogens are divided into categories based on their genetic makeup. Those that cause disease include bacteria, viruses, fungi, protozoans, and parasites. Nosocomial infections are caused by different types of bacteria, viruses, and fungi that are "resident" pathogens, meaning they are normally found in the environment. They can be deadly to animals that have a weakened immune system which includes animals that have undergone major surgery, have cancer or another disease, are old or very young, or are extremely stressed. These sick or injured animals are susceptible to **secondary infections** from *Staphylococcus*, *Streptococcus*, and other bacteria that are commonly found in veterinary facilities.

Many animal diseases are **species-specific**. For example, feline leukemia virus (FeLV) can only infect cats, and canine parvovirus can only infect dogs. This is important to know because some hospitals do not have a **quarantine** area large enough to handle major outbreaks, but you could house a cat with FeLV in the dog ward or a dog with parvovirus in the cat ward if necessary.

Some pathogens that cause diseases in animals can spread to humans: this is called **zoonosis**. There are over 200 **zoonotic** diseases that can be passed from animals to humans. There are also diseases that can be passed from humans to animals; this is called **anthroponosis** or anthroponotic diseases. For example, human influenza can be transmitted to ferrets.

What steps need to be taken to prevent nosocomial infections?

1. Everyone needs to do their part in keeping the facility clean, orderly, and well organized. Being each other's safety net is important to safeguard the patients, clients, and staff from becoming infected by a pathogen. A valuable and competent veterinary assistant is one who not only maintains the immediate environment of the patient, but also looks at the surrounding areas, identifies and corrects potential issues. He/she will also be able to extend the cleanliness to all areas inside and outside of the facility.

Treat every animal as if it is harboring *every* pathogen known to man! It can take days for an animal to show signs of an illness or condition so it is important to follow some basic rules after taking care of every animal.

   - When in doubt, consider it contaminated. Clean or change out everything that came into contact with the animal before it is used on another. This includes otoscope, stethoscope, clippers, scissors, exam tables, bedding, cages, kennels, and so on.
   - Gloves must be put on before touching any potentially contaminated surface, whether animate or inanimate. They must be removed and disposed of properly to reduce contamination to skin and environment.
   - Clean, washable clothing is worn to protect "street clothes." Scrubs, coveralls, aprons, or lab coats are worn in the clinic and must be changed if visibly or known to be contaminated. Utilize a roller brush to remove loose hair from one patient before going on to the next. The use of these items of clothing prevents diseases from leaving the clinic.
   - The use of footbaths or disposable booties prevents tracking pathogens into sterile zones or out of sick wards.

Reflection

Explain what a nosocomial infection is and how it is transferred to a lay person.

In order to control pathogens, an understanding of how they survive in the environment and respond to disinfectants is important. Most pathogens are highly susceptible to sunlight, heat, cold, oxygen, and chemicals. **Aerobic organisms** die quickly when exposed to any of these conditions. **Anaerobic organisms** have adapted to surviving extreme conditions; they thrive in environments that are dark, moist, and low in oxygen. Some bacterial pathogens are **spore-forming** which are able to

withstand extreme weather conditions and can live for a long time. Both anaerobic and spore-forming organisms are very difficult to destroy.

Viruses are different in that they require a living host to multiply. Many are short lived outside of a host, but some are tougher and can survive for 24–72 hours outside of a host. Most viruses are destroyed by the body's immune system which develops antibodies that attach to a virus and destroys it by a chemical process. This is brought about by the body's ability to recognize the antigens that are on the surface of the virus. These antigens are recognized by lymphocytes which produce and release the antibodies. Vaccinations induce the lymphocytes to recognize the antigens and that is why we vaccinate for rabies, distemper, parvovirus, feline leukemia, and other contagious viruses.

In defense against these pathogens we have in our arsenal disinfectant agents and sterilizing techniques that can destroy the various pathogens. Agents that kill pathogens will have the suffix *-cidal* affixed to the root word that describes the pathogen:

Bactericidal = destroys bacteria

Viricidal = destroys viruses

Fungicidal = destroys fungus

Sporicidal = destroys spore-forming bacteria

Bacteriostatic or **virostatic** are examples of agents that prevent further replication. The suffix *-static* is attached to the root word. These agents are chemical compounds that will destroy several different pathogens. If they are formulated to destroy every pathogen they are referred to as broad-spectrum disinfectants. When choosing a disinfectant, read the label. Look for what it destroys and if, for example, the bottle reads "bactericidal and viricidal only" it will not destroy fungi or spore-forming bacteria. Most clinics will opt for a broad-spectrum disinfectant that will destroy everything.

These chemical agents are only as good as the person using them. They must be appropriately diluted and applied properly. Read the label; it will be very specific on how the agent should be diluted and how long it should be in contact with the surface that needs to be disinfected. This is called **contact time** and will vary depending on the surface being cleaned and the product being used. Dilutions must be precise because too dilute and it will not destroy the pathogen and if too strong it may damage equipment or be toxic to the person using the product.

Reflection

Explain what the difference is between a *-cidal* and a *-static* disinfectant. Explain how disinfectants are only as good as the person using them.

There are three levels of cleaning: cleaning, disinfecting, and sterilizing.

Cleaning

Cleaning is when we mix a detergent like dish or clothes soap with water. It lifts the soil and debris from the surface. The water then carries the soil and debris to the bucket, or wash tub via a mop or cloth. Cleaning reduces microbes but not sufficiently to prevent nosocomial infections. Cleaning is carried out prior to disinfecting because many disinfectants do not penetrate through heavily soiled or debris-filled surfaces. Many are also deactivated if they come into contact with organic material. When cleaning it is important to use clean cloths, mops, or paper towels. Paper towels are the best choice as they are used once and disposed of. Wash cloths and mops, if allowed to get dirty or contaminated with debris like feces or vomit, become saturated with microbes and become fomites.

Disinfecting

Disinfecting is the use of specific chemicals that reduce the number of microbes substantially on inanimate or animate surfaces. There are two types of disinfecting chemical compounds:

Disinfectants used only on inanimate objects
Antiseptics used only on living tissues

Disinfectants require accurate dilutions to be safely used. Carefully measuring the disinfectants as they are put in spray bottles, or added to mop buckets, washing machines, and sinks is very important for them to work well. They usually do not do well if an area is extremely grimy or full of debris. Surfaces should be cleaned with detergent and water to remove the visible contaminates. Then the area is sprayed or mopped with the diluted disinfectant and allowed to air dry for the necessary time to destroy pathogens. Some disinfectants need less time, but you must wait the entire amount of contact time before wiping it dry with paper towels. Contact times can vary from 1 minute to 30 minutes depending on the pathogen of concern. For example, spore-forming bacteria are the hardest to kill and so require more contact time.

Contact time is determined using the phenol coefficient; this is the "kill strength" of a disinfectant. For example, if a disinfectant product has a phenol coefficient of 50 it is capable of destroying half of the microbes compared to the same number destroyed by phenol.

Several disinfectants are used in a veterinary facility. If unfamiliar with them read the label and Material Safety Data Sheets (MSDS) to find out what pathogens they destroy, how to dilute them properly, what the contact time is, and if they are affected by time, temperature, pH, or organic materials. Let's look at four of the most common disinfectants.

1. Chlorine (sodium hypochlorite) or bleach is an excellent disinfectant; bactericidal (regular and spore-forming, i.e., yeast), viricidal, and fungicidal. Bleach has a phenol coefficient of 40. For general use it is diluted 1 : 32 but needs to be stronger to destroy ringworm fungus so it is diluted at 1 : 10 if ringworm is suspected. Bleach is deactivated by organic material, sunlight, and time. Diluted bleach is only effective for 24 hours. To use it properly, clean up visible debris with a detergent and water combination, then spray with bleach and allow to air dry. It is important to make sure the surfaces are completely dry before allowing a pet onto the surface as bleach, even diluted, is harmful to skin.

2. Quaternary ammonium compounds (quats) – Parvosol II™, and Roccal-d™ – are very effective against bacteria and viruses, good against fungi, amoebas, and enveloped viruses. They are not very effective against endospores or non-enveloped viruses. Dilutions vary with each product so read the labels or MSDS carefully. Quats are commonly used to soak sharp surgical instruments like scissors. However, they lose their efficacy if coming into contact with organic material like blood. It is important that instruments are cleaned and rinsed well before soaking them in a quat.

3. Hydrogen peroxide – Rescue™ is a 4.25% hydrogen peroxide. Hydrogen peroxide is usually considered an antiseptic, but at 4.25% it is a broad-spectrum disinfectant of inanimate objects. Contact time varies with the pathogens it kills; the longer it stays on the surface, the more types of pathogens it destroys. The average time is 5 minutes, but a stronger dilution can destroy pathogens in 3 minutes. Rescue™ can be purchased as ready-to-use wipes, ready-to-use spray bottles, or concentrates. There is also a shampoo version that can be used on animals with skin infections.

4. Benzalkonium chloride is a broad-spectrum disinfectant effective against coliforms, gram-positive and gram-negative bacteria, and yeasts. It is non-corrosive to metals, eco-friendly, biodegradable, and tissue friendly. It comes in a highly concentrated form that can be used for cleaning and disinfecting surfaces throughout the clinic.

5. Alkalis (lye) and formaldehyde are extremely toxic agents that are *not* used as standard disinfectants. However, lye is used to treat soil contaminates, especially if the contamination is animal carcasses. Formaldehyde is a fixative that stops the maturation process in living tissue. Both agents are highly dangerous to use and are carcinogenic. Respirators

and working under a vented hood is recommended when dealing with these products.

6. Glutaraldehyde is a chemical sterilizing agent that is broad-spectrum in nature. It is used on endoscopic instruments but will damage living tissues. It must be double rinsed with sterile water before contact with living tissues.

7. Phenols are potent disinfectants and antiseptics – Lysol and essential oils like tea tree oil – should never be used around or on cats as they are toxic.

Antiseptics are disinfecting chemicals that are used to reduce the number of microbes on living tissues. Often you will hear people refer to a surgical scrub on an animal as being "sterile." It really isn't sterile; it is very clean but not sterile. If you were to "sterilize" tissue, it would die. Antiseptics can have a detergent mixed in with the chemical to produce suds. This is used to tell where you have scrubbed and where you have missed! Many are a broad-spectrum disinfectants meaning they can destroy almost all pathogens depending on contact time. Some will be used full strength and others will need to be diluted. Remember to read the label! Some commonly used antiseptics are as follow.

1. Alcohol (isopropyl or ethyl) is used at 70% concentration. It is purchased at this strength or it can be purchased at 90–100% in which case you would have to dilute it to 70%. Alcohol destroys bacteria and viruses by dehydrating them. It is a good degreaser and is used to disinfect thermometers, injection sites, and to dry surgical sites. Hand sanitizers are made up of 70% ethyl alcohol and are effective on 99.9% of the bacteria on hands 30 seconds after application and 99.99–99.999% in 1 minute, demonstrating that contact time is important when using antiseptics.

2. Povidone-iodine is used at 2% dilution. It is a broad-spectrum antiseptic that is used for surgery. There are two preparations: a scrub solution that will suds up and is used to scrub the skin before a surgical procedure; and a thinner solution that is further diluted 1:10 and sprayed or painted on intact skin before surgery starts. It can also be used at 0.35% dilution (17.5 mL of 10% povidone-iodine in 500 mL of normal saline) as a lavage for wounds. It is a brown color and stains fur, is deactivated by organic debris and alcohol, so it has fallen out of favor in some veterinary clinics. Residual effects last 4–6 hours.

3. Chlorhexidine – Nolvasan™, Hibiclens™ – both come in scrubs or solutions. It is not deactivated by alcohol or organic materials; it is inhibited by soaps and pH changes. It is used full strength as a surgical scrub, diluted 1:40 to lavage wounds, and has a 2-day residual effect. It can be used as a broad-spectrum antiseptic on inanimate objects at a 3 oz per gallon dilution. It can be corrosive to surgical instruments, so a detergent made to clean instruments is recommended.

4. Chloroxylenol at 3% is an antiseptic used when patients are allergic to povidone-iodine or chlorhexidine. It is used as a surgical scrub, oral mouth wash, and a wound lavage agent. It is bacteriostatic for 6 hours after application. It is non-toxic to avians and mammals.

5. Hydrogen peroxide – 3% hydrogen peroxide, Rescue™ 4.25% concentration. At 3%, hydrogen peroxide is a mild antiseptic. It is often used to flush out wounds when first presented. The bubbling action is caused by the enzyme catalase, found in blood and cells which converts hydrogen peroxide into water and oxygen. Usually a onetime application as studies have shown that it can destroy healthy tissue. Hydrogen peroxide is also a bleaching agent that will remove bloodstains from hair and clothing.

Sterilization is the destruction of microbes, achieved with autoclaves or gas. Autoclaves are machines that use pressure, steam, and time to kill microbes; gas sterilizers utilize ethylene oxide, humidity, and time. More information about sterilization techniques can be found in Chapter 14 on surgical techniques. Maintenance information on the autoclave is given later in this chapter.

Learning Exercise

From the list of disinfectants and antiseptics select the most appropriate one for the scenario described in the table. You may use more than one.

Scenario	Disinfectant or antiseptic
Disinfecting sharp surgical instruments	
Scrubbing surgical site on a patient	
Disinfecting a kennel	
Lavaging a wound	
Sterilizing endoscopic equipment	
A good degreaser or drying agent	

Hospital Waste – Non-Hazardous versus Hazardous

Veterinary practice can generate a great deal of waste. It is usually divided into two categories: non-hazardous and hazardous. Hazardous waste is anything that can harm humans, animals, and the environment. Both are further divided; non-hazardous into recyclable or non-recyclable, and hazardous into medical, chemical, or biologic waste. Each are handled in specific ways.

Non-hazardous recyclable waste is usually paper, plastics, and glass. Many municipalities have "single stream" recycling programs, meaning everything goes into one recycling bin. However, in a veterinary facility not all waste is safe to recycle. To know what to recycle, compare the waste generated in a home to the same types of waste that is generated in a hospital. If the waste is the same as in a home it can go into the recycling bin. For example, water and soda bottles, cardboard boxes, magazines, and paper. If it is different from what is found in a home, the decision needs to be made based upon the item. A guideline is to ask if it is safe for humans, animals, and the environment. For example, an empty or half used bag of Ringer's lactate solution in a plastic bag needs to be thrown away. Ask yourself, is it recyclable? Yes, it is plastic, the solution is non-hazardous to humans, animals, and the environment, so it is a safe product to throw into the recycle bin. An example of hazardous waste could be an outdated bottle of formaldehyde. Ask yourself, is it recyclable? Yes, the bottle is glass. However, the contents are extremely toxic to living tissues and the environment, so it is hazardous and *not* recyclable. It will need to be disposed of as a chemical hazard, which we will discuss shortly. If in doubt about an item's suitability for recycling, ask someone or look it up on the internet.

> **TIP BOX 4.1**
>
> When dealing with hazardous materials, select the appropriate personal protective equipment (PPE) to protect yourself from injury.

Mechanical, chemical, and biologic hazards are those items that will cause harm to humans, animals, and the environment. Examples of mechanical hazards are needles and broken glass contaminated with body fluids. These items are usually captured in specific containers for "sharps" (Figure 4.1). The container is usually red and made of a heavy puncture-proof plastic. It is designed to hold needles and syringes that have been used for giving injections or drawing blood. It is used to protect workers from accidently being poked by needles that have an infectious organism or agent. Needles come with a cap but it is advised to never recap a needle once the cap is taken off. After an injection or blood draw the syringe is placed directly into the sharps container and the needle cap disposed of with the syringe packaging into the waste can. Some municipalities require glassware such as used microscope slides and any blood collection tubes to be contained in a sharps container too. The containers are picked up and incinerated instead of going to the landfill. These items are never thrown into

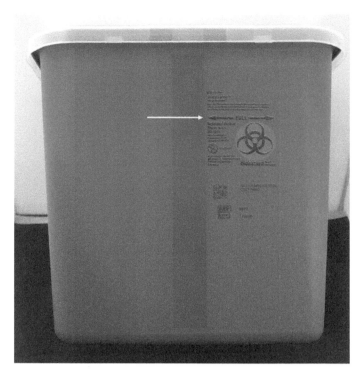

FIGURE 4.1 Sharps container.

the regular trash as they can poke or cut the custodial staff when taking the trash out.

Chemical wastes are those items that are of danger to living beings and the environment. The veterinary clinic has a few of these items. For example, formaldehyde used to "fix" tissues for diagnostic analysis, radiographic fixer solution, chemotherapy medications, pesticides, anesthetic gas, and some vaccines. Product bottles and outdated products need to be disposed of properly. That may mean that they are placed into a special container, picked up and incinerated, or, in the case of the fixer solution, picked by a company that recycles the silver. The MSDS will tell you how to dispose of the product so when in doubt check those. If a chemical is spilled, an absorbable material like kitty litter is poured on top of the spill, swept into a dustpan, and dumped into the trash which must be taken to the dumpster immediately. Chemotherapy medications, and anything that has come into contact with them, are placed into a yellow biohazard container which is picked up for incineration.

Biologic hazards are anything with blood, feces, or urine on or in them, microbiologic cultures, laboratory samples, vaccine bottles, isolation waste, and patient tissues or in some cases entire bodies if what killed them was zoonotic. Biohazard waste should be emptied into bags that are marked "biohazard" and are picked up for incineration. Newsprint that has been used in kennels is not recycled; it can be put into the trash for the landfill. This is no different from putting human diapers in the landfill.

Cleaning Techniques When Caring for Hospitalized Animals

Providing patient comfort and safety are the underlying principles in caring for hospitalized patients. Keeping them clean, safe, fed, and comfortable is often delegated to the veterinary assistant. By keeping a clean and healthy environment you are not only reducing the risk of nosocomial infections, but the result is a patient that will heal faster, a happier client, and a successful clinic. This chapter discusses the proper cleaning techniques; patient requirements are discussed in Chapter 10.

Order of Cleaning

Before starting into the wards you should have a cleaning cart that can be stocked with supplies.

1. Clean water dishes and food dishes (paper trays) which will have to be filled for each pet depending on the type of food given in the hospital or whether on a special diet. Check the patient records to confirm the type of food and amount.
2. Detergent and water spray bottle
3. Small scrub brush for kennel doors – large long-handled brush for runs
4. Disinfectant diluted in spray bottle
5. Paper towels
6. Newsprint and/or clean towels and blankets for bedding
7. Disposable gloves – switched between contagious pets *and* after handling feces/urine
8. Replacement litter, clean litter boxes, litter scoop if needed
9. Large garbage can with liner for trash – another can for dirty laundry
10. Pheromone spray for cats, enrichment toys for dogs and cats (boarding animals only)
11. Brooms – small one for tight spaces, large one for large rooms or hallways, dust pan
12. Dust mop
13. Mop bucket with squeeze mechanism to remove excess water. Fill with disinfectant measured out to the proper dilution, clean mop head and squeegee and/or a second mop and bucket filled with water.

Start cleaning the least contaminated kennel working to the most contaminated or infectious kennel. This is true in every ward and usually the surgery ward is considered the cleanest and the quarantine ward the dirtiest. The goal is to minimize cross-contamination and maximize patient comfort. Once in the wards if you have a choice between a pet that has not soiled its cage, has slept nicely on the bed provided, and not tipped its water over, and the pet that has soiled its cage, walked in it, spread it from top to bottom, has a soaked blanket and food tipped over and smeared all over, take care of the neat pet first! This seems wrong because we want to provide dry, comfortable kennels for all animals but the few minutes it takes to care for the neat pet versus the messy pet won't matter. Also, it always seems that if a pet is highly anxious and pawing at the cage, it will tip its water over before you are even able to leave the ward! Thus, you will have to start over again! If there is room, you could move the messy pet to an empty run to get them out of the dirty kennel but save cleaning that one until last as it is the most contaminated.

Some clinics do not deep clean a kennel or run if the patient is tidy. Refreshing the water and food, fluffing up the towel or blanket is thought to be less stressful for the pet than moving it into one cage while cleaning its assigned cage, then moving it back. If the animal is boarding, encourage the owner to bring a towel, blanket, or bed from home. The morning or day before they are to go home wash the item, so it looks and smells good. Pets appreciate a stroll outside to relieve themselves and stretch their legs. A few good pats and some kind words will also go a long way in keeping them from becoming depressed.

If the kennel is messy, gently remove the pet, placing dogs in a run and cats in a holding kennel. Then remove all the items inside the kennel. If there is visible debris in the kennel, spray the detergent and water mixture then wipe with paper towels to remove it from the cage surfaces. Again, clean from the least dirty part of the kennel to the dirtiest. The cleanest will be the ceiling, then sides, bars, and floor of the kennel (Figure 4.2).

If there is not much debris or once it has been removed, spray the kennel surfaces with disinfectant and wait for the contact time to elapse before wiping dry with a paper towel. While waiting you can start on another kennel if there is room to move the next animal. Once

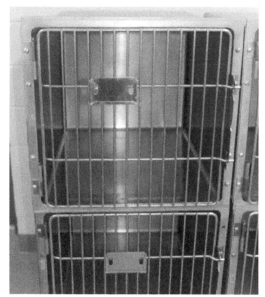
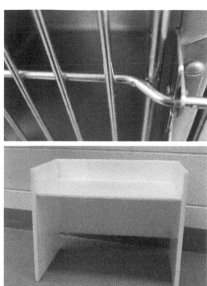

FIGURE 4.2 Kennel: note the cage card holder, door showing latch and crossbars, and kitty perch.

the contact time has elapsed, replace the bedding; this may be layers of newsprint and/or towels or blankets. Place clean water and food dishes in a place where they are not easily tipped inside the kennel. If there is a litter pan, scoop the feces and urine out, remove visible debris on the sides with detergent and water mixture, spray with disinfectant, wait for contact time, then dry with a paper towel. If utilizing paper litter pans, dump everything in the large trash can and put a newly filled paper litter pan in the kennel. Some clinics will spray a pheromone onto a cat's bedding to reduce anxiety. If the bedding is clean, leave it in the cat's kennel as studies have shown familiar smells are of comfort to the animal.

Put the animal back into its original kennel, making sure the door is latched. Accidental escapes and injuries have occurred because the kennel door wasn't closed properly. If the dog has relieved itself in the run, pick up feces, hose down urine, squeegee dry, spray with disinfectant, wait for contact time to elapse, and then it is ready for the next dog. If the dog did not relieve itself, perhaps a trip outside is required before putting it back into its original kennel. For cats, after putting them back in their original kennel, spray the holding kennel with disinfectant, wait for contact time to elapse, wipe dry with a paper towel, and then it is ready for the next cat.

Note that the dog and cat were carefully placed back into their *original* kennel. This is very important for a couple of reasons: (i) it is the kennel that has been assigned to the pet on the computer or in the file so when treatments are required or the owner has come to collect the pet it is important to get the right pet; and (ii) if the animal is contagious you don't want to spread it to another animal by putting it in the wrong kennel.

Cage cards and ID collars should be used to keep track of what animal goes where (Figure 4.3). Cage cards can range from simple to complex. Some cage cards have blank columns in which the staff fills in the observations along with the date and time of the observation. Others have circled abbreviations to choose from or they can be as simple as a place to write the name of the patient, date admitted, and the potential reason. Some clinics also use a clean/dirty cage card; this can help prevent accidental exposure of patients to contagious diseases.

ID collars are paper bands that can be written upon and have a sticky end to fit the collar so they cannot be pulled off, much like a hospital band around a human's wrist only these go around the animal's neck. The name of patient, last name of owner, and kennel number should be on the ID collar before it is attached to the patient. If for some reason there are no cage cards or ID collars, keep a notebook on the cart or in your pocket and mark which animal goes where as you take them out for cleaning.

Some clinics provide raised beds or mats for dogs to sleep upon (Figure 4.4) and perches that allow cats to be raised away from the litter box (Figure 4.2, lower right). These should be checked and cleaned as necessary while the patient is in the hospital. Once the patient goes home, raised beds need a thorough deep clean with disinfectant and a scrub brush used to get into all the nooks and crannies. Part of the cage and run that is often overlooked when cleaning is the door. It is difficult to clean doors with a spray bottle and paper towel. They should be inspected regularly and lifted off their hinges and scrubbed thoroughly with a disinfectant as necessary. The corners of the bars and where the bars or wires meet are often caked with feces or litter if the pets liked to paw at the doors. Run walls should be scrubbed down with a long-handled brush, especially if intact male dogs were being housed in them.

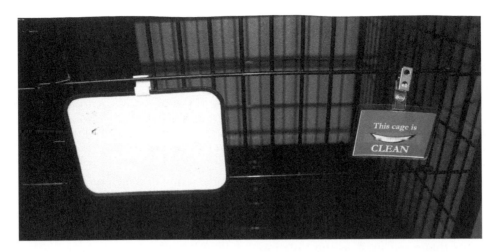

FIGURE 4.3 Cage cards.

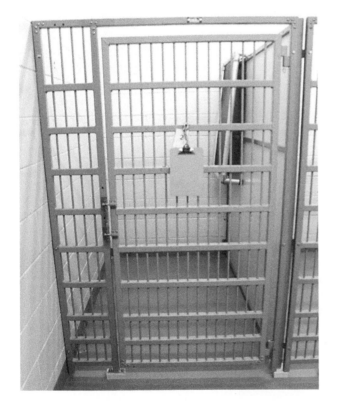

FIGURE 4.4 Run with raised bed – hanging from side wall ready for next patient.

If the clinic only uses newsprint for bedding, check to see what to use for white animals. The newsprint tends to rub off and white animals will turn gray! If possible, all boarding animals should have a bath on the morning of their departure.

Once the kennels in the ward are all cleaned, the room itself needs to be cleaned. Pick up any feces that are on the floor, sweep up any debris and put it in the large trash bucket. Dunk the mop into the disinfectant then squeeze the mop head lightly, mop an area on the floor as far as you can reach standing in one position,

then rinse the mop by dunking it a couple of times, squeeze and repeat as many times as needed to clean the entire floor. Then either rinse and really squeeze the water out of the mop head and "dry" mop the floor or use a squeegee to remove as much water as possible. Repeat in the runs if necessary. Some clinics will want you to spray the runs down with warm water before mopping so you don't smear feces and urine around! The last things to clean are the light switch, doorknob, front and back of the door, and the window to the ward.

Some clinics will use a second mop bucket filled with just water and each time the mop needs to be rinsed it is rinsed in the clear water and squeezed first before going into the bucket of disinfectant. This method reduces the amount of organic material introduced to the disinfectant solution. This is only an issue if the disinfectant being used is deactivated by organic material. When finished with the wards, the mop head should be removed and put in the laundry. Hot water, detergent, and bleach should be used as per your washing machine instructions to launder the mop head. The area where the mop bucket is left should also be cleaned and disinfected. The mop bucket should be refilled with properly diluted disinfectant and a clean mop head placed on the mop. This is so it will be ready for the next cleaning and for taking care of messes made by patients in the reception area or exam room. If it has been used for that purpose during the day, it should be emptied out and replenished before starting the next cleaning as it would bring contaminates into the surgery recovery room.

The cart is then straightened up and replenished for the next time. Spray bottles are refilled, litter pans, food dishes, newsprint, and towels are replaced as necessary. Secure the large trash bag closed with a tie, tape, or knot and take it to the dumpster. Do not leave feces-filled trash cans in the clinic for any length of time as the smell tends to permeate through the building! Replace the trash can liners.

A few words about contagious pets. We don't always know whether a pet is contagious, so it is always best to consider every pet to be a walking disaster waiting to happen! Don't put pets into runs or cages together, never put a "healthy" patient with a surgical patient, and don't put patients into runs that have not been cleaned in between occupants. If the isolation ward is full, remember some diseases are specific to specific animals. If you have a puppy with parvovirus and there is no room in the dog isolation ward, put it in the cat room. If you have a cat with feline leukemia, put it in the dog ward. This is not ideal as far as stress levels are concerned but at least you won't be spreading these contagious diseases! Remember to switch gloves, change boots or booties, leave lab coats that were used in the isolation ward there or put them straight in the laundry. Never walk into the isolation ward with your everyday scrubs and bare shoes! You could spread disease to the rest of the patients you work with that day or take it home to your own pets.

Reflection

After reading the section on order of cleaning kennels describe in your own words which room you would start with, how you would handle each animal and how you would clean, care for, and provide comfort to the animals in that room.

Facility Maintenance

The entire veterinary facility must be cleaned on a regular basis. There may be someone hired to do the daily janitorial work, but that person may be the veterinary assistant! If that is the case, all rooms need daily attention.

1. Stock a cleaning cart with detergent and water spray bottles, disinfectant diluted and in a spray bottle, window cleaner, and paper towels.
2. Large trash can with a liner and extra trash can liners – varying sizes to fit the trash cans.
3. Mop bucket that is reserved for the public areas of the practice. Reception, exam rooms, lab, offices, and so on.
4. Extra paper towels to fill dispensers.
5. Hand soap and/or hand sanitizer to refill dispensers.
6. Brooms – a small one for corners and tight spaces, a large one for hallways, and a dustpan.
7. Dust mop, dusting cloth, and furniture polish if necessary,
8. Toilet bowl brush and cleanser,

Start in cleanest room and move through to the dirtiest. Start high and work your way down to the floor.

Offices and the lunch break room are usually only used by the staff, so empty trash, vacuum if carpeted or sweep and mop. Wipe down the lunch table and dust the desk in the office. Wipe the light switch, doorknob, and front and backs of the door.

TIP BOX 4.2

Time saving tip: when replacing garbage can liners, put a few extra liners in the bottom of the can, then put the new liner on top. If the garbage can gets full or contaminated during the day you don't have to run for a liner as one is there waiting!

Repeat for the reception desk area, wiping down the desk and if there is a patient ledge or counter wipe that off with disinfectant. Move to the reception area and the exam rooms. Start by dusting or wiping down the furniture, counters, and chairs with the products that are made to clean those surfaces. Wood furniture will need polish, counters will need disinfectant spray, and bookshelf or coffee tables perhaps just a dust cloth. If the chairs in the reception area are cloth covered, use a vacuum to remove hair and then wipe them down with a towel sprayed with disinfectant. Remove the trash either by dumping it into the large trash can or by removing the liner and replacing it with a new one. Check the wall around the trash cans for splatter, use the detergent and water spray bottle to wash that area, followed by the disinfectant spray. Replenish paper towels, refill disinfectant spray bottles in the exam rooms, and refill hand soaps/sanitizers. Wipe the doorknobs, light switches, and doors with disinfectant. If there are windows clean those with a window cleaner. Use the dust mop to capture hair and dust bunnies, then the broom to sweep them into the dustpan. Follow by mopping the floor as described in the kennel cleaning section.

TIP BOX 4.3

Look at what you are going to clean and choose the cleaner suitable to the object!

The laboratory and bathrooms are next. Wipe off counters and clean the sink with disinfectant. For bathrooms, clean mirrors with window cleaner, apply toilet bowl cleaner to the bowl then brush clean and flush, wipe the seat top, bottom, and base with disinfectant and paper towels, and replenish toilet paper as needed. For both rooms, remove the trash and replace liners if necessary, replenish paper towels, soap/sanitizer, and disinfectant spray bottle in the lab. Wipe off the light switch, doorknob, and front and back of the door. Sweep and mop the floor.

When you have a "moment in time" clean out a drawer or cupboard. These are often neglected and fill quickly with hair, debris, and sometimes partial rolls of tape and bandage wrap. Remove everything, even the drawer from the cabinet if you can. Decide what is still usable or if it can be moved to another area for use and discard the rest. Either wipe the drawer clean or tip it to one corner and dump the debris into a trash can. If you cannot remove the drawer, vacuum it to get it clean. Wipe down with a disinfectant spray and replace the items neatly and move on to another drawer if you have time. To clean cabinets, remove all the items, wipe the shelf with disinfectant spray, and replace items neatly. Always remember to check items for expiration dates before putting them back. Restock items as necessary.

Organizing bins are available in all sizes, shapes, and colors. They are very useful for organizing supplies into like items or per procedure in drawers and cabinets. Check for an inventory card that lists the items that should be in the bin or drawer. This is a great time saver for restocking drawers so if there isn't one ask for permission to make them up for the drawers. If possible, laminate the card so it can be tucked to one side, easily found but not easily destroyed.

Storeroom shelves should be dusted and floors swept and mopped on a weekly basis. If the clinic uses pallets to keep food off the ground, take advantage of empty pallets between food orders to lift them up and sweep under them. Hair and dust bunnies love to congregate beneath pallets. If you notice rodent droppings report it to the office manager to get traps or poison supplies.

Refrigerators and freezers are another often neglected area in the facility. Refrigerators should be wiped down with a disinfectant on a weekly basis. Check everything for expiration dates before putting them back. If there is a refrigerator for human use in the break room, be the designated person to check through it and toss items that are moldy or old. Wipe the surfaces with disinfectant spray. *Never* place human food into refrigerators that are storing vaccines, medications, or laboratory supplies and samples. This is not healthy and could cause some serious issues with human health!

Hospital Laundry

Laundry rooms tend to be neglected and are often one of the dirtiest places in the facility! The dryer dust, lint, debris from bedding, and splatter from the mop buckets all add to the mess. Stay on top of the mess by wiping down the laundry machines, cleaning the lint trap after each load, sweeping and mopping the room daily.

Laundry itself is a daily, sometimes all-day chore! Wet piles of contaminated bedding or scrubs cannot be allowed to sit for any length of time. The piles are sources of disease and potential mold that becomes airborne when finally sorted out and washed. Sort laundry into four piles: surgical items, scrubs or lab coats, towels and bedding are sorted into dry and wet/contaminated. Wash from cleanest to dirtiest.

Surgical items must be washed first as these are the "cleanest." Pretreatment of bloodstains on wraps and gowns require a soak in cold water before placing them into the wash. If the washing machine has a presoak option, place all items with blood on them in the wash, add a presoak detergent that contains hydrogen peroxide, set it on cold water, and turn it on. Once the presoak cycle is completed and if there is room add the other surgical wraps and gowns and wash in hot water with regular detergent measured out as per label instructions. Do not put towels in with the surgical items, because the lint from the towels will stick to the cloth and can fall into the surgical incisions causing a foreign body infection. Make sure the lint trap is clean on the dryer, add the surgical items and a fabric softener sheet if used, and start the drying cycle.

Scrubs, lab coats, and coveralls are washed next. Check all the pockets for items and for stains on the material; pretreat if necessary. These items can be washed on warm or cool water settings with regular detergent if not contaminated. Read the labels; if some of your items require cold water it is important to follow the directions otherwise they may be damaged. If items are contaminated, use a disinfectant for the presoak cycle then wash in the appropriate water temperature with detergent, and dry with a fabric softener sheet.

Dry towels and blankets are washed after the scrubs. They are shaken out over the trash can to remove any litter or feces. If there were feces on the material put that item in with the wet/contaminated load. Place the water setting on hot, add detergent, and if available set for heavily soiled on the machine. This setting will take a bit longer and the agitation is a bit more robust. Place into the drier and add a fabric softener sheet. Repeat for as many loads of dry bedding items as need to be washed. Remember to clean the lint trap between loads. Hair and lint collected in the trap will decrease the effectiveness of the dryer, resulting in longer drying times and a backlog of wet wash waiting for the dryer.

> **TIP BOX 4.4**
>
> If necessary, set a timer on your phone to remind you to check the laundry throughout the day. Sometimes we get so busy we forget and get behind!

Wet/contaminated bedding, mop heads, and cleaning towels need to be handled carefully and last. A mask, goggles, gloves, and waterproof apron is suggested PPE. Shake the items out over the garbage can to remove any feces or litter that may be clinging to the item. Place them into the washer and adjust the machine to a hot water temperature, presoak, heavily soiled setting, add a disinfectant and turn on the machine. When the presoak cycle is finished, add detergent, leave settings the same other than wash and turn on the machine. Dry with a fabric softener sheet.

When laundry is finished, run the washing machine a final time without any items. Add bleach and/or detergent and set for hot water wash. This cleans the machine so it is ready for the next day's surgical scrubs. There are attachments for a vacuum cleaner that can reach into the lint trap area. Vacuuming this once a week will pick up the lint, dirt, and hair that escapes the lint screen as if left to build up it could cause a fire.

> ### TIP BOX 4.5
>
> Do *not* overload washing machine or dryer! Doing so decreases the effectiveness of the machine's action and will end up costing more time and money.

Fold all the laundry as it comes out of the dryer and store in the proper locations. Once laundry is finished for the day, clean the tops of the machines, sweep and empty the trash, and mop if necessary.

Reflection

Now that you have some idea of how much work goes into keeping a facility clean, how could you help the janitorial staff in the clinic or even at your school throughout the day?

Equipment Maintenance

There are many pieces of equipment that require constant cleaning between patients. A veterinary assistant must be capable of thoroughly cleaning each piece in order to have it ready for the next patient. Remember that inanimate objects can be fomites and our job is to make sure they don't become one! There are also other instruments or pieces of equipment that require certain maintenance procedures, which are covered in the individual chapters later in this textbook. The following are instructions for general cleaning or maintenance of common pieces of equipment found in the veterinary hospital.

The most notorious potential fomite is the hair clipper. This piece of equipment is utilized to trim or shave the hair from animals. The hair clipper has two parts: the base which houses the motor and driving piston, and the clipper head which is the part that removes the hair. It is to be hoped that the clinic has kept an owner's

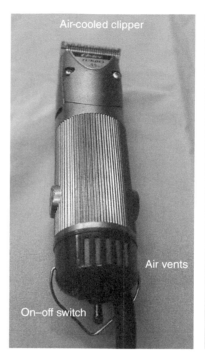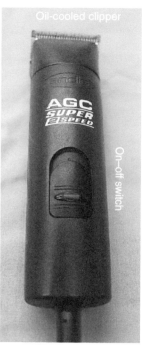

Air-cooled clipper

Oil-cooled clipper

Air vents

On–off switch

On–off switch

FIGURE 4.5 Air-cooled and oil-cooled hair clippers.

manual that can be consulted for the clipper body maintenance. If not, you may be able to find instructions online for the major maintenance of the body. The following needs to be done daily and sometimes throughout the day if the clipper is heavily used.

Determine if the clipper is an air-cooled or oil-cooled clipper. An air-cooled clipper will have air vents or air intake screens on the end or near the end of the body. Oil-cooled clippers do not have these vents (Figure 4.5). Make sure these are not plugged with hair or debris as this will make the clipper overheat. These clippers also require the clipper blades to be sprayed with a lubricant cooling agent when in use. It is sprayed onto the clipper blades while the clipper is on and applied as the handle gets warm (Figure 4.6). You should hear the motor run faster and louder as you apply the spray. If you don't lubricate the blades, the clipper body will get too hot to handle.

Oil-cooled hair clippers require the clipper blades to be oiled first thing before use and at regular intervals while in use. The oil is applied at the junction of the blades (Figure 4.7). Again, if this isn't done the handle will get too hot to hold.

Both types of clippers will need to have the blade heads cleaned in between patients. The heads can be removed by pushing up on a small lever at the base of the clipper head (Figure 4.8a). While pushing the lever up, ease the clipper head away from the clipper body (Figure 4.8b). When the clipper head is pushed all the way back it should slide off the clipper pin (Figure 4.8c). The blades can be cleaned by pushing the top blade over approximately half way, then using

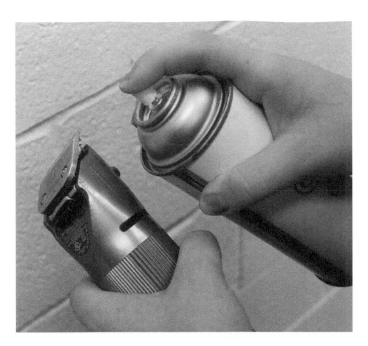

FIGURE 4.6 Air-cooled clipper head being lubricated.

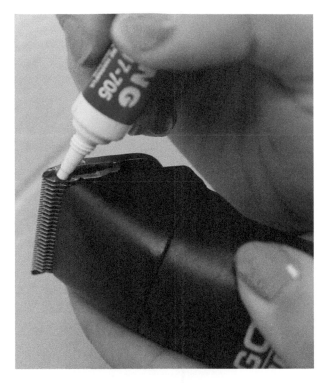

FIGURE 4.7 Oil-cooled clipper head being oiled.

a brush clean the hair from the surfaces. When finished on that side, push the blade back the other way until it is half off and clean that end (Figure 4.8d). If you should accidently slide the top blade all the way off, use a screwdriver to lift the springs that hold it in place and slide the blade back on to the blade base (Figure 4.9). *Never* loosen or remove the screws on the back of the clipper head (Figure 4.10). These hold the spring clips in place and are adjusted at the factory to apply optimal pressure for removing hair.

With the clipper head off, use a small brush to remove the hair inside the driver compartment. This tends to get full of hair and will eventually pack in there so hard that the driving arm does not work properly.

If the clipper should be dropped it can break the drive lever. This is an easy part to replace on an Oster™ clipper (as shown in Figure 4.11). This compartment is accessed by removing the two Philips screws on the front panel of the clipper. This compartment is also where you grease the clipper every 6 months. Older models will also become packed with hair and it is a good practice to check the compartment every few months and clean it out with a cotton swab.

To reattach the clipper head to the clipper, slide the clipper onto the pin (Figure 4.9). Then plug the clipper in and start it by flipping the switch on the end or pushing the button on the body forward. Then push the clipper head back into place and if the top blade does not move press the head in a bit more. Spray disinfecting spray made for clippers on to the running blades followed by cooling spray for the air-driven clippers or oil right at the junction of the blades for the oil-cooled clippers (Figure 4.12). The clipper is now ready to be used on another patient.

You don't always have to take the clipper head off, especially if a patient has short hair. You can get away with just brushing the clipper blades off and then spraying with disinfectant spray followed by the lubricant. However, if there is any chance that this short-haired animal has anything contagious the full out clean is best.

Even with the best of care blades get dull and need to be replaced. Clinics usually have a few extra clipper heads available for replacing dull blades. These blades can be re-sharpened so don't throw them away. You should ask where the replacement blades are and pay attention as there will most likely be a "dull" box, a "sharp" box of used blades, and new blades in their shipping containers. Whether using a re-sharpened blade or a new blade there is a shipping oil applied to the blades that needs to be removed before they are used. Find the blade wash, read the directions on the container, and proceed to wash the blade (Figure 4.12). Blade wash can also be used if the clipper has been run through bloody or pus-filled hair.

There are companies that repair clippers and sharpen blades for less than it takes to buy new. A quality clipper that will last years, if taken care of, will cost between $150 and $200. The blades are about $25–$30 each. Most clinics will have two sizes of clipper heads available. A size 40 clipper head will take the hair off down to the skin. This one is used for shaving surgical, wound, and IV catheter sites. A size 10 clipper head will leave about 1/4 of an inch and is used to trim out mats (Figure 4.13). Notice the length of the teeth when comparing the size 10 to the 40. There are a few different sized clipper heads

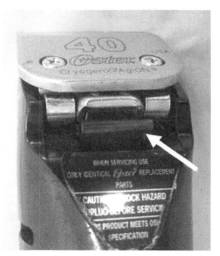

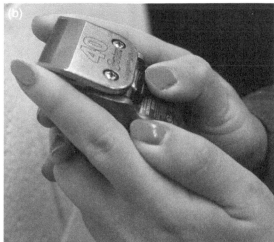

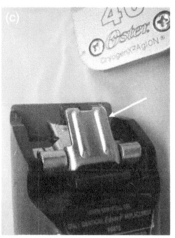

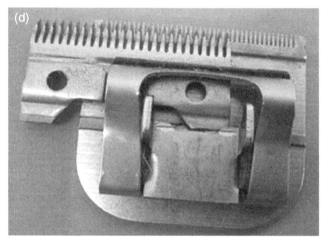

FIGURE 4.8 Clipper head removal and cleaning.

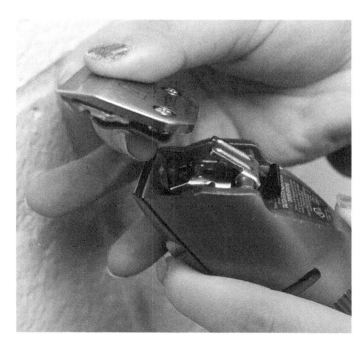

FIGURE 4.9 Putting top blade back onto blade base.

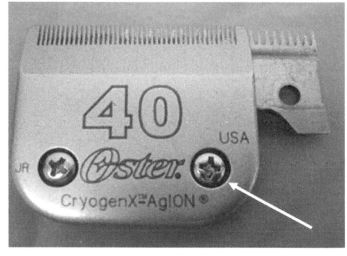

FIGURE 4.10 Screws on back of clipper head.

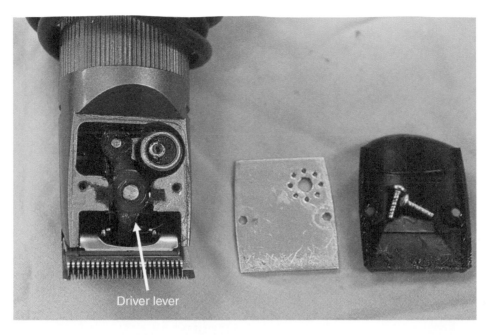

FIGURE 4.11 Inside driver compartment – driver lever.

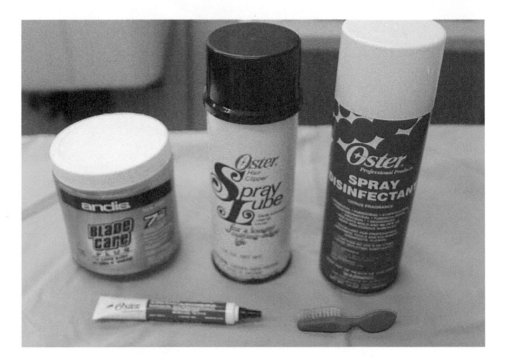

FIGURE 4.12 Blade wash, spray lube, spray disinfectant, blade oil, cleaning brush.

that are used by groomers to get different lengths of hair. If a clipper has been dropped, check the clipper head for missing teeth. Replace the clipper head because the missing teeth will cause gouges in the skin when shaving. Check the clipper body housing and if cracked take it to the inventory manager for repair.

Toenail Clippers

There are several types of toenail clippers available to the veterinary staff (Figure 4.14). Figure 4.14a shows a scissor-like trimmer which comes in four sizes to fit the size of pet you are trimming. The one shown is a medium size, with one size bigger and two sizes smaller available. Figure 4.14b shows a guillotine trimmer; you place the toenail through the oval, then squeeze the handles which pushes the blade forward slicing off the nail. Figure 4.14c shows a White's nail trimmer. It is used when a toenail has overgrown in a complete circle and is protruding into the pad. The hooked jaws can be placed around the nail to cut it short. These trimmers become dull and are hard to sharpen again and so they are

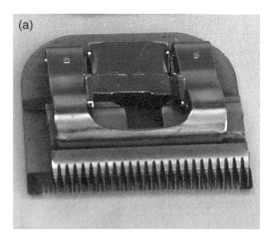
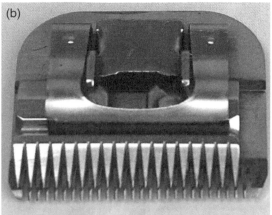

FIGURE 4.13 Clipper head sizes: (a) size 40 blade; (b) size 10 blade.

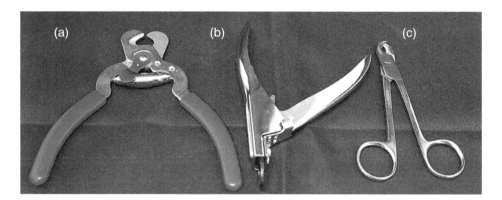

FIGURE 4.14 Toenail trimmers.

usually replaced. The guillotine trimmer has replacement blades that are easy to replace. The only cleaning that needs to be done on these is if a blood vessel was accidently cut. If this should happen, clean the tips of the blades off with alcohol or the spray disinfectant and wipe dry with a paper towel.

Otoscope

The otoscope has several cannulas that are of different sizes for different sized pets (Figure 4.15). This instrument is used to look into ears, but it can also be used to look up a nostril or into the vaginal vault. Whatever the reason for its use the cannulas tend to become full of wax or body fluids. If they are not disposable, they need to be cleaned. First rinse them under warm to hot water, then spray with a disinfectant spray, use a cotton swab to clean and dry the inside of the cannula and a paper towel to dry the outside.

Vacuums

Vacuums are used in the surgery prep area to pick up hair that has been shaved from a surgical site. There is also one used in the facility for carpeted areas and

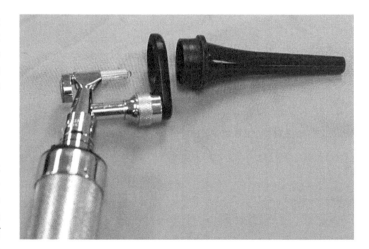

FIGURE 4.15 Otoscope and cannula.

furniture. Some clinics will have a central vacuum system. The maintenance for a vacuum is usually to make sure the vacuum collection container is emptied. Central vacuum systems have a large collection bin and you may be asked to do a weekly or biweekly check to empty the bin. Otherwise, a clinic will have a canister or small portable vacuum in the surgery prep area. This will have to be emptied daily or the hair gets into the

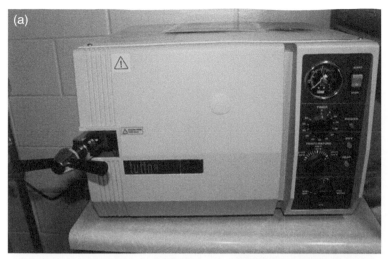

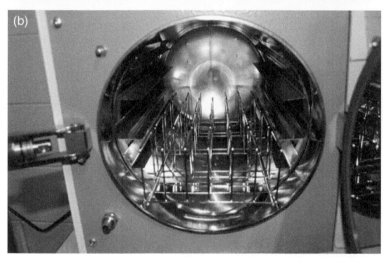

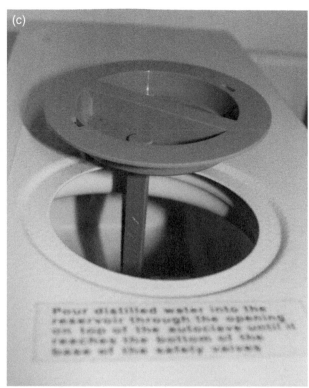

FIGURE 4.16 Autoclave: (a) exterior; (b) interior; (c) water fill.

casing and can clog up and stop the motor. The vacuum for the facility will usually be an upright model that may require bags to be changed when full. Often these machines will have an indicator light that will turn on when the bag is full. Many of the modern-day vacuums have dust or allergy filters that also need to be changed on a regular basis. Setting up a monthly check of the filters is a good way to remember to change them. Remember to let the inventory manager know that you need more bags and filters when you take the second to last one.

Autoclaves

An autoclave is used to sterilize surgical instruments, gowns, and drapes for surgery. It is probably one of the most neglected pieces of equipment in the hospital. It requires distilled water to produce clean steam; however, many clinics use tap water. When tap water is converted to steam it leaves behind minerals naturally occurring in the water on the machine surfaces, conduits, and filters. This is doubled when the steam saturates surgical wraps and the detergent used to clean them becomes aerosolized adding to the buildup of minerals. If you see a buildup of white crusty material in the chamber and/or in the water tank that is what has caused it (Figure 4.16). This buildup of minerals is deposited upon the surgical instruments and can cause corrosion.

Duraline Biosystems Inc. (http://www.duralinesystems. com/blog/show/how-to-care-for-autoclave-steam-sterilizer), a maker and seller of autoclaves, recommends weekly cleaning of trays and racks with a non-scratch scour pad and a mild non-abrasive detergent such as Bon-Ami™. Rinse the racks well to remove all of the detergent. Drain the water from the reservoir and replenish with distilled water. Perform a biologic live spore test to check that the autoclave is working properly. Monthly, clean the chamber and flush the lines with an autoclave cleaner. Read the directions on the label for the cleaner's specific steps. Inspect the electrical cord and plug for any signs of overheating. Yearly, have your autoclave inspected, cleaned thoroughly, tested, and calibrated.

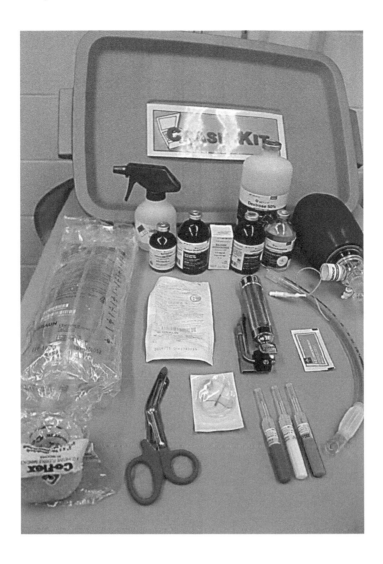

FIGURE 4.17 Crash cart items.

Crash Cart

Crash carts are used to help animals that have stopped breathing, are choking, or their hearts have stopped beating (Figure 4.17). Most clinics will assign the upkeep of this cart to the veterinary technician; however, the veterinary assistant may be assigned to do it. A good practice is to replace the crash cart items with new each week or month and use any "short-dated" or older products in the clinic so you aren't throwing anything away because it has become outdated. Replace any item that you have removed or has become outdated and ask the inventory manager what to do with those products that have become outdated.

Radiograph Processors

Processors that develop radiographs are often referred to as automatic processors (Figure 4.18). They require cleaning and refreshing or replacement of the developing and fixing chemicals. Each make of automatic processor is a little different but all will have rollers that need to be wiped down on a regular basis. The machines also require

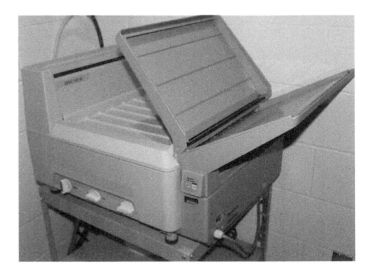

FIGURE 4.18 Automatic processor.

a full shut down and clean out on a regular basis. If you are assigned this task, read the manufacturer's manual and set up a schedule for the required maintenance. The restocking of chemicals will be dependent on the number

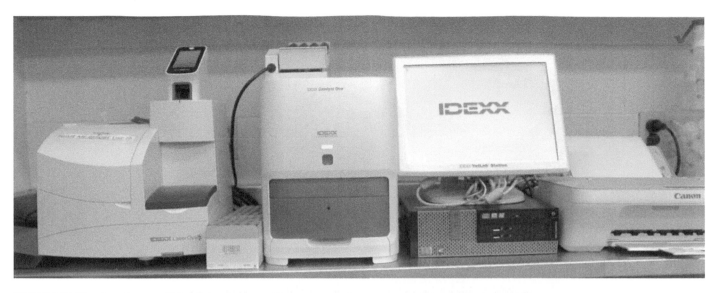

FIGURE 4.19 Blood analyzer and blood chemistry machine, connected to computer station and printer.

of radiographs taken. The chemical levels should be checked daily in the morning so that the tanks can be replenished before the day's patients start to arrive.

Blood Analyzers and Blood Chemistry Machines

The maintenance on these machines varies with each brand. These are very expensive machines and usually it is a task the veterinary technician will handle (Figure 4.19). However, if you are asked to "prime" a machine the instructions should be available and easy to follow. Some clinics have contracts with the machine's manufacturer to carry out the routine maintenance.

Centrifuges

Centrifuges are used to spin laboratory samples: blood, urine, and feces. Each centrifuge will have a head that accommodates tubes of various sizes (Figure 4.20).

When the centrifuge is turned on the head spins at speeds of 1000–1500 r.p.m. The very nature of this machine is a biohazard spill waiting to happen! Tubes break or splatter body fluids into the head and chamber of the centrifuge. Allowing that to sit without cleaning it up will often unbalance the centrifuge causing more body fluids to be spilt. Goggles, gloves, and mask or face shield are the PPEs required when cleaning the centrifuge.

The centrifuge labeled A in Figure 4.20 is a hematocrit centrifuge. It often breaks the tubes or they are put in the wrong way, which results in blood being sprayed all over the inside cover. Soap and a brush will be required to clean the blood off and then it should be sprayed with disinfectant and allowed to air dry. The centrifuge labeled B in Figure 4.20 holds tiny tubes and is

remarkably good in that it doesn't break the tubes very often. If it should become contaminated it doesn't come apart. So, twisting a paper towel up to fit inside the tube holes is the only way to clean them out. You will need one to soak up the spill and another sprayed with disinfectant. The centrifuge labeled C in Figure 4.20 has tube holders that can be removed for cleaning. Dump any fluid or debris down the sink. Then, using a brush, hot water, and soap, clean the tube thoroughly. Spray with disinfectant, wait for the contact time, and then wipe with a paper towel. Replace the tubes, then spray the head and inside surfaces housing the head with a disinfectant spray and wipe dry after the designated contact time has elapsed. There is often sprayed feces or urine and so the PPE required are goggles, mask or face shield, and gloves.

Microscopes

Microscopes are delicate pieces of equipment that are used every day in the clinic's laboratory. Many microbes require a magnification of 1000 times. The 100× objective is the one that magnifies to 1000 but requires an immersion oil to work properly (Figure 4.21). This oil is placed on a microscope slide and the objective tip is then put into the oil. This oil is difficult to clean off without damaging the objective or the other parts on the microscope. To clean the objectives and light lens use lens cleaner and a lens paper. These are formulated to clean without scratching. Add a couple of drops to the lens paper and then gently clean the tip of the objective and the surface of the light lens. To clean other areas of oil or dust, you can use lens cleaner and Kimtech wipes™ which are a little more abrasive, so they are only used on areas of hard plastic or metal. A paper towel is too big to get into nooks and crannies and too abrasive for the lens.

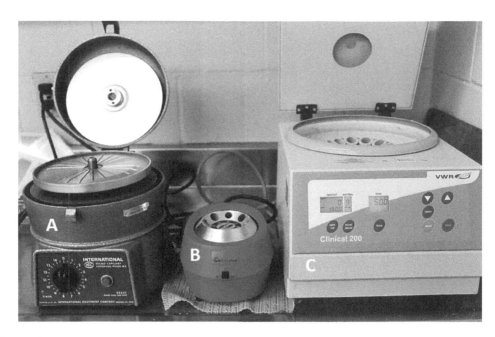

FIGURE 4.20 Centrifuge station.

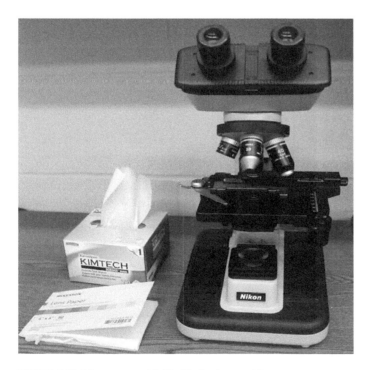

FIGURE 4.21 Microscope with KimTech wipes and lens paper.

Mobile Veterinary Units

These vehicles should be as clean as any brick and mortar clinic facility. Not only the outside, but the inside of the different compartments need to be cleaned out on a

> **TIP BOX 4.6**
>
> When you overhear a client asking the vet to give his horse a tetanus shot after a health certificate examination because the vet truck is filthy, it is time to clean the truck!

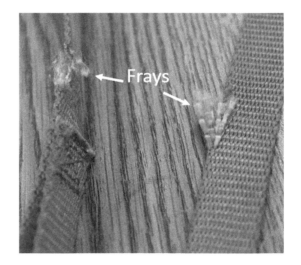

FIGURE 4.22 Frayed leash.

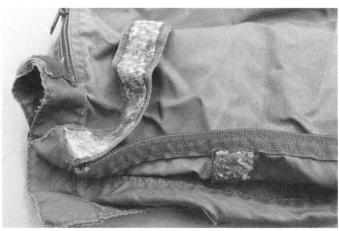

FIGURE 4.23 Feline restraint bag.

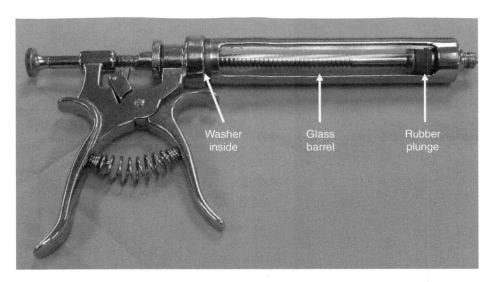

Washer inside

Glass barrel

Rubber plunge

FIGURE 4.24 Automatic dose syringe.

regular basis. Some vets will do it themselves as a stress reducer but some never get around to it because they are so busy or exhausted! Utilizing "moments in time" even if it is just to go through the medications and check them for outdates and/or clean out one compartment at a time is better than never! Use a vacuum to remove the big chunks and then spray each compartment with disinfectant and wipe dry with a paper towel after the contact time has elapsed. Restock the compartment as necessary.

Halters, Ropes, Leashes, and Harnesses

Check all of these for tears or fraying (Figure 4.22). If they have metal pieces, check for cracks. If damaged, consult with the inventory manager as to what to do with the damaged items. It is dangerous to use these items when frayed, torn, or cracked as they can break unexpectedly.

Feline restraint bags and nylon muzzles can be laundered in the washing machine. Do not put them in with towels as the self-sticking straps get full of lint (Figure 4.23). Plastic muzzles can be sprayed with a disinfectant and wiped dry after the contact time has elapsed. All of these should be washed between patients.

Automatic Dosing Syringes

These "guns" come apart and the glass or plastic tube can be cleaned with hot water and soap and rinsed thoroughly (Figure 4.24). The rubber gasket under the cap is checked. It should bend easily and not feel hard. If it does, change it for a new one. The plunger has a rubber or silicone tip that can be changed if cracked and hard. A little mineral oil on the plunger stopper is OK if it is difficult to put into the glass tube when reassembling it. Check these each time you clean the dose syringe.

Reflection

With so many pieces of equipment to take care of, how do you envision learning more about the ones discussed and others that you may be exposed to in a veterinary clinic?

Chapter Reflection

This chapter is all about cleaning and maintaining the facility and equipment in a veterinary practice. Share your thoughts about why the clinic and equipment have to be maintained at such a high level and how do you see yourself participating in this monumental task.

Anatomy and Physiology

Anatomy is the study of body structures that are visible to the naked eye. Physiology is the study of body functions and how the body works together as a whole. Without solid knowledge of anatomy and physiology, the rest of the information about animals, diseases, conditions, medications, and laboratory tests will be harder to comprehend. Consider it a foundation of your understanding of veterinary medicine. Veterinarians and veterinary technicians "speak" anatomy and physiology all day, every day. If you don't understand what they are talking about, how can you be helpful?

"Speaking" Anatomy

There are several types of terms associated with anatomy; there are directional terms and common anatomic terms for external and internal body parts. We start with common anatomic terms and then move to the directional terms. This is followed by a discussion of the individual body systems. For each system we cover both parts and function.

Animal anatomy is similar to human anatomy; however, most animals walk on four legs! That is why they are

Tasks for the Veterinary Assistant, Fourth Edition. Teresa F. Sonsthagen.
© 2020 John Wiley & Sons, Inc. Published 2020 by John Wiley & Sons, Inc.
Companion website: www.wiley.com/go/sonsthagen/tasks

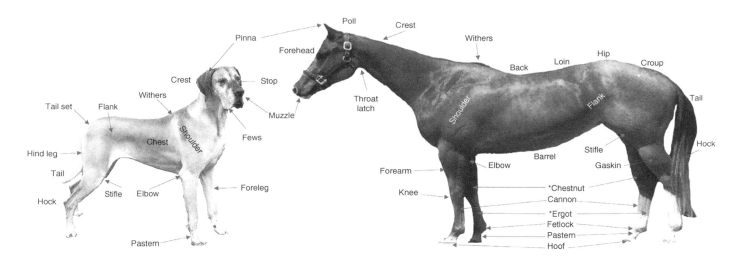

FIGURE 5.1 Dog and horse body parts. *Chestnuts and ergots are small "horny" growths not seen on this photo. Their locations are indicated by arrows.

called quadrupeds and humans and birds are bipeds. For that reason, we must adjust our thinking to accommodate those legs. There are those animals that allow us to ride or pack stuff on them and so some of their parts are a bit different and need to be learned as well. Figure 5.1 shows the common landmark terms used; some for all animals, with a few differences marked on both the dog and horse.

Learning Exercise

Practice naming the parts using pictures of dogs and horses from the internet.

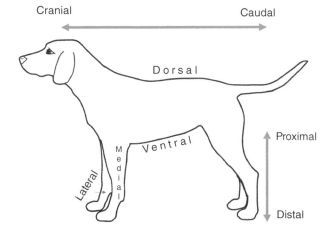

FIGURE 5.2 Directional terms.

Directional terms are used by veterinarians to write in medical records, to identify the specific location of a lesion or injury that may not be obvious. He/she will use it to request a radiograph of a specific body part or for an ultrasound treatment on a certain part of a leg. Learning the directional terms will speed up the process of taking care of animals because you can read what is written in the medical record rather than tracking the veterinarian down to ask.

Most animals are quadrupeds, meaning they stand on four legs. This makes describing where their "front" or their "back" is difficult if you compare them with humans. Is the back their spine or rump? Is the front the head, chest, nose, or belly? To eliminate this confusion veterinary medicine uses terms to describe the various directions and surfaces on an animal.

The most commonly used terms to describe direction are left and right. To be clear when reporting left or right, it is as if the animal is facing the same way as you, so your left is its left and vice versa. The following are the

commonly used, more specific directional terms (Figure 5.2):

Cranial – towards the head

Rostral –used for locations on the head or in the mouth that means towards the nose

Caudal – towards the tail from the point of reference

Proximal – closest to the point of attachment

Distal – a point further away from the point of attachment

The most commonly used terms to describe surface:

Dorsal – the surface area encompassing the length of the spinal column

Ventral – the surface area encompassing the abdomen or belly

Lateral – towards the middle – the inside of the leg is closest to the middle of the body

Medial – away from the middle – the outside of the leg is away from the middle of the body

Learning Exercise

Practice directional terms by finding pictures on the internet of an animal standing, lying down, and sitting. It can be a bit challenging when the animal is not in a standing position!

Body Systems

The body is made up of 11 systems: skeletal, muscular, integumentary, nervous, cardiovascular, pulmonary (respiratory), immune, digestive, urinary, reproductive, and endocrine. But first a brief discussion about the molecular level of the body. The body is composed of cells that combine to make the larger structures. Cells are made up of a **nucleus** to control the activity of the cell. **Cytoplasm** encircles the nucleus and is made up of fine fibers and **organelles** that take care of energy production and waste elimination for the cell. The cell itself is surrounded by a membrane or cell wall that protects the integrity of the cell. Cells can be single entities like blood cells that make up the body's immune system, which we will discuss later, or they combine to make up the tissues in the body. There are four types of tissues that make up the body structures.

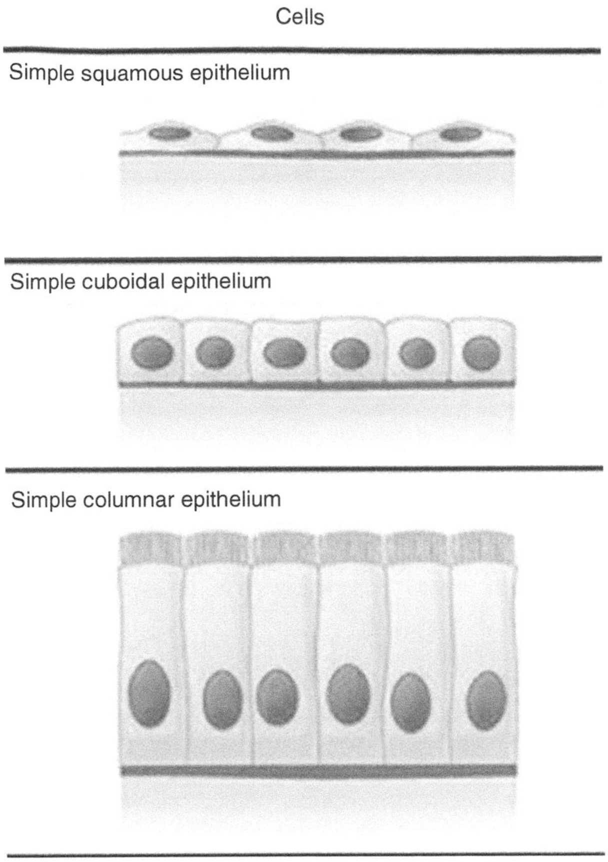

Learning Exercise

For the following body systems find pictures of the structures without labels and practice naming the parts. Make flash cards of the diseases on one side, the organ it affects and what the causative agent is for that disease.

Epithelial tissues are composed of cells that line or cover the body and its organs. There are three types: squamous, cuboidal, and columnar (Figure 5.3). These are further differentiated to accommodate the function of the various organs, but that is beyond what you need to know.

Connective tissue is made up of cells and a matrix that provide structure to the body. There are two different types of cells: fibroblasts (or fibrocytes) include cells that make up bone, ligaments, tendons, cartilage, and blood; adipocytes make up the adipose tissue also known as fat. The matrix itself can be fluid, semi-fluid, gelatinous, or ground substance, and protein fibers known as collagen.

Muscle tissue is made up of cells that are bound together in sheets and fibers. There are three types of muscle tissue: skeletal, cardiac, and smooth.

Cells

Simple squamous epithelium

Simple cuboidal epithelium

Simple columnar epithelium

FIGURE 5.3 Epithelial cells. Adapted from Wikimedia Commons.

Nervous tissue is made up of neurons that conduct messages throughout the body.

Histology is the study of tissues. A veterinarian will take tissue samples and examine them under a microscope to determine if the tissues are diseased. If unsure of the diagnosis, they may send these samples to a diagnostic laboratory for examination by veterinary **pathologists**. These are veterinarians that have specialized in finding the cause of diseases.

As previously mentioned, the body is made up of 11 systems. Let's look at each system individually.

Skeletal System

The skeletal system provides the framework, support, and protection for the body and is made up of bones. Bones are produced by cells called osteoclasts, the bone cell itself is called an osteocyte, and new bone cells are produced by osteoblasts. Bones have an inner cavity called the endosteum that contains the bone marrow where blood cell production takes place. The outer covering of bone is called the periosteum. All the bones combined make up the skeletal system. It is divided into two parts: the **appendicular** skeleton are the bones of the

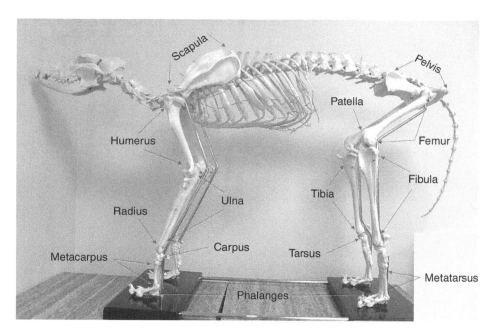

FIGURE 5.4 Appendicular skeleton.

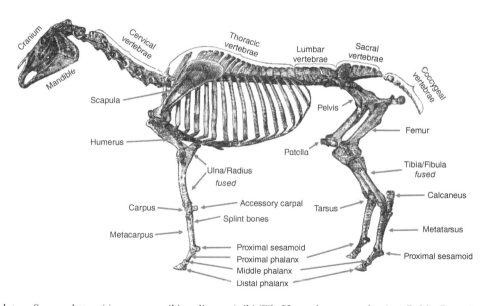

FIGURE 5.5 Horse skeleton. Source: https://commons.wikimedia.org/wiki/File:Horse_bones_ugglan.jpg. Public Domain.

limbs and the **axial** skeleton are the bones that make up the trunk and head of the body. Bones are attached to each other by **ligaments**.

Dogs, cats, ferrets, and rodents all have similar appendicular skeletons. The bones of the front legs starting from proximal to distal include the scapula, humerus, radius, ulna, carpals, metacarpals, and digits or phalanges (Figure 5.4). The bones of the back legs from proximal to distal include the pelvis, femur, patella, tibia, fibula, tarsus, metatarsus, and digits or phalanges.

Livestock limbs have evolved a bit differently in that the bones have elongated, and some have fused together (Figure 5.5). In horses, the front limb bones go in order from proximal to distal and include the scapula, humerus, radius/ulna (fused), carpus (knee), metacarpus (cannon bone), proximal (pastern), middle (fetlock), and distal (coffin bone) phalanx.

On either side of the metacarpus are the second and fourth metacarpal bones fused to the third metacarpal bone; these are called splint bones. On the dorsal side of the leg behind the carpus is the accessory carpus and on the distal end of the metacarpus is the proximal sesamoid bone. The rear limb bones going from proximal to distal include the pelvis, femur, tibia/fibula (fused), tarsus, metatarsus (cannon bone), and the same list of phalanges as for the front leg. On the dorsal side just

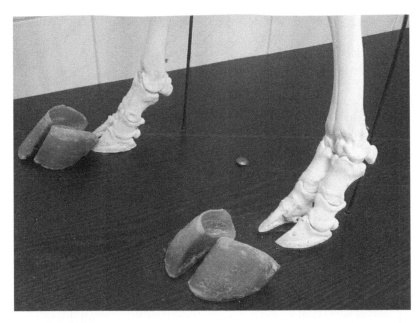

FIGURE 5.6 Cow lower forelimb – modified by TF Sonsthagen. Source: https://commons.wikimedia.org/wiki/Category:Cattle_hooves_and_feet#/media/File:Ro%C3%9Fthal_2010_Schulfest_11.jpg. Public domain.

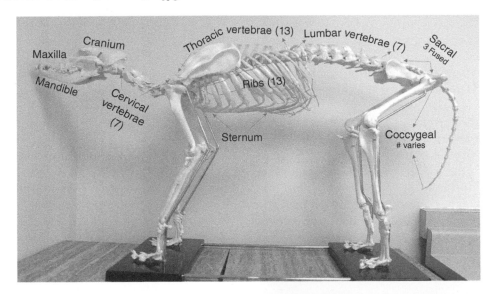

FIGURE 5.7 Axial skeleton.

above the metatarsus sits the calcaneus (hock). Between the femur and the tibia on the ventral side of the leg is the patella or knee cap.

Cattle, sheep, goats, and pigs have the same leg bone structure as horses, but the proximal, middle, and distal phalanx are split into two giving them a **cloven** or divided toe. The last two phalanxes are enclosed in the hoof (Figure 5.6).

The axial skeleton consists of the skull, vertebral column, and thoracic cage (Figure 5.7). The skull has many bones but the three of concern for us are the **cranium** which contains and protects the brain, the **maxilla** and **mandible** make up the jaws and hold the teeth. Figure 5.8 demonstrates where the horns grow from the head of a goat.

The vertebral column is made up of individual vertebrae. They protect the spinal column and act as an

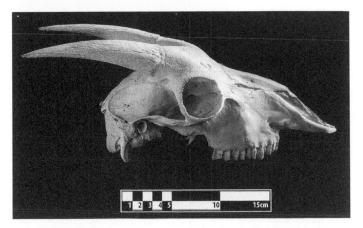

FIGURE 5.8 Goat's head. Source: Wikimedia Commons. Used under CC BY-SA 4.0, https://commons.wikimedia.org/wiki/File:Goat_skull_(MAV_FMVZ_USP).jpg.

anchor point for the skull, thoracic cage, and the appendicular skeleton. The vertebral column is divided into five sections (Figure 5.7).

The cervical vertebrae make up the neck and have seven individual bones including the atlas which connects to the skull and the axis which connects to the atlas cranially and the third cervical vertebrae caudally (Figure 5.7). There are 13 thoracic vertebrae that span the length of the thoracic cage. Seven lumbar vertebrae connect to the thoracic vertebrae at the thoracic–lumbar junction. This is often referred to as the TLJ when veterinarians are asking for radiographs of that area. The next three vertebrae are fused together and make up the sacral vertebrae or the sacrum. The last section is the coccygeal vertebrae; the number of these can vary depending on whether the animal has a natural or surgical dock of the tail.

The thoracic cage is made up of 13 pairs of ribs; one attaches to each side of the thoracic vertebrae. Ribs 1–12 are held in place by the sternum, the last rib is called a "floating" rib and only attaches at the vertebra. The caudal end of the sternum is called the xiphoid process. It is usually palpable and is a landmark for various procedures in surgery and radiography.

Diseases that can affect the skeletal system include **arthritis,** an inflammation of the joints which involves swelling and pain. **Osteoarthritis** is the degeneration of joint cartilage causing pain, stiffness, and sometimes the growth of bone spurs. Vertebral disk disease can happen at any time but like arthritis is often associated with age deterioration. **Cancer** of the bone, or osteosarcoma, is seen frequently in older, large breed dogs. Bones can have **congenital** abnormalities, which include hip and elbow **dysplasia**, which are poorly formed hips and elbows. A young animal may experience **panosteitis**, which is inflammation of the bones. **Osteochondritis** and **osteochondritis dissecans** (OCD) are developmental diseases that occurs in large and giant breed puppies if not fed properly.

Muscular System

Muscles are made up of bundles of fibers that are covered with a thin sheet of fibrous material called **fascia**. The physiology of muscles is that they contract and relax from nerve impulses. This contraction and relaxation mechanism provides locomotion of the body itself. Muscles also work in other body functions; moving blood, food, air, and waste products through the body. There are three types of muscles to assist in making these functions happen.

Skeletal muscles are those attached to bones. They are voluntary muscles which means an animal has to "command" the muscle to contract and relax via the central nervous system. Skeletal muscles contract to lift,

extend, contract, or retract to move a body part, and then relax so the body part can return to "normal." Think about walking. It may not seem like a voluntary movement, you just walk, right? Wrong, even if you are not aware of it, when your leg starts the movement of a step you have either consciously or subconsciously commanded it to do so. Skeletal muscles are attached to bones by **tendons**.

Smooth muscles are involuntary muscles that contract and rest without conscious thought. This is stimulated by the autonomic nervous system. Smooth muscle lines organs such as the gastrointestinal tract, to move food or waste through the digestive system. Muscles in the uterus contract to expel a baby. There are muscles in the urethra and bladder for the expulsion of urine. Blood vessels are lined with muscles to help move the blood through them and bronchi have muscles to pull air in and push it out of the lungs with the help of the diaphragm.

Cardiac muscle is also involuntary and is autorhythmic, which means it generates its own action potential. Once the muscle contraction starts it moves through the organ without stopping. It is fueled by blood vessels that bring in oxygen and nutrients and carry away waste products generated by the contraction and relaxation of the muscle tissue. We will spend more time on the cardiac muscle when we discuss the cardiovascular system.

Veterinary assistants need to know the names and locations of the skeletal muscles. These are the muscles that are used for locomotion and some of these are used for injections because of their size. It is interesting to note that the names of muscles on four-legged and two-legged animals are very similar, and that includes people! The size and length may be a bit different based upon how the animal developed. Figure 5.9 shows a dog and Figure 5.10 a horse with the underlying muscles outlined.

Muscles can be affected by disease and trauma. **Myopathy** is a general term for muscle disease. **Polymyositis** is an inflammation of many muscles. **Degenerative myopathy** causes weakness in the affected muscles. More common occurrences of muscle trauma are strains where the muscle is overstretched. Sprains occur when the ligament is overstretched. Sometime these ligaments tear because a leg twists or bends wrongly. A common torn ligament seen in animals is the anterior cruciate ligament. **Tendonitis** is when the tendons have become inflamed from repetitive overuse.

Cardiovascular System

Analogy:

Think of the cardiovascular system as a highway system that serves a major city. The "heart" of any town is the downtown area, it is connected to the suburbs by high speed roads called "arteries" and slower, smaller "veins" called streets. Arteries are

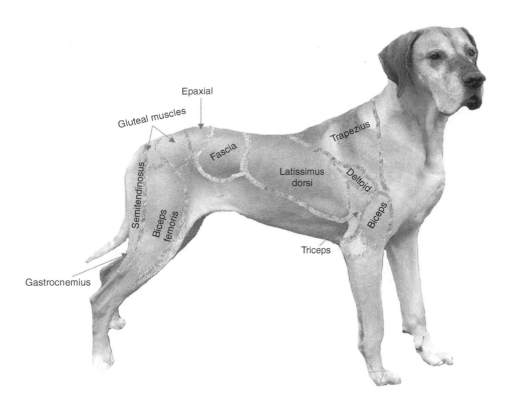

FIGURE 5.9 Muscles of a dog. Adapted from Wikimedia Commons.

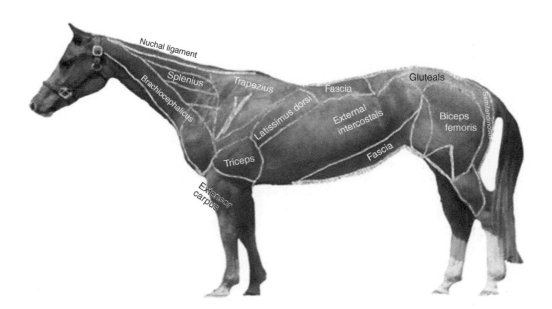

FIGURE 5.10 Muscles of a horse. Adapted from Wikimedia Commons.

built to handle many cars, have few stop signs, and are the main means of transporting vital supplies downtown. The veins handle lighter traffic and have multiple stop signs throughout the city, but eventually you can make your way back downtown. These streets and roadways are connected by ramps (capillaries) that allow one car to enter or exit at a time.

The heart is a hollow, four-chambered muscular organ that is divided into right and left sides (Figure 5.11).

From the exterior you can see the two upper chambers called the **atria** (singular, atrium), and lower chambers called **ventricles**. There are four major vessels attached to the chambers of the heart. Two of them bring blood to the heart: the superior vena cava and the pulmonary veins. Two allow blood to leave the heart: the aorta and pulmonary artery.

All four chambers have valves that control the direction of the blood flow as the heart beats (Figure 5.12).

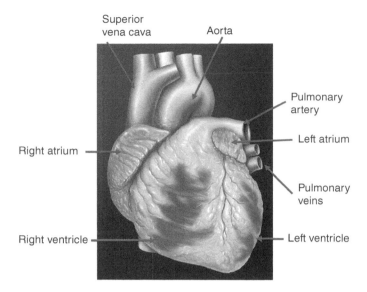

FIGURE 5.11 Heart – exterior structures. Source: Wikimedia Commons. Used under CC BY 2.5, https://commons.wikimedia.org/wiki/File:Heart_anterior_exterior_view.jpg.

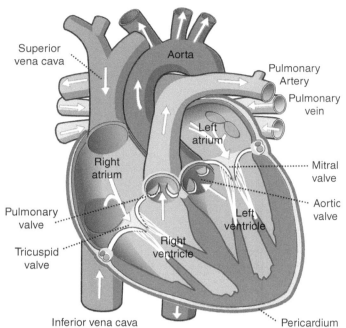

FIGURE 5.12 Heart – interior and path of blood through the heart. Source: Wikimedia Commons. Used under CC BY-SA 3.0, https://en.wikipedia.org/wiki/Heart#/media/File:Diagram_of_the_human_heart_(cropped).svg.

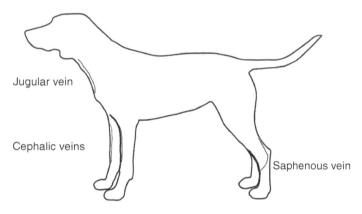

FIGURE 5.13 Vein schematic: dog.

The right side of the heart receives the blood from the superior vena cava, which brings deoxygenated blood from the body into the right atrium. It enters the right ventricle through the **tricuspid valve**. The right ventricle pushes the deoxygenated blood into the **pulmonary artery** via the **pulmonary valve** to the lungs. The lungs oxygenate the blood and it is circulated back to the heart via the **pulmonary veins**, which dump into the left atrium. The oxygenated blood leaves the left atrium through the **mitral valve** to the left ventricle. The left ventricle pushes the oxygenated blood through the **aortic valve** into the **aorta** which branches off at the aortic arch to feed the top and lower parts of the body. The left ventricle is larger than the right because it must push the blood all the way through the body.

The aorta branches into many **arteries** to take blood and nutrients to the tissues and organs of the body. It also picks up waste produced by the tissues. In order to get to all the tissues, the arteries need to branch into even smaller vessels called **arterioles**. These arterioles branch yet again into **capillaries**. Capillaries are so small that only one blood cell at a time can pass through their walls. The capillaries drain into **venules**, which are small veins. **Veins** carry deoxygenated blood and other materials into larger veins that flow into the largest vein called the **vena cava**. The vena cava carries the blood back to the heart.

Arteries tend to be thick walled to handle the pressure of the blood being pushed through them by the heart. **Systolic** blood pressure is a measurement of the blood being pushed through the arteries. **Diastolic** blood pressure is the amount of pressure that remains in the arteries after the "wave" has passed.

Veins are thinner and have small valves to keep blood from pooling. Veins are used to draw blood from because the pressure is lower in them than in the arteries. They contain the same blood cells, nutrients, minerals, and salts as arteries. Sometimes the arteries and/or veins become blocked. A blockage in the circulation to the rear part of the animal is known as a **saddle thrombus**. This may cause acute paralysis of the hind limbs, pads on feet may be blue from deoxygenation and the animal may cry out in pain.

When the veterinarian listens to the heart, **auscultates**, with a stethoscope it is to check the rhythm of the heart. The characteristic "lub-dub" is made by the sounds of the valves closing as the heart contracts. The "lub" is the mitral and tricuspid valves closing and is the start of systole and the "dub" is the closing of the aortic and pulmonary valves at the end of systole. **Heart murmurs**

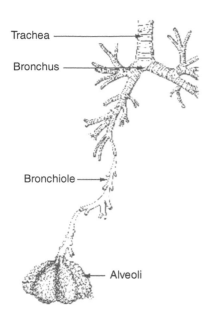

Trachea

Bronchus

Bronchiole

Alveoli

FIGURE 5.14 Lung anatomy. Source: https://en.wikipedia.org/wiki/Respiratory_tract#/media/File:Illu_quiz_lung05.jpg. Public Domain.

are also detected upon auscultation; these are caused by imperfections or damaged valves in the heart. An ultrasound of the heart can show the valves opening and closing, a radiograph may be taken to check for enlargement of the heart, and an **electrocardiogram (ECG)** may be used to study the electrical impulses of the heart.

The blood vessels commonly used for **venipuncture** are the cephalic veins, jugular and saphenous on dogs and femoral on cats (Figure 5.13). Jugular veins are used when blood collection is needed for tests. The other veins are usually saved for IV catheterization as they are smaller and tend to collapse during blood draws. On livestock, blood draws and IV injections or catheterizations are almost always done on the jugular vein.

Disease, congenital defects, and age can cause the heart not to pump as well. Some common diseases are **chronic heart failure (CHF)** which is often an age-related disease; however, it can occur if the blood vessels that feed the heart are blocked, or it can be caused by cardiomyopathy. **Dilated cardiomyopathy** occurs when the heart muscles stretch out reducing the strength of the beat. **Hypertrophic cardiomyopathy** occurs when the heart walls enlarge making the chambers smaller so less blood is pumped. Dysfunction of the heart's electrical system, which stimulates the heart to beat properly, causes **arrhythmias** (abnormal heart beats) and **atrial fibrillation** (rapid fluttering of the atria).

Respiratory System

The respiratory system is how oxygen is transferred to the blood. The start of the respiratory system is the nose and mouth. Most animals breath through their nose and occasionally through their mouth (Figure 5.14).

The area behind the mouth and nose is called the **pharynx** which splits into the trachea and epiglottis. The trachea starts with the **larynx** or voice box. The larynx has a flap called the **epiglottis** that covers the **trachea,** to prevent food from going into the trachea. The trachea is a tube with cartilaginous rings along its length to keep it open so air can move into the lungs. The lungs consist of four lobes. The trachea splits into right and left **bronchi** entering the two largest lobes to the right and left sides. Each bronchus further divides into multiple **bronchioles** throughout the lobes of the lungs. These bronchioles branch out and end at an **alveoli,** or air sacs.

Alveoli are surrounded by pulmonary venules filled with deoxygenated blood. The carbon dioxide is exchanged for oxygen in the alveoli and moves into the pulmonary arterioles. These vessels eventually meet at the pulmonary veins taking oxygenated blood into the left side of the heart for broadcasting to the rest of the body.

Diseases of the respiratory tract include **pneumonia**, which is a buildup of fluids inside the lungs. This can be the result of infection or secondary to another disease like kennel cough (caused by *Bordetella bronchiseptica*) or aspirating vomitus when the animal is unconscious or anesthetized. **Plural effusion** is a condition of fluid in the thoracic cavity surrounding the lungs. It is caused by a disruption in the normal production or removal of fluid in the thoracic cavity. This disruption could be from a tumor, overhydration, or chronic congestive heart failure for example. **Asthma** is a constricting of the bronchi and/or bronchioles. The trachea can become compromised by either congenital or mechanical collapse. This collapse can be complete where the animal turns **cyanotic** or it can be partial where the animal coughs or gasps for breath. Either symptom is an emergency and the animal should be seen as soon as possible.

The veterinarian will evaluate the lungs using a stethoscope. The sound should be clear whooshing sounds, if crackles, squeaks, wheezing, or no sound is heard he/she may ask for a radiograph to see if there is fluid inside or around the lungs.

Immune System

The following explanation of the immune system is *very* rudimentary. Immunology is a subject unto itself and a few paragraphs about it cannot cover the intricacies of this vital body function. It is a fascinating subject which is being understood more and more each year. The study of immunology has given us the means to not only fight off bacterial and viral infections, but is also now being used in the fight against cancer. The following is the immune system "in a nutshell."

The immune system is responsible for protecting the body from pathogens that cause diseases and infections. There are two systems that can respond to a pathogen found in the body. The **innate** system is often the first line of defense and is composed of white blood cells known as granulocytes; neutrophils, eosinophils, and basophils, and the white blood cell known as a monocyte. These blood cells circulate through the body and take care of bacteria, parasites, allergens, and viruses as they come upon them or are called to the location by cells in the tissues known as mast cells. These cells will destroy pathogens either by ingesting them or by releasing granules that destroy chemically.

The other response is from the **adaptive** system. The adaptive system is largely made up of white blood cells called lymphocytes. Lymphocytes are unique because they can adapt to whatever the body needs in the way of defense against a pathogen. They are the cells that produce long-term immunity to diseases. For example, one type of lymphocyte will produce a receptor to detect **antigens** that are unique to a pathogen the body has dealt with before. That lymphocyte will stimulate another type of lymphocyte to produce **antibodies** against the pathogen. These lymphocytes are very long lived and will take care of that pathogen at any time it enters the body.

Another type of lymphocyte roams throughout the body and attacks non-self cells like cancer and new pathogens. If this occurs that lymphocyte will call for reinforcements and the different types of lymphocytes will come to its aid. This lymphocyte can kill non-self cells and pathogens by releasing a chemical.

One way that innate and adaptive immune systems work together is by monocytes presenting antigens to lymphocytes. Monocytes **phagocytize** a pathogen, meaning they encircle and destroy it. In the process they take a piece of the pathogen, called an antigen, and poke it through their cell wall. They then travel to the **lymph nodes** where the lymphocytes hang out, and a specific type of lymphocyte will intercept the monocyte, take the antigen, and produce a receptor for that specific antigen. This lymphocyte will then move into the body looking for that pathogen. When it finds it, it will attach to the pathogen and destroy it, or signal that it needs help. More lymphocytes will converge on the area. Some will replicate and produce more lymphocytes with that receptor to kill more of the pathogen and others will produce lymphocytes that can produce antibodies for future use. These are the lymphocytes used to produce immunity against diseases by **vaccinations**. A small amount of antigen for a specific disease is introduced to the body. The lymphocytes that produce antibodies become involved in the destruction of the "pathogen."

Lymphocytes are produced in the bone marrow like the other blood cells; however, they are released early in their maturation which allows them to change or to replicate themselves. They circulate in the bloodstream and tissues, but most are sequestered in the lymph nodes. This allows large numbers to be deployed when needed. There are thousands of lymph nodes throughout the

body, with a few that are superficial enough to be felt if enlarged. The **popliteal** lymph node is found caudal to the knee; the **axillary** is found in the armpit; the **inguinal** is found in the groin; and the **submandibular** is found beneath the jaw.

Diseases of the lymph system include **lymphoma**, a type of cancer that is systemic and fatal. A biopsy of a swollen lymph node can determine if it is cancer or some other **lymphadenopathy** or disease of the lymph node. Cancers of the bone marrow can affect the production of white and red blood cells, either too few or too many or cells that don't do their jobs correctly. **Autoimmune** conditions make the blood cells attack "self" or normal body cells because they don't recognize it as being part of the body.

Digestive System

The role of the digestive system is to take in food and extract the nutrients to nourish the body and then eliminate the waste or unusable remainder. In the animal kingdom, some animals have one-compartment stomachs called **monogastric**, or there are **ruminant** animals with four-compartment stomachs. Cats, dogs, pigs, horses, and most pocket pets are monogastric. Cows, sheep, goats, deer, and camelids are ruminants.

The digestive system starts with the mouth and the taking in of food or **prehension**. Every animal has some teeth; Table 5.1 shows the dental makeup and number for each animal.

The teeth are used to break the food down into smaller parts. The tongue assists with keeping it in the mouth and rolls the food around as it mixes with saliva. The chewed food is swallowed and moves down the esophagus to the stomach. In the monogastric stomach the food is exposed to stomach acids that break it down further (Figure 5.15).

Peristaltic waves move the material from the stomach into the small intestine where the nutrients are absorbed. The small intestine has three parts: the duodenum, jejunum, and ileum. Finally, the undigestible material continues to move into the colon or large intestine. The colon also has three parts: ascending, transverse, and descending colon. In the colon, water is removed and feces formed. The feces move into the sigmoid flexure and finally into the rectum. The anal **sphincters** control the passage of feces into the environment which is called **defecation** or **defecating.**

In ruminants, the chewed food goes to the **rumen** where it is exposed to bacteria to ferment the cellulose in foliage to break it down, then it goes into the **reticulum** (Figure 5.16). The remaining solids are regurgitated and chewed again, this is referred to as cud. The finer food particles move into the **omasum** for further processing. The final stop is in the **abomasum** or true stomach where digestive **enzymes** breaks the food into its

TABLE 5.1

Dental Formulas per Animal

Animal Total #	Incisors (I)[a]	Canines (C)	Premolars (P)	Molars (M)	
Dogs – 42	2	1	3	2	× 2
	2	1	4	3	
Cats – 30	2	1	3	1	× 2
	2	1	2	1	
Rabbits – 28	1[b]	0	3	3	× 2
	1	0	2	3	
Horses – 40 (42)	3	1	3	3 (4)	× 2
	3	1	3	4	
Cattle – 32	0	0	3	3	× 2
	4	0	3	3	

[a] The top number indicates the number of teeth in the top jaw, on one side, bottom number indicates the number of teeth in the lower jaw, on one side. The × 2 indicates the two sides of the mouth.

[b] One "peg" tooth sits behind the incisors of the upper jaw.

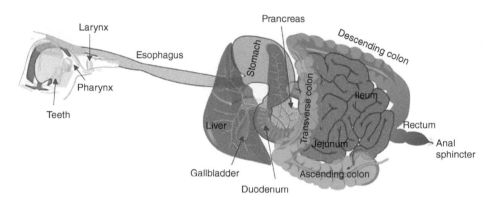

FIGURE 5.15 Monogastric digestive tract. Source: https://commons.wikimedia.org/wiki/File:Digestive_system_without_labels.svg. Public Domain.

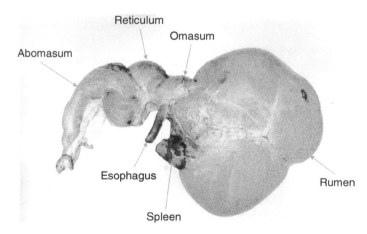

FIGURE 5.16 Ruminant stomach. Source: Wikimedia Commons. Used under CC BY-SA 4.0, https://commons.wikimedia.org/wiki/File:Ruminant_Stomach.jpg.

nutrients and then it follows the same path as described for monogastric animals.

There are three more organs that assist with digestion: the **liver, gallbladder,** and **pancreas** (Figure 5.17).

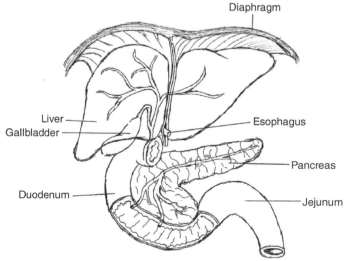

FIGURE 5.17 Liver, gallbladder, and pancreas. Source: Wikimedia Commons. Used under CC BY-SA 4.0, https://commons.wikimedia.org/wiki/File:Liver_Gallbladder_SI.jpg.

The liver's main function is to filter toxins from the blood, metabolize drugs, and produce bile which is stored in the gallbladder. The bile is used in the digestion of fats. The pancreas produces digestive enzymes which are excreted into the duodenum. It also secrets insulin which breaks down sugars.

Diseases that affect the gastrointestinal system often cause vomiting and/or diarrhea. There are many reasons for vomiting and diarrhea including stress, dietary indiscretion, bacterial toxins, or foreign bodies blocking part or all the digestive tract. **Gastric dilation volvulus (GDV),** also known as bloat, is the dilation or expansion and twisting of the stomach. The stomach fills with gas or too much food which causes it to expand and then twist, or flip over. This twisting blocks the passage of food cuts off the blood supply causing **necrosis** and, if not caught and treated early, death. **Gastritis** means an inflammation of the stomach and is usually brought on by eating inappropriate food. **Ileus** is the paralysis or cessation of normal intestinal movement. **Irritable bowel disease (IBD)** is a condition where the intestines are overly sensitive to food and/or stress. **Pancreatitis** is inflammation of pancreas brought on by ingesting rich or highly salty food like ham. **Parasites** can cause diarrhea and vomiting if the adult worm load is high. **Parvovirus** will also cause extremely watery and bloody diarrhea.

Fecal samples are tested for parasites in order to find the causative agent. Radiographs of the abdomen may be ordered to check for a blockage. This will often involve giving the animal a contrast medium to make items visible. Endoscopy can also be utilized to directly visualize the interior of the gastrointestinal tract. Ultrasound can be used to indirectly visualize structures in the abdominal cavity such as the liver and gallbladder.

Urinary System

The job of the urinary system is to filter the blood of waste products and maintain the balance of water in the blood. The main organs are two **kidneys**, one on each side of the spinal column on the cranial end of the abdominal cavity (Figure 5.18). The kidney is made up of millions of **nephrons** which filter the blood as it flows through the kidney producing urine. Urine flows out of the kidney through a tube called a **ureter** which ends at the **bladder**. The bladder is a hollow organ that can expand to accommodate the urine. The bladder has a sphincter that controls when it releases the urine to the outside through the **urethra**. This is called **urinating** or **micturition.**

Diseases that effect the kidney are seen more often as the animal ages. **Chronic renal failure** is when the kidney can no longer filter properly or regulate the amount of fluids in the blood. **Acute renal failure** is a sudden onset

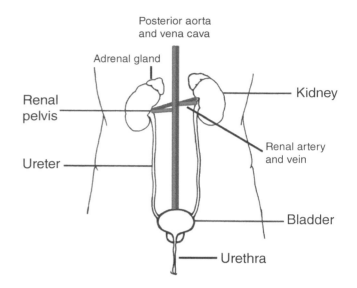

FIGURE 5.18 Urinary system. Source: Wikimedia Commons. Used under CC BY-SA 3.0, https://commons.wikimedia.org/wiki/File:Bladder_stone_ruler.jpg.

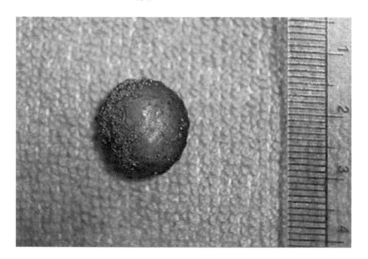

FIGURE 5.19 Urolith.

from toxic overload or poisoning. The bladder can also become diseased. **Incontinence** is the failure to hold urine. This can be caused by hormonal changes, often seen in older unspayed female dogs, structure, or muscle weakness. **Feline lower urinary tract disease (FLUTD)** symptoms include frequent trips to the litter box with or without urine being expelled, straining to urinate, or bloody urine. It can be caused by several factors: blockage of the urethra with crystals, bacterial infections, anatomic defects, tumors, or **idiopathic** cystitis. FLUTD can lead to blockage of the urethra and is considered a medical emergency. The urine continues to be produced by the kidney and can eventually backup into the kidney causing the animal to become toxic because the kidneys cannot work properly. **Urinary tract infections (UTIs)** are usually caused by a bacterial infection and can happen to both cats and dogs. **Uroliths** or bladder stones can form and cause bloody urine, straining to urinate,

Cross-section of testicle

Bull testicle

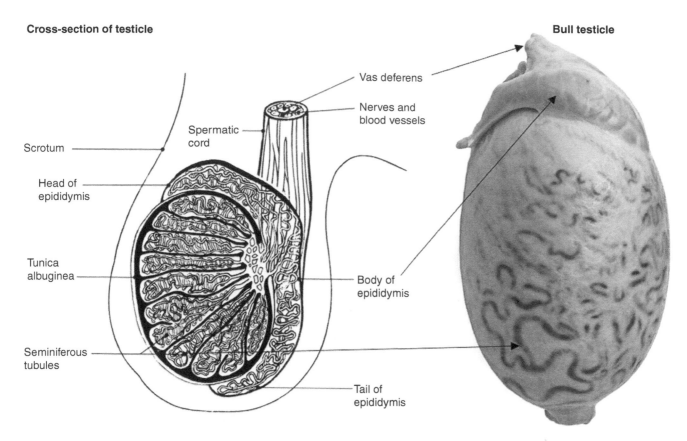

Vas deferens

Nerves and blood vessels

Spermatic cord

Scrotum

Head of epididymis

Tunica albuginea

Body of epididymis

Seminiferous tubules

Tail of epididymis

FIGURE 5.20 Cross-section and intact bull testicle. Adapted from Wikimedia Commons.

frequent urination, and pain upon urination (Figure 5.19).

The veterinarian will request a **urinalysis** to check for a UTI. Radiographs with a contrast agent may be ordered to check for bladder stones. An ultrasound is used to visualize the kidney and bladder. Blood samples may be taken, and blood chemistries performed to check for kidney function.

Reproductive System

The reproductive systems of males and females combine to create life and sustain the species. The male reproductive system is consistent across the different species. The male reproductive tract consists of the **testes**, which contain the seminiferous vesicles, epididymis, vas deferens, **urethra**, **prostate gland,** and **penis**.

Sperm is produced in the seminiferous vesicles (Figure 5.20). The epididymis is where sperm is stored. When the male is aroused the sperm leaves the epididymis through the vas deferens, fluid from the seminiferous vesicles and prostate gland are combined with the sperm as it travels into the urethra and out, inseminating the female.

The female reproductive tract varies depending on the number of offspring the species produces. The

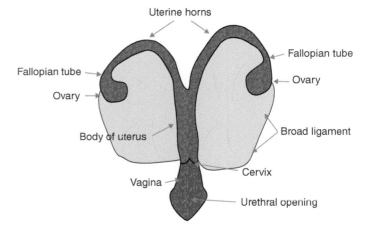

Uterine horns

Fallopian tube

Fallopian tube

Ovary

Ovary

Body of uterus

Broad ligament

Cervix

Vagina

Urethral opening

FIGURE 5.21 Female reproductive tract.

uterine horns are longer to accommodate multiple fetuses (Figure 5.21). However, the process of egg fertilization is the same in all species. Eggs are produced in the **ovaries**, hormones released by the pituitary gland stimulates the release of eggs into the fallopian tubes. This is called **ovulation**. Fertilization of the egg occurs in the fallopian tubes, and the fertilized ovum moves and implants in the uterus. An **embryo** begins to grow into a **fetus**. The life support system for the fetus is the placenta. It supplies nutrients, oxygen, and blood

TABLE 5.2		
Number of Offspring and Gestation Periods of Animals		
Animal	Offspring (no.)	Gestation period
Dog	Small 1–4 Medium 4–6 Large 8–12	58–68 days 63 average
Cat	3–5 average 8+ often	63–69 days
Horse	1 rarely 2	340 days
Cow	1 rarely 2	279–287 days 283 average
Sheep	1, often 2	150 days
Goat	1, 2, or 3 are common	145–154 days 150 average
Pig	8–12 average	114 days
Rabbit	1–14 6 average	29–35 days 30 average
Ferret	1–6	35–45 days
Guinea pig	1–8 2–4 average	59–73 days 63 average
Hamster	6–12 average	16 days
Rat	10–12 average	21–23 days

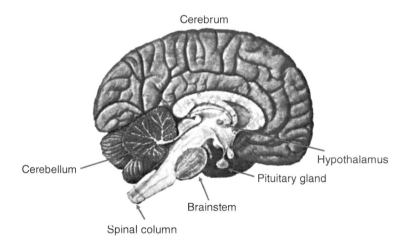

FIGURE 5.22 Brain. Adapted from Wikimedia Commons.

and carries away waste material. The amount of time it takes for a fetus to mature enough to sustain life independently of its mother is called the **gestation period.** Gestation periods vary widely between species. See Table 5.2 for the gestation periods and number of offspring for companion animals, pocket pets, and livestock.

Parturition, or giving birth, occurs at full term and begins with muscular contraction of the uterus. If the species delivers more than one baby a short rest between deliveries is normal. **Dystocia** is when an animal has trouble and cannot deliver on its own or there is an extended period between births with straining but no results. Dystocia is an emergency and the animal must be

seen immediately. Often dystocia leads to a **cesarean section** or surgical removal of the fetus. If a cesarean section or c-section is required a full team will be assembled to take care of the infants as they are removed. They are often groggy from the anesthetic the mother is under and need to be stimulated to breathe. A brisk rubbing of the body and a little upside-down hold to drain fluids is sometimes necessary.

Nervous System

If the circulatory system is a major city's highway, think of the nervous system as the phone and internet network.

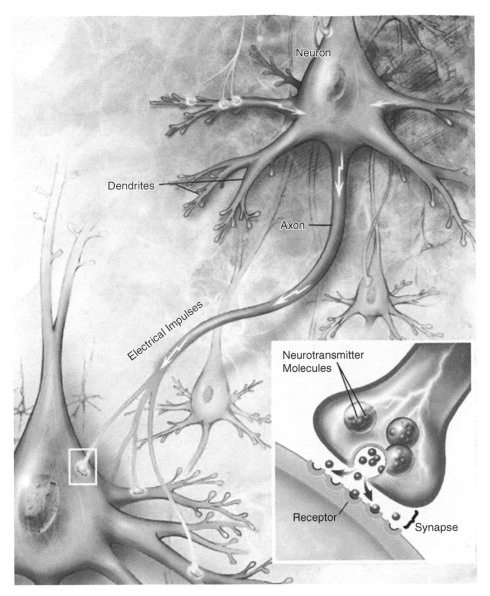

FIGURE 5.23 Neurons and synapses. Source: https://commons.wikimedia.org/wiki/File:Chemical_synapse_schema_cropped.jpg. Public Domain.

The **central nervous system (CNS)** is made up of the brain and spinal column (Figure 5.22).

The brain is made up of the cerebrum, cerebellum, and the brainstem. The cerebrum, the largest portion of the brain, is responsible for the higher functions which include the senses, movement, and learning. The cerebellum is smaller and coordinates muscle movement, posture, and balance. The brainstem is the relay center connecting the other two parts to the spinal cord. It is responsible for the body functions of heart rate, breathing, digestion, body temperature regulation, wake–sleep cycles, swallowing, coughing, vomiting, and so on. Deep underneath the cerebrum is the hypothalamus which is home to part of the nervous system called the **autonomous nervous system (ANS)** which responds in times of stress. The ANS has two systems of its own. Most of the time the **parasympathetic nervous system** is

running the animal's body keeping everything going at a normal pace. Normal heart beat and breathing, muscles moving when told, digestion working properly, and so on. However, life isn't always normal!

Think of a mouse minding its own business searching for food. When suddenly a big cat pounces. Without thinking, the mouse jumps away, running at full speed, trying to get away. If caught or cornered, it would fight by biting and screeching at the cat.

The mouse has demonstrated the **sympathetic nervous system** taking over as it responds to the stress of almost being eaten. This is called the fight or flight response. The heart is stimulated to beat faster, breathing speeds up, and the body gears up for a flight or fight in a blink, no need for thought or decision. If the mouse gets away it would probably find a safe spot to calm down, returning to normal when operations of the body are switched back to the parasympathetic nervous system.

How does all these things happen? How do muscle move? What prompts a swallow? The CNS is made up of millions of neurons (Figure 5.23). The neurons of the spinal cord branch off through the body and this is referred to as the **peripheral nervous system**. The process of nerves bringing or sending signals to and from an area of the body is called **enervation**. Enervation can come from the CNS or it can come from the peripheral nerves back to the CNS. Impulses sent along the neurons are carried by chemical messengers called **neurotransmitters**. Neurotransmitters are serotonin, dopamine, acetylcholine, norepinephrine, gamma-aminobutyric acid, and glutamate. Each has a different job; for example, serotonin is responsible for sleep, mood, appetite, temperature regulation, sensory perception, and pain suppression. The neurotransmitter travels along the axon (branch) of a neuron, when it reaches the end of the axon it jumps a space or **synapse** between it and the next neuron and the impulse continues along.

Disease, trauma, and drugs affect the CNS. When the nerves are not functioning properly a variety of symptoms appear. **Ataxia** is uncoordinated movement; the front legs cross and the animal staggers. **Conscious proprioception** is when the animal doesn't know where its feet are, almost like it doesn't have feet. Vertebral disks can push on the spinal column leading to ataxia, pain, and paralysis. **Seizures** or convulsions are a continuous random firing of nerves and indicates a nervous system disorder. Diseases such as **distemper** can cause seizures, tremors, and limb weakness from its effects on nerves. **Vestibular** disease is caused by an inner ear infection or a tumor in the brain. Symptoms include head tilt, circling, and **nystagmus**, a rapid flicking motion of the eyes. The veterinarian will carry out proprioception tests, examine the eyes, and order radiographs or an MRI to confirm or rule out tumors.

Endocrine System

The body is controlled by several hormones that are produced by glands and make up the endocrine system. The master gland is the **pituitary** which it is located beneath the brain (Figure 5.22). It controls the actions of the other glands located throughout the body. One of which is the **thyroid** gland located on the dorsal side of the neck. Its main function is metabolism which is the chemical processes required to sustain life. Calcium regulation is controlled by the **parathyroid** located on the thyroid gland. The **adrenal glands** found on top of the kidneys have two roles (Figure 5.18). One is to control inflammation and body functions. The other is to produce the adrenaline hormone which is used in times of stress to facilitate the flight or fight response. The **pancreas** is a gland that produces insulin to maintain blood sugar levels. Not enough insulin leads to **diabetes mellitus**. The **gonads** are sex glands that produce the hormones a male and female need to be able to reproduce.

Diseases of the glands cause **hypothyroidism** or **hyperthyroidism**, too little or too much thyroid hormone. Too much adrenal hormone or **hyperadrenocorticism** leads to Cushing's disease. Too little adrenal hormone or **hypoadrenocorticism** leads to Addison's disease.

Blood tests can determine which hormone is missing, low, or elevated and the veterinarian is usually able to treat the animal with medication to control the disease process. However, that animal may be on a medication for life.

Integumentary System

The integument is the skin and its primary role is protection. The skin is made up of three layers (Figure 5.24). The first layer is the **epidermis**, which is made up of 4–5 layers of epithelial cells, called keratinocytes. They produce keratin, a protein that gives hair, nails, and skin their hardness and waterproof qualities. The topmost layer of keratocytes are dead and slough away being replaced by cells from the deeper layers. The second layer of skin is called the **dermis**. The "living layer" contains blood and lymph vessels, hair follicles, sweat glands (if the animal has sweat glands), nerves, and other structures. It is composed of two layers of interconnected elastin and collagenous fibers providing elasticity to the skin. The deepest layer is the **hypodermis**, more commonly referred to as

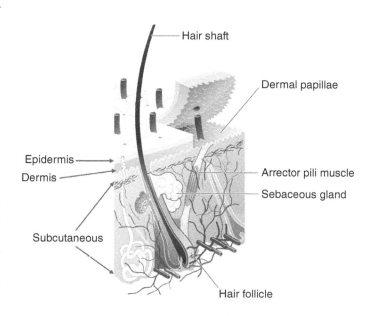

FIGURE 5.24 Layers of the skin. Source: Wikimedia Commons. Used under CC BY-SA 3.0, https://commons.m.wikimedia.org/wiki/File:Ctenocephalides canis.jpg#mw-jump-to-license.

the **subcutaneous** layer. It connects to the underlying fascia of muscles and bones. It consists of well-vascularized, loose **areolar connective tissue** and **adipose** tissue (fat). This fat provides a cushion and insulation.

Hair, horns, claws, and hooves are accessory structures in the integumentary system which are made of keratin and other proteins. Hair is made of protein filaments that grow from follicles found in the dermis. Horn grows from a core of live bone. Dehorning animals requires the removal of the horn "bud" to keep the horn from growing back. Claws, hooves, and spurs also grow from a "bed" and if these are damaged or removed (declawing) they do not grow back, or they grow back deformed.

Diseases that affect skin are infections, allergens, parasites, and trauma. Animals with infections may present with small bumps of pus called **pustules**. They can also present with hot, red, weeping skin. These are often called **hot spots**. Animals with allergens present with hives, raised red itchy areas. Parasites of the skin, like mite infestations, can look like hives. Some parasites are visible to the naked eye, like ticks, fleas, and lice, and are known as **ectoparasites**. **Ringworm** is a fungus that presents as round red raised areas that may be itchy.

Veterinarians carry out several tests to determine what is wrong with the skin. Skin scrapings to check for mites involves scraping the skin with a scalpel blade and looking at it under the microscope. To test for fungus, hairs on the edge of the infected area are collected and added to a growth medium or looked at under the microscope. If it turns out to be an allergen, medication to reduce the inflammation is given. Alternatively, they may run tests to see what is causing the allergic reaction. Areas infected by bacteria may be cultured.

Chapter Reflection

Think about the different body systems and write one sentence (or more) about what you learned about each system that surprised you or something you didn't know about until now.

Suggested Reading

Biology Dictionary. 2019. Muscle tissue. https://biologydictionary.net/muscle-tissue/ (accessed July 12, 2019).

Chhabra T. 2018. Types of connective tissue. Sciencing. https://sciencing.com/7-types-connective-tissue-8768445.html (accessed July 12, 2019).

Hines T. 2018. Anatomy of the brain. Mayfield Brain and Spine. https://mayfieldclinic.com/pe-anatbrain.htm (accessed July 12, 2019).

McDougal W. Connective tissue: types, functions and disorders. Study.com. https://study.com/academy/lesson/connective-tissue-types-functions-disorders.html (accessed July 12, 2019).

Rice University. Anatomy and Physiology: Chapter 5 Layers of the skin. BCOpenTextbooks.https://opentextbc.ca/anatomyandphysiology/chapter/5-1-layers-of-the-skin/ (accessed July 12, 2019).

Rutgers. Nervous tissue. https://bio.rutgers.edu/~gb102/lab_6/605am-nervous.html (accessed July 12, 2019).

Shah SM. 2018. Sperm release pathway. Medline Plus. https://medlineplus.gov/ency/anatomyvideos/000121.htm (accessed July 12, 2019).

Socratic. 2016. Where are sperm created? Where are they stored? https://socratic.org/questions/where-are-sperm-created-where-are-they-stored (accessed July 12, 2019).

University of Washington. 2001. The O' cells. https://depts.washington.edu/bonebio/bonAbout/bonecells.html (accessed July 12, 2019).

Introduction to Animals

Scientific Classification of Animals

The Linnaean System of Classifications is a **cladistics** system, based on evolutionary differences in the genomes. Originally, it classified animals by the way they moved. Refinements were made with the discovery of more species and recognition of evolutionary classifications. Developments in sequencing **deoxyribonucleic acid (DNA)** has led to further refinement of this system.

Scientific classification groups life forms into increasingly smaller groups based on increasingly similar characteristics. Classification and scientific names were developed to make it easier to describe and provide specific information about an animal. All living things are divided into six kingdoms: animals, plants, fungi, protozoa, archaea, and bacteria. (Viruses and prions cause disease but they do not meet the criteria to be considered living.) Each kingdom is further divided until each organism is classified by genus, then species, and finally by breed or variety. The classifications groupings are as follows:

Kingdom

  Phylum
    Class
      Order
        Family
          Genus
            Species
              Breed or variety

In veterinary medicine you may see the scientific name of animals being used. This includes the genus

Tasks for the Veterinary Assistant, Fourth Edition. Teresa F. Sonsthagen.
© 2020 John Wiley & Sons, Inc. Published 2020 by John Wiley & Sons, Inc.
Companion website: www.wiley.com/go/sonsthagen/tasks

TIP BOX 6.1

A mnemonic for remembering the Linnaean System of Classification:

Kings **P**laying **C**ards **O**n **F**ine **G**old **S**eats
Kingdom, **P**hylum, **C**lass, **O**rder, **F**amily, **G**enus, **S**pecies

and species and is usually written in italics. For example, the domestic dog's scientific name is *Canis* (genus) *familiaris* (species). Note the genus is always capitalized, and the species follows starting with a small letter. Table 6.1 shows the genus and species names of the companion animals and livestock commonly seen in veterinary practice. Also included in the table is the signalment term used under species in a medical record. The signalment term is not italicized nor does it always have to be capitalized.

In addition to the signalment term for genus and species there is a term for each male, female, and offspring of the species. To further clarify an animal's identification, specific terms are used for neutered or castrated animals. Table 6.2 shows a list of terms for males, females (altered and unaltered), and offspring.

Within each genus of animal there are several species as developed by nature based upon environmental circumstances. For example, let us compare an Arctic fox with a red fox (Figure 6.1). Both are in the order *Carnivora*, family *Canidae*, both are the same genus but are different species. The Arctic fox is *Vulpes lagopus* and the red fox is *Vulpes vulpes*. Both look like foxes, both act like foxes, but they are uniquely different. The Arctic fox has a gray to black coat in the summer and a white coat in the winter. The red fox stays red all year long. The Arctic

fox has a denser hair coat than the red fox because of the environment in which it lives. There are many varieties of fox around the world and each has its own species, whereas a dog is *Canis famililiaris* whether it is a Great Dane or a Chihuahua. This is because all dogs came from one genotype but were bred selectively by humans for various desirable traits. By selecting certain genetic traits or mutations based on **phenotype** or external characteristics (coat length, color and texture, length of legs, shape of head, ears, and tail), humans also selected for behavior or an innate ability to perform a job and so developed hundreds of breeds of dogs. Dog still exists within its genus but looks and behaves in a myriad of ways. The following are some examples of how breeds were developed using phenotypes, function, and behaviors.

Phenotypes

Specific coat pattern – Angora rabbits (long hair) over New Zealand Whites (short hair)
Coat colors – Appaloosa (spotted coat) over a chestnut horse (solid colored coat)
Looks – English Bulldog (brachiocephalic face) over a Greyhound (**dolichocephalic** face)
Function – Clydesdale draft horse over a thoroughbred race horse
Behaviors – Working dogs (German Shepherds) over non-sporting dogs (Poodles)

All these characteristics and behaviors can be brought about by the manipulation of genetic traits.

TABLE 6.1

Genus Species and Signalment Term of Companion Animals and Livestock

Animal	Genus	Species	Common term
Dog	*Canis*	*familiaris*	Canine
Cat	*Felis*	*domesticus*	Feline
Rabbit	*Oryctolagus*	*cuniculus*	Lagomorph
Ferret	*Mustela*	*putorius furo*	Ferret
Guinea Pig	*Cavia*	*porcellus*	Cavi
Hamster	*Mesocricetus*	*auratus*	Hamster
Gerbil	*Meriones*	*unguiculatus*	Gerbil
Mouse	*Mus*	*musculus*	Mucadae
Rat	*Rattus*	*norvegicus domestica*	Rattus
Horse	*Equus*	*caballus*	Equine
Cattle	*Bos*	*taurus*	Bovine
Sheep	*Ovis*	*aries*	Ovine
Goat	*Capra*	*aegagrus hircus*	Laprine
Pig	*Sus*	*scrofa domesticus*	Porcine
Bird	Many names		Avian

TABLE 6.2

Signalment Terms for Males, Females, and Offspring

Animal	Male	Female	Altered	Offspring
Dog	Dog	Bitch	–	Pup, puppy
Cat	Tom	Queen	–	Kitten, kitty
Rabbit	Buck	Doe		Kits
Ferret	Hob	Jill	Female – sprite Male – gib	Kits
Guinea pig	Boar	Sow	–	Pup
Hamster	Buck	Doe	–	Pup
Gerbil	Buck	Doe	–	Pup
Mouse	Buck	Doe	–	Pup, pinkie
Rat	Buck	Doe	–	Pup, pinkie, kitten
Horse	Stallion, stud	Mare, dam	Male – gelding	Foal Male – colt Female – filly Up to 2 years
Donkey	Jack	Jenny	Male – gelding	Same as adults
Mule	John	Molly	Male – gelding	Mule colt Mule filly
Cattle	Bull	Cow Heifer – before first calf	Male – steer	Calf
Sheep	Buck, ram	Ewe	Male – wether	Lamb
Goat	Ram, billy	Doe, nanny	Male – wether	Kid
Pig	Boar	Sow Gilt – before first litter	Male – barrow	Piglet
Chicken	Rooster, cock	Hen Pullet – >1 year of age	Male – capon	Chicks
Turkey	Tom	Hen	–	Poult
Duck	Drake	Duck, hen	–	Ducklings
Goose	Gander	Goose, hen	–	Gosling
Llama/alpaca	Sire	Dame	Male – gelding	Cria

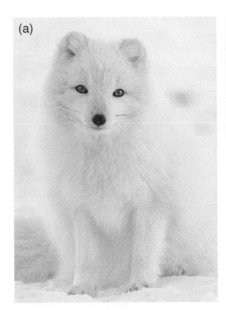
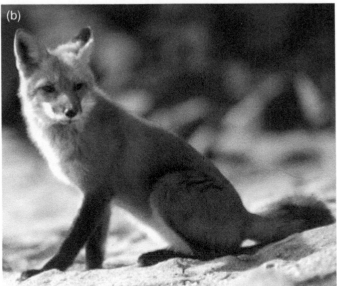

FIGURE 6.1 (a) Arctic fox and (b) red fox. Source: https://commons.wikimedia.org/wiki/File:Iceland-1979445_(cropped_3).jpg and https://commons.wikimedia.org/wiki/File:Vulpes_vulpes_sitting.jpg. Public domain.

Reflection

Now that you know every animal has a scientific name, look up what humans are called, then think about how the name for our species describes us.

Introduction to Genetics

Examples of genetic traits are specific hair coat length or color, different length leg or back, or an ability to produce more milk. Each of these traits is determined by a specific site on a gene called an **allele**. Genes are the genetic code made up of DNA that is contained within every cell in the body. An allele is made up of a pair of genes, with one gene coming from each parent. The way each allele or pair of genes interact or express themselves determines an animal's characteristics. **Dominant genes** within an allele are those that are always expressed visually and can mask **recessive** genes within the allele. **Phenotype** refers to how the animal looks visually, a green colored budgerigar or a blue one will have green and blue phenotypes, respectively. **Genotype** refers to what alleles the animal carries and what alleles they can contribute to offspring. An animal has a specific dominant phenotype, but its genotype may carry alleles that are recessive (carriers or "split to" alleles). The split to or carrier recessive characteristic may be noted after a slash such as Dominant trait/recessive trait or Green/blue. Green is a naturally dominant gene in budgerigars and blue is a recessive gene. As the gene characteristics are carried in pairs (alleles) an animal can appear (phenotypically) to be one color (dominant) but carry another color (recessive) that is not expressed or seen. So, a budgerigar that appears green colored has a green allele, but it can be a "split to" or be a "carrier" of a blue allele without any visual sign.

The parents of any individual contribute one gene to their offspring, half of their allele. By only contributing half of their genetic material to their offspring they do not multiply the genetic code within their offspring. Which allele the parent contributes is statistically a 50–50 chance. So, a budgerigar that is green split to blue (G/b) could contribute a dominant green allele (G) or a recessive blue allele (b) to its offspring. This is better demonstrated using a **Punnett square** which can assist with predicting phenotype of genotype of offspring by combining the parents' alleles or genes.

Dominant alleles are designated with a capital letter, and recessive alleles are designated with a small letter. The letters are chosen based on the first letter of the dominant trait. An animal is **homozygous** when the same genes make up an allele. An animal designated as a "split to" or "carrier" of a recessive allele is termed **heterozygous**. For

TABLE 6.3

Punnett Square for Breeding Green Homozygous Cock (GG) Bred to a Green Homozygous Hen (GG)

	G female	G female
G male	GG	GG
G male	GG	GG

The offspring of this breeding will be 100% phenotypically green and genotypically homozygous for the dominant trait of green.

TABLE 6.4

Punnett Square for Breeding Blue Homozygous Cock (gg) to a Blue Homozygous Hen (gg)

	g female	g female
g male	gg	gg
g male	gg	gg

Remembering that Green is the dominant allele, the letter for a recessive blue is a small g. The homozygous recessive trait would be designated as (gg) for a blue homozygous budgerigar. The offspring from this mating would be 100% blue.

TABLE 6.5

Punnett Square for Breeding a Homozygous Blue Cock (gg) to a Homozygous Green Hen (GG)

	G female	G female
g male	Gg	Gg
g male	Gg	Gg

All of the young from this breeding will appear phenotypically green but will be heterozygous or split to blue genotypic.

example, a homozygous dominant green bird would be designated as (GG), a heterozygous green split to blue bird would be (Gg), and a homozygous blue bird would be (gg). When we utilize the Punnett square, we can determine statistically the probable phenotypic and genotypic outcome of the breeding of two animals.

The Punnett squares in Tables 6.3, 6.4, 6.5, 6.6, and 6.7 demonstrate the different combinations of alleles expressed in the offspring by breeding green and blue budgerigars together of differing dominant and recessive traits. The Punnett square is filled in across the top and down the left side by half of the allele from each parent. Traditionally, the female's allele is across the top and the male's down the side. The female's allele is filled in the square first, followed by the male's.

TABLE 6.6

Punnett Square for Breeding a Homozygous Blue Cock (gg) to a Heterozygous Green/Blue Split Hen (Gg)

	G female	g female
g male	Gg	gg
g male	Gg	gg

Because the heterozygous green budgerigar appears like a homozygous green budgerigar, mating a green bird to a blue bird will determine if the parent is homozygous (GG) or heterozygous (Gg) as in this breeding. Because green is dominant, a blue offspring can only be obtained from the breeding if the green parent is split to blue or heterozygous to the blue color.

TABLE 6.7

Punnett Square for Breeding a Heterozygous Green/Blue Cock (Gg) to a Heterozygous Green/Blue Hen (Gg)

	G female	g female
G male	GG	gG
g male	Gg	gg

Both parents are phenotypically green birds but are split to blue. The outcome of this breeding would be 25% green homozygous, 50% heterozygous green split to blue, and 25% blue homozygous.

TABLE 6.8

Punnett Square for Breeding Heterozygous Green/Blue, Homozygous Black-Wing Cock (GgBB) to a Heterozygous Green/Blue, Homozygous Gray-Wing Hen (Ggbb)

	Gb female	gb female	Gb female	gb female
GB male	GGbB	gGbB	GGbB	gGbB
gB male	GgbB	ggbB	GgbB	ggbB
gB male	GgbB	ggbB	GgbB	ggbB
gB male	GgbB	ggbB	GgbB	ggbB

Offspring would look like this:
Homozygous dominant Green, Heterozygous Black wing = 2
Homozygous recessive Blue, Heterozygous Black wing = 6
Heterozygous Green/Blue, Heterozygous Black wing = 8

Another Punnett square shows how more than one dominant or recessive trait can be inherited by the offspring (Table 6.8). We once again use our heterozygous green/blue split (Gg) budgerigar male and female, but let's add in a wing tip color. Normal wing tips are homozygous dominant black, expressed as (BB), there is also a homozygous recessive gray wing tip, expressed as (bb). Now we have four possible combinations of alleles from each parent. Every combination is used across the top and the side of the Punnett square.

The gray winged hen's phenotype is no match for the male's homozygous dominant gene for black wings. Of the 16 possible offspring only 6 of them will be blue with black wings and 10 will be green with black wings. As can be seen by this chart, the more genetic factors that an individual has the more difficult it becomes to predict the outcome of the breeding. However, if you took the GgBb offspring (heterozygous green/blue with heterozygous black/gray) and mated that with another of the same phenotype you would get a different mix of offspring again!

Unfortunately, breeding for phenotype over function and behaviors has developed specific genetic-based diseases or conditions, some of which have been passed on to other animals within the species. Examples would be the long backs and short legs of the Dachshund. The long back is prone to hyperflexion when the dog jumps from the couch or bed to the floor. The jarring impact causes the disks to become luxated which can cause paralysis. When a Dachshund is crossed with a dog with a normal length back the offspring will have an elongated back, telling us that the gene for long backs is dominant. Breeding Bulldogs with their brachiocephalic faces has led to dogs that can't breathe very well and so are prone to heat stroke and hypoxia when the weather is hot and humid. Also, because of the size of their heads, they cannot give birth easily, if at all, by themselves. Cesarean sections are how most bulldogs have puppies. The big head and chest also prevent them from swimming well or for very long. This is just a few examples of breeding for a type. There are numerous textbooks that cover genetic conditions in animals that can be passed on to offspring.

Learning Exercise

Play around with the Punnett square using your family as an example. Do you have a mom with brown hair and a dad with black hair? Look at your siblings. How many have black hair? Is it a mix? Or use eye color or use height. Can you figure out the dominant and recessive genes responsible? Plug it into the Punnett square and see what the odds were that you would have been born with a different eye or hair color or height.

Breeds of Animals

It is important to learn a bit about what a purebred animal is, who is responsible for the registration of these animals, and how to recognize the breed traits to help you identify breeds of dogs, cats, and pocket pets. This is a synopsis of what you need to know and your instructor will lead you in how to find out about the different breeds or varieties.

A purebred animal is one that breeds true, meaning when breeding a Poodle to another Poodle you get a Poodle that meets the breed standard. A breed standard describes the animal from head to toe and is used to judge if the animal is "of standard" if shown or if deciding to use it for breeding. For dogs, the American Kennel Club (AKC) is a registration organization with each breed having an organization or club. The Cat Fanciers Association (CFA) and individual breed clubs do the same for cats. Horses, cattle, sheep, and pigs have breed associations for each species.

Reflection

Now that you know what a purebred animal is, discuss the "breeders" that mix breeds like Labradors and Poodles and call them Labradoodles and charge thousands of dollars for a "designer" breed. What are people paying for? Are these breeders hurting the original breeds by doing this cross-breeding? Will Labradoodles ever become a purebred dog?

The AKC has separated all dogs into seven groups: herding, hounds, non-sporting, sporting, terriers, working, and toys. Each of these groups, except for the non-sporting group, have similar characteristics, not only in body shape, but in what they were bred to do for humans. It is beyond the scope of this book to go into all 190 breeds the AKC recognizes, but we will talk about each group and point out some traits to use as identifiers.

Herding Group

The herding group is made up of those dogs that like to herd and or keep other animals in a group. The largest are the Shepherds, the hairiest are the Old English Sheepdogs, and the smallest are the Corgis (Figure 6.2).

When you look at the group as a whole you see similar body types in all but the Corgis. The common body type is long legs, deep chests, and thick hair coats to protect them from cold weather and thorns. Some have shorter hair coats because of where they were developed (e.g., Australian Cattle Dogs). Old English Sheepdogs have a **double hair coat** which means they have a thick, dense underlayer with long **guard hairs** protruding through that to protect them from snow and rain. There are several breeds that have double hair coats of varying lengths and densities. The short legged Corgi was developed to move the neighbor's livestock off their owner's pastures, so they didn't need the extra leg length to move through or climb to Alpine meadows.

All the dogs in the herding group are extremely intelligent and hard working. If they are to be pets, they must have an activity to keep their minds active like fly ball, agility courses, or getting out for long runs with their humans. Herding dogs are very affectionate to their owners, will herd children and keep an watchful eye on them. As a whole, they are a bit wary of strangers but that makes them good watch dogs, as part of their behavior to sound off when "danger" is near.

Hound Group

Hounds were developed to hunt different animals in a variety of terrains. Because of this the group can be divided into **sight hounds** and **scent hounds**. Sight hounds were developed to see and chase after fast prey like antelope, gazelle, and rabbits. They have very long legs, lean bodies with deep chests for speed and endurance (Figure 6.3). Some have longer hair like the Afghan Hound and others have extremely short hair like the Greyhound. The tallest of all dogs are Irish and Scottish Wolfhounds. They are more muscular than their cousins and were developed to hunt bear, boar, and of course wolves. The sight hounds tend to be more of a one-person dog and a bit aloof and sedate when around a stranger. They will tolerate handling but don't usually give you that happy, wagging tail.

The scent hounds were developed to hunt rabbits, fox, badgers, and racoons. Most of them have short hair coats, a couple have a wire coat (medium length and harsh to the touch) or long hair. The largest of the scent hounds are the Bloodhounds and the smallest are the Miniature Dachshunds. Bloodhounds have a renowned sense of smell and are credited with being able to pick up a scent many hours old. They are often trained as search and rescue dogs. Beagles, Foxhounds, and Harriers are very similar in color, being mostly "hound colored" which is a combination of tan, white, with hints of black short hair. The differences between them are height. Beagles are 13 or 15 inches at the withers whereas Foxhounds and Harriers are 20–25 inches. They were all developed to chase fox or rabbits in a pack. Because of this these dogs are usually not happy living alone; they need a pack for entertainment. Dachshunds are a breed that has been heavily manipulated by humans. They

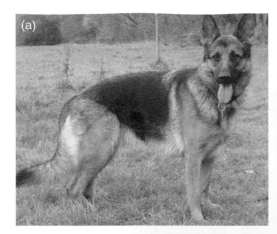
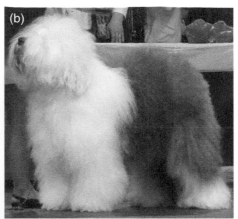
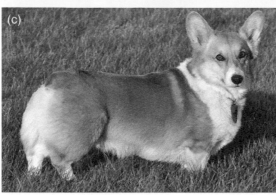

FIGURE 6.2 Herding group: (a) German Shepherd, (b) Old English Sheepdog, and (c) Welsh Corgi Pembroke. Note the ears on both the Shepherd and the Corgi; they are naturally *erect* ears. Both the Sheepdog and Corgi are naturally *bobtailed*. Source: Wikimedia Commons. Used under CC BY-SA 3.0, https://commons.wikimedia.org/wiki/File:DSHwiki.jpg; https://commons.wikimedia.org/wiki/File:Welchcorgipembroke.JPG; https://commons.wikimedia.org/wiki/File:Bobtail_in_Riga_4.JPG.

were originally developed to hunt badgers so their bodies were selected for short crooked legs to fit into badger holes, sharp pointed noses to grab onto the badger's nose, and heavily muscled hindquarters to drag the badger out of the hole. They come in two sizes (standard and miniature) and three hair coats (smooth, wire, and long). The scent hounds tend to be easy keepers, meaning that they get fat on regular-sized rations. It is always a good idea to keep them lean by measuring their food and weighing them regularly. Scent hounds are usually more gregarious than their sight hound cousins. All of them love their people and will be lap dogs if you let them, which is fine with a Miniature Dachshund but not so great with a 120 lb Irish Wolfhound!

Non-Sporting Group

The non-sporting group is basically a catch-all group. They don't have a specific group, body type, hair coat length, or job they like to do. This group ranges from Poodles (four sizes) with tight curly hair, Dalmatians with spotted short hair, to Chows with super thick double coats (Figure 6.4). The faces are **brachiocephalic** or "smashed in" like the Bulldog, Boston Terrier, and Lhasa

Apso or **mesocephalic** with regular length noses like the Dalmatian, Schipperke, or Shiba Inu. They tend to be very attached to one person and can be standoffish and aloof with strangers. Approach all these dogs with caution, as some are known to bite without warning. As a group they do not make the best pets if children are in the home, unless the owner knows how to maintain their dominance and the dog knows where it stands in the "pack" (family).

Sporting Group

The sporting group is made up of dogs used for hunting birds (Figure 6.5). There are four types of dogs based upon the type of bird or the type of hunting humans liked to pursue. **Setters** are large dogs with long hair, which come in three colors. Irish Setters are red, English Setters are white with black or brown spots, and Gordon Setters are black and tan. The Setters are used for upland game like pheasants and grouse. **Retrievers** are heavier built dogs than a Setter and have either short or long hair. Two of the retrievers are very popular dogs; the Labradors which come in black, yellow, or chocolate colored short hair and the Goldens that range from a light

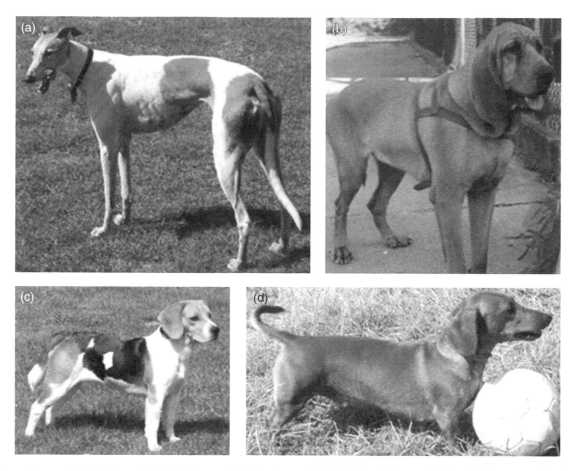

FIGURE 6.3 Hound group: (a) Greyhound, (b) Bloodhound, (c) Beagle, and (d) Dachshund. Source: Wikimedia Commons. Used under CC BY-SA 3.0, https://commons.wikimedia.org/wiki/File:GraceTheGreyhound.jpg; https://commons.wikimedia.org/wiki/File:Bloodhound-Female.jpg; https://commons.wikimedia.org/wiki/File:Beagle_Faraon.JPG; https://commons.wikimedia.org/wiki/File:20080821_%D0%A4%D0%B5%D0%B4%D1%8F_%D0%BD%D0%B0_%D0%BF%D1%80%D0%B8%D1%80%D0%BE%D0%B4%D1%96.JPG

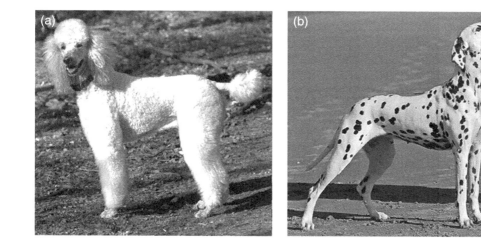
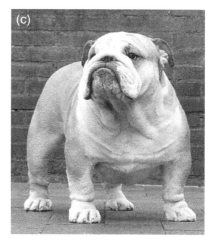

FIGURE 6.4 Non-sporting group: (a) Poodle, (b) Dalmatian, and (c) Bulldog. Compare the mesocephalic faces of the Poodle and Dalmation with the brachiocephalic face of the Bulldog. The Poodle and Dalmation have *hanging* ears, and the Bulldog has a *rose* ear. The Poodle has a *docked* tail. Source: Wikimedia Commons. Used under CC BY 2.0, https://commons.wikimedia.org/wiki/File:Standard_poodle_apricot.jpg; https://commons.wikimedia.org/wiki/File:Binka_10_06.jpg; https://commons.wikimedia.org/wiki/File:BulldogAnglais.jpg.

yellow to a dark red long hair. They are used for upland game and duck retrieval and both are known for their "soft mouths," meaning they won't injure the meat when bringing birds to their owners. **Pointers** are large dogs with short hair coats that come in white with black or brown patches, brown roan, red, gray, or tan. They may have long tails or tails that are docked. There are a number of breeds including the English Pointer,

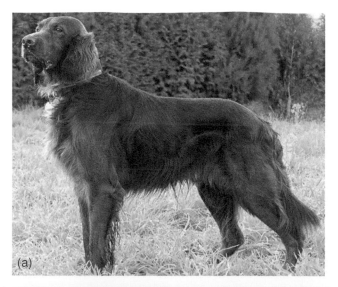
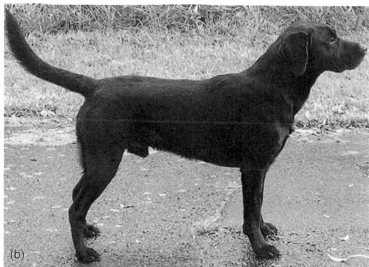
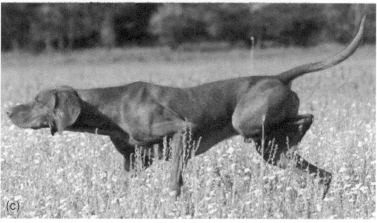
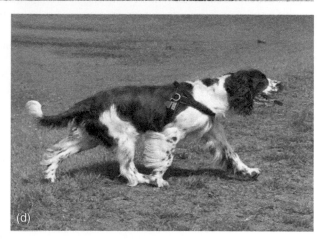

FIGURE 6.5 Sporting group: (a) Irish Setter, (b) Labrador Retriever, (c) Vizsla, and (d) English Springer Spaniel. Source: Wikimedia Commons. Used under CC BY-SA 3.0, https://commons.wikimedia.org/wiki/File:Can_Setter_dog_GFDL.jpg; https://commons.wikimedia.org/wiki/File:Perfect_Side_View_Of_Black_Labrador_North_East_England.JPG; https://commons.wikimedia.org/wiki/File:Vizsla_r%C3%A1h%C3%BAz_a_vadra.jpg; https://commons.wikimedia.org/wiki/File:English-Springer-Spaniel.jpg.

Weimaraner, Vizsla, and German Shorthair to name a few. They indicate an upland bird (pheasant or grouse) in the bush by "pointing" with their nose, often with a front leg bent and tail straight out. This is an instinctual behavior that was created by humans using selective breeding. The fourth type of sporting dog is the **Spaniel**. These are medium-sized dogs that usually have a thick wavy or straight coat although there is one with a short coat. The group is made up of the English Springer, English Cocker, American Cocker, and Brittany Spaniels to name the most common breeds. They are good at retrieving both upland birds and waterfowl; however, they have mostly been relegated to family pet, but many retain the instinct to search for birds. Spaniels usually have their tails docked and require professional grooming to keep the hair coat in check.

Sporting dogs are very friendly and want to please their owners. They are gregarious dogs that like everyone including children, although Spaniels have a history of being snappish in old age. They will bark at strangers but will immediately become friends with almost everyone. Of course, this is a general statement as there will be some individuals that do not like strangers or are unapproachable.

Terrier Group

The Terrier group of dogs was bred to take care of vermin like mice, rats, and weasels (Figure 6.6). They are tenacious dogs that are intelligent, tend to have a mind of their own, and will frustrate the novice owner! This group has it all from large to small in stature, and your choice of short, wire, or long hair coats. They can be friendly and outgoing or reserved and aloof until they know you are family or friend. They like to bark, making them good watch dogs. They can be full of energy with some seeming to have springs for legs like the Fox Terrier! Some of the best family dogs are found in the Terrier group and these would be the West Highland (Westy), Scottish

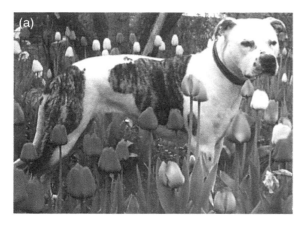
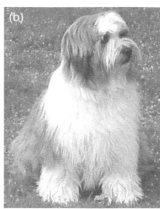
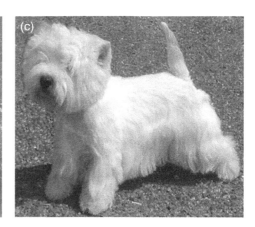

FIGURE 6.6 Terrier group: (a) American Staffordshire, (b) Tibetan, and (c) West Highland White Terrier. Source: Wikimedia Commons. Used under CC BY-SA 3.0, https://commons.wikimedia.org/wiki/File:Roc_1_copie.jpg; https://commons.wikimedia.org/wiki/File:American_Staffordshire_Terrier.jpg; https://commons.wikimedia.org/wiki/File:Tibetan_Terrier_Image_001.jpg.

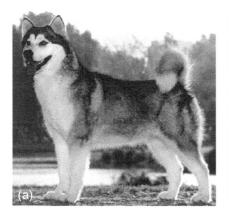
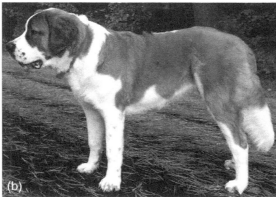
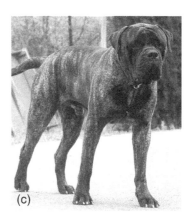

FIGURE 6.7 Working group: (a) Alaskan Malamute, (b) St. Bernard, and (c) Bullmastiff. Note the *sickle* tail on the Malamute, the *flews* on the St. Bernard and the Bullmastiff, and the *brindle* hair color of the Bullmastiff. Source: Wikimedia Commons. Used under CC BY-SA 3.0, https://commons.wikimedia.org/wiki/File:Alaskanmalamute0b.jpg; https://commons.wikimedia.org/wiki/File:St_Bernard_Dog_001.jpg; https://commons.wikimedia.org/wiki/File:Bullmastiff_Junghund_1_Jahr.jpg.

(Scotty), and the Cairn Terriers. They all have a similar profile with medium to long hair coats that require professional grooming, and weigh about 14–24 lb. Tails are often docked on Terriers and they either have an **erect, bat** ear, or a **cropped** ear. Examples of long-haired terriers are the Tibetan and Bedlington. Some of the dogs in this group have gotten a bad name because of indiscriminate breeding and little to no socialization or training. Those breeds are the "pit bull" type of dog that include the Staffordshire, American Staffordshire, and the American Pit Bull Terriers. All three make good pets with careful socialization and training. They do have the instinct to chase and kill but virtually all Terriers do, so concentrating on training to "leave it" and "drop it" for *all* Terriers is a must. The reason Pit Bull Terriers get into trouble is they are medium to large-sized dogs that weight between 35 and 70 lb and can do a lot of damage in a short period of time.

Working Group

The working group of dogs was developed to assist humans in various ways. One group was developed to pull carts and/or sleighs, another was developed for rescuing people in snow, water, or rough terrain, and the third was developed for protection or police work. Generally, these dogs are large breeds and have short to long double coats depending on the job they were bred to perform (Figure 6.7). The sled dogs are Huskies, Malamutes, and Samoyeds to name a few. All have similar body types: prick ears, ring, sickle, or squirrel tails, and double hair coats. They range in weight from 60 to 90 lb. It may take time to make friends with these dogs but once you do you are a friend for life. The rescue dogs include St. Bernards, Newfoundlands, and Great Pyrenees. These dogs can weigh well over 100 lb, have double coats and large heads and long lips called **flews**.

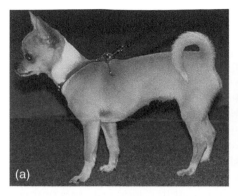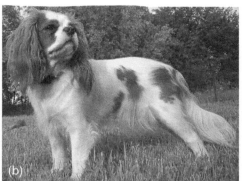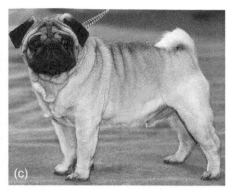

FIGURE 6.8 Toy group: (a) Chihuahua, (b) Cavalier King Charles Spaniel, and (c) Pug. Source: Wikimedia Commons. Used under CC BY-SA 3.0, https://commons.wikimedia.org/wiki/File:Chihuahua_01_K.jpg, https://commons.wikimedia.org/wiki/File:Betty_Verdure.Photo_Ph.BRIZARD.JPG, https://commons.wikimedia.org/wiki/File:Mops_oct09.jpg.

They are gentle giants that tolerate piles of children with aplomb and are very protective of their little people! Most drool a little and some drool a lot! The protection and police dogs include Rottweilers, Dobermans, Great Danes, Boxers, and Mastiffs. Mastiffs were used to develop most of the dogs in this group. Their large size and deep voices deter even the most foolhardy burglar. Luckily, these dogs are truly gentle giants and their bark is worst than their bite. All of these are great dogs and make good family pets.

Toy Group

The toy group of dogs was developed to fit into pockets or satchels to be carried and pampered by royalty across Europe and Asia (Figure 6.8). For the most part they still think of themselves as royalty and expect to be treated as such, meaning don't touch me unless you want to be bitten! Luckily, they weigh between 8 and 20 lb so they don't cause massive damage when they bite, but it still hurts! Again, there is a wide range of hair coats and sizes available in this group. They are usually one person's pet and they may not tolerate the rest of the family. The smallest toy is the Chihuahua coming in at 3–6 lb and they can have short or long hair coats. Their distinguishing feature is their "apple dome" head, the rounded skull offset by **prick** ears. The next smallest is the Yorkshire Terrier, with long flowing gray gunmetal hair. They are often seen in the veterinary clinic with the initials BD/LD in the record which means "big dog injured little dog." However, it was most likely the Yorkie that picked the fight! The Pomeranian rounds out the smallest toys, being a double-coated puffball with a squirrel tail. The larger long-haired toys include Cavalier King Charles Spaniels, Maltese, Papillon, Pekingese, and Shih Tzu. The larger short-haired toys include Pugs, Chinese Crested, and the Italian Greyhound. Again, there are individuals in this group that are notorious for biting but then there are delightful individuals that are fun to get

to know and love. If children are to be in the mix it is better to raise this group with the child rather than getting one when the child is a toddler. Having said that, it is important to teach the child to respect the dog and the dog to respect the child.

Learning Exercise

As you go about your day and see different breeds of dogs, see if you can guess their breed by the descriptions provided above. Perhaps by starting a "scrapbook" or quiz card app on your phone, take a picture and use it to help you learn the breeds.

Cat Breeds

Cats have been domesticated for thousands of years; they have been worshipped as gods, declaimed as spawn of the devil, and loved as part of the family. Most of the cats seen in the veterinary clinic will be of the "domestic type" meaning that they are not purebred cats. They come in all shapes, hair coat lengths, and colors. The medical record will often show under breed the abbreviations DS for domestic short hair, DL for domestic long hair, or DM for domestic medium hair. There is one breed of cat that has a dominant gene for its hair coat, eye color, and color pattern and that is the Siamese (Figure 6.9). The Siamese is a solid-colored cat ranging in body color from ivory to a seal brown with **points** that include a mask, paws, and tail in a darker shade of brown, and brilliant blue almond-shaped eyes. This **color pattern** is called a seal point and is homozygous dominant (SS) or homozygous recessive (ss). So, when a purebred Siamese mates with a regular domestic cat often all or most of the offspring will have blue eyes and a seal

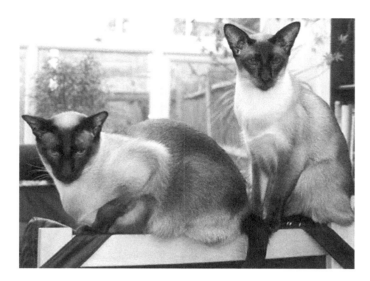

FIGURE 6.9 Siamese cat. Source: Wikimedia Commons. Used under CC-BY-SA 2.0; https://commons.wikimedia.org/wiki/File:Two_Siam_Seal_Point.jpg.

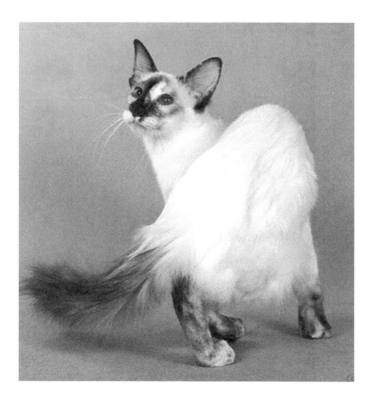

FIGURE 6.10 Balinese Torte Point. Source: Wikimedia Commons. Used under CC-BY-SA 3.0; https://commons.wikimedia.org/wiki/File:Balinese-cat-2.jpg.

point color pattern. In this case the medical record could indicate that the cat is a Siamese Cross.

The Siamese cat is one of two cat breeds that have been heavily manipulated by humans. Their original body style was of a medium-sized cat, with a round head and a coat color as described earlier. However, this cat underwent a transformation. A longer, leaner **oriental** body was developed, with a sharply triangular head and the color points

are now Seal, Blue, Chocolate, Flame (red), and Lilac! The oriental body shape has been used to develop other breeds of cat like the multicolored Oriental Shorthair, the solid colored Burmese, the Tonkinese that is somewhat reminiscent of the old-fashioned bodied Siamese or the Balinese Torte Point (Figure 6.10). The other full breed short hair cats are the Bengal, Korat, Russian Blue, British, American, and Exotic Shorthairs.

Other shorthaired cats with rather unique coats are the Devon, Cornish, and Selkirk Rex cats. They were developed from spontaneous mutations of the hair coat. Instead of a straight hair shaft it comes out curly or wavy. These cats have an oriental body with large ears and round eyes (Figure 6.11). Another spontaneous mutation was used to develop the Scottish Fold; this cat's pinnas are folded over so that the ear canal is not accessible (Figure 6.11).

Medium hair-length purebreds include Birmans, Angoras, Maine Coon cats, American Bobtail or Wirehair, and the Turkish Van to name a few. These cats have hair coats in multiple colors. The Maine Coon is the largest cat and has very distinctive tuffs of hair on the ears and between the toes, as well as a very impressive mane. They often weigh in at 12–18 lb, are often 40 inches long and 10–13 inches tall (Figure 6.12).

The last group of cats are the longhairs. The most popular of these and the most common is the Persian. This is the second most manipulated cat breed in that its face wasn't always so very "pushed in" or classified as a brachiocephalic face (Figure 6.13). Persians have a thick double coat made up of dense, soft fur beneath long guard hairs. The soft fur gets matted very easily and so requires daily brushing to prevent these mats. Unfortunately, many Persians are grumpy about this and rarely sit still or enjoy the attention. So, we see them in the veterinary clinic because there is a "hot spot" or bacterial infection under the mats. These areas must be shaved in order to treat them and so often the client opts to have the entire cat shaved.

The color point version of the Persian is called a Himalayan. They have the color points on the head, tail, and paws. Ragdolls are also a color point; however, they have white markings, and the Norwegian Forest cat can come in any color.

Learning Exercise

Distinguishing cat breeds can be difficult. Utilize the internet to learn of any cat shows coming up in your area. If possible go to the show and visit with the owners. Most will gladly allow photos if you ask nicely and tell them why you are taking them. Build a scrapbook or reference book with cat breeds.

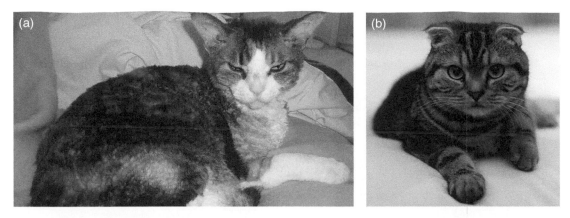

FIGURE 6.11 (a) Devon Rex, note the wavy coat and calico color pattern; (b) Scottish Fold, note the pinna bent over and brown tabby color pattern. Source: https://commons.wikimedia.org/wiki/File:Drex.jpg. Public Domain.

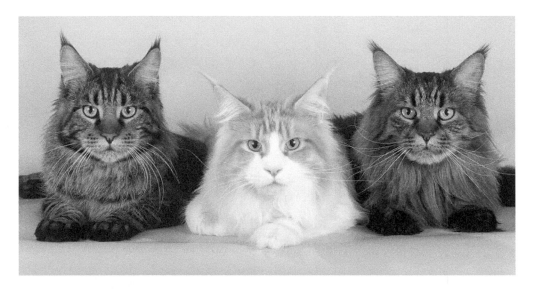

FIGURE 6.12 Maine Coon cats, orange tabby with white markings between two brown tabbies. Source: https://commons.wikimedia.org/wiki/File:%D0%A4%D0%BE%D1%82%D0%BE_%D0%BA%D1%83%D0%BD%D0%BE%D0%B2.jpg. Public Domain.

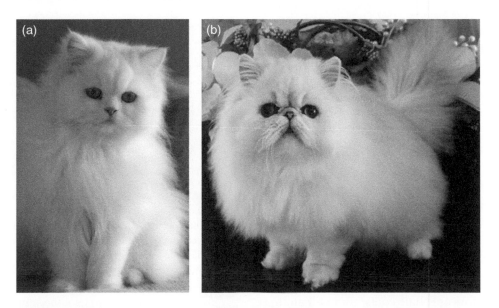

FIGURE 6.13 (a) Old Style Persian with white coat and (b) New Style Persian with silver color pattern. Source: Wikimedia Commons. Used under CC BY 3.0, https://commons.wikimedia.org/wiki/Filc:Shaded_silver_Persian_Cat_Missionhill Cosmic_Rainstorm.jpg, https://commons.wikimedia.org/wiki/File:SnowyandHazy.jpg.

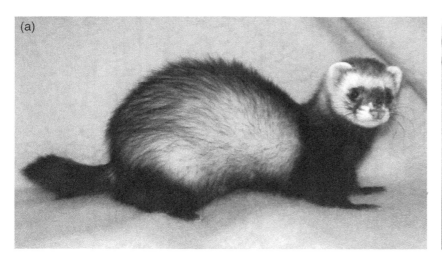

FIGURE 6.14 Ferrets: (a) polecat color pattern and (b) albino. Source: Wikimedia Commons. Used under CC BY-SA 3.0, https://commons.wikimedia.org/wiki/File:Coco_4074.JPG, https://commons.wikimedia.org/wiki/File:Ferret_2008.png.

Pocket Pets

The pocket pets that we see in the clinic include ferrets, rats, mice, gerbils, hamsters, guinea pigs, chinchillas, and rabbits.

Ferrets

Ferrets are part of the weasel family and in certain states they cannot be kept as pets. Female ferrets are induced ovulaters and if not bred when they come into season can become extremely sick. This is considered an emergency and they should be seen immediately. Ferrets come in two colors: natural or polecat and albino (Figure 6.14).

Rats

Rats are used in research and kept as pets. The Long–Evans or hooded rat is the variety most people keep as pets as they are usually gentle, highly intelligent, and seem to appreciate companionship. They come in a multitude of colors, thanks to manipulation by humans. As rats age they can develop cancerous growths on their bodies which some clients will ask to have removed (Figure 6.15).

Mice

Large numbers of mice are utilized in research every day. There are numerous types of mice that have been developed to facilitate research; however, we will not be covering those varieties of mice. There are mouse fanciers in the world and because mice produce quickly and often, their phenotypes have been manipulated. We now have a myriad of colors and hair coats; they call all these mice "Fancy"! Unfortunately, mice don't live very long so we don't often see them in the clinic (Figure 6.16).

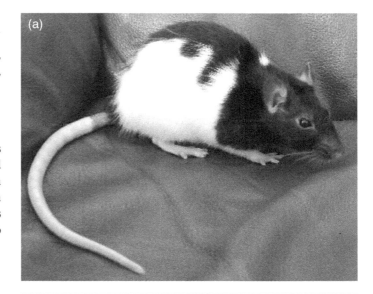

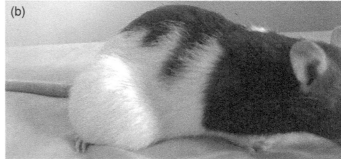

FIGURE 6.15 Hooded rat. Note the tumor on the hind quarter (b), you can barely make it out in (a). Source: https://commons.wikimedia.org/wiki/File:Twinkle_the_brown_hooded_rat.jpg, https://commons.wikimedia.org/wiki/File:Brown_hooded_rat_with_a_large_tumor.jpg. Public Domain.

Gerbils

Native to the desert, gerbils are **nocturnal**, meaning they are active at night. They are voracious diggers and rearrangers

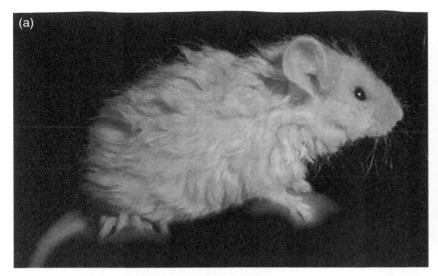
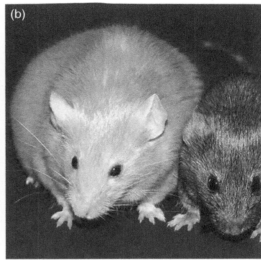

FIGURE 6.16 Fancy mice: (a) angora and (b) agouti. Source: Wikimedia Commons. Used under CC BY 3.0, https://commons.wikimedia.org/wiki/File:Agouti_Mice.jpg, https://commons.wikimedia.org/wiki/File:Fancy_angora_lab_mice.jpg.

and to keep them happy at least 2–3 inches of substrate must be provided in their cages. Gerbils can have a condition that is epilepsy-like. If suddenly startled they can go into a seizure-like episode. Usually, it passes with time and the gerbil is fine; however, occasionally the seizure lasts for a long period of time at which point you may see them arrive at the clinic. Putting them in a semi-darkened room with no noise until they can be seen is how to handle this urgent visit. Gerbils are also amazing jumpers and if they should leap from a hand and land on the floor a broken leg is not unheard of, they do well with splints and so you may also see them in the clinic for this urgent care visit (Figure 6.17). Gerbils can also "slip" their tail. It is a survival mechanism so if a person grabs for a gerbil but only gets the tail, the skin will come off the vertebrae. These need to be snipped off so they don't catch on items inside the cage. The gerbil will be fine, just a little short in the tail department.

Hamsters

Hamsters tend to be healthy little critters (Figure 6.18). They are prone to a gastrointestinal disturbance called **proliferative ileitis** or wet tail. The causative agent is the bacteria *Lawsonia intracellularis* which is spread by contaminated food and water. Contributing factors include weaning, transportation, overcrowding, and rapid dietary changes. Some varieties of hamster seem more susceptible than others, with the Teddy Bear hamster being one of the most susceptible. These animals need to be treated within 24–72 hours of seeing the clinical signs of a wet hind end and tail. The golden hamster is the one found in nature; humans have developed several different varieties including miniatures.

Guinea Pigs

Guinea pigs are larger than other pocket pets and are very gregarious (Figure 6.19). They chirp and holler at their people when it is time for food, or you've arrived home from work. They are **crepuscular** in nature, meaning their awake times are dawn and dusk. A unique trait is that they will grow to fit their enclosure – the bigger the cage the bigger the guinea pig! There are three scenarios for which you may see them in the veterinary hospital. One is rickets. This is a disease caused by a lack of vitamin C. They do not synthesize it from their food and so need to have daily supplements. Without they will present with swollen sore joints and lameness. The second is if they are going to be bred it is important to do it just as they mature at about 2–3 months of age. Otherwise, the female's pubic bones fuse often causing **dystocia**. The third issue is constipation from pine chip bedding. They eat the bedding and it blocks their intestinal tract. Use recycled newspaper or other types of bedding to avoid this issue. Guinea pigs have been manipulated by humans and the American Rabbit Breeders Association recognizes 13 breeds of **cavy**! The English guinea pig is the natural occurring one; others that are seen commonly are the Peruvian with its 6 inch long hair, the Abyssinian with its "rosettes" or "cow licks," the Silkie with long thick hair, the Texel with wavy medium-length hair, and the Teddy with fluffy soft short hair.

Chinchillas

Chinchillas were originally raised for the soft fur market but make entertaining pets (Figure 6.20). They are healthy animals if fed and housed properly. They must have a daily dust bath to keep their fur clean and tidy. Otherwise they will lose hair in clumps and it may look as if they have a

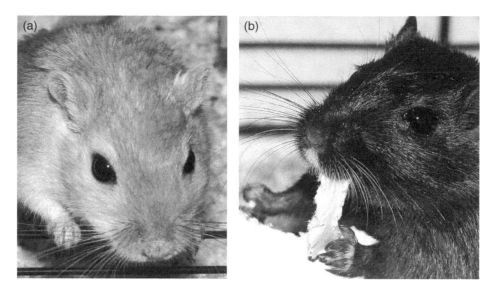

FIGURE 6.17 Mongolian gerbil: (a) natural color and (b) manmade black. Source: Wikimedia Commons. Used under CC-BY-SA 4.0, https://commons.wikimedia.org/wiki/File:2008-02-16_Mongolian_gerbil.jpg; https://commons.wikimedia.org/wiki/File:2008-02-16_Mongolian_gerbil_eating_toilet_paper_roll.jpg.

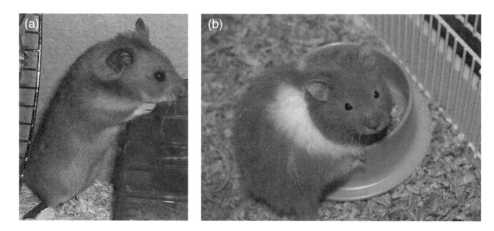

FIGURE 6.18 Hamster: (a) Golden and (b) Teddy Bear. Source: Wikimedia Commons. Used under CC BY-SA 2.0, https://commons.wikimedia.org/wiki/File:Hamster_(1).jpg; https://commons.wikimedia.org/wiki/File:Guarding_the_food_(449725625).jpg.

skin disease. Chinchillas can develop bacterial infections but if the cage is kept clean the chance of this is greatly reduced. The natural color is grey with a white belly, but silver, black, violet, beige, white, sapphire, and ebony are a few of the color mutations developed by humans.

Rabbits

Rabbits have been raised for meat, fur, and exhibition for centuries. The American Rabbit Breeders Association recognizes 49 breeds of rabbits. All rabbit breeds can be used for all three purposes, although raising them for exhibition is more popular than the other two. Rabbits come in three size ranges: miniatures or dwarfs at 2.5–4 lb, standards at 8–10 lb, and giants are any breed over 10 lb (Figure 6.21). Rabbits are also hardy and do well indoors or out. If kept outside, it is important to keep their drinking water clean and plentiful. On a hot day it is not unheard of that one rabbit will drink a gallon or more of water! Long toenails are often a reason for a trip to the veterinary clinic. They get caught on fencing and get ripped off. This is urgent but not an emergency although they do bleed a lot! Another reason for a clinic visit is ear mites, a small parasite that causes extreme itchiness and sores. If not breeding the rabbits it is a good idea to get them spayed and/or neutered which can reduce the number of fights but does not guarantee it! Stitching up the loser of these fights is another reason you will see a bunny at the clinic.

Determining the Sex of Companion Animals

Sexing an animal is an important skill for assistants and technicians alike. It is common for an owner to rescue an animal, either a stray or by private purchase, and not know the sex of the animal. This is very important to prevent accidental breeding. This tends to be more of an issue with immature cats and pocket pets. Another important reason to be able to determine the sex of an

animal is when getting them ready for neuter or spay surgery!

Dogs are easy to determine. Males will have a prepuce and penis on the ventral side of the abdomen and testicles on the ventral caudal end. However, cats are often a bit more difficult. Always check the sex of every cat in for spay or neuter surgery. Many a tom cat has been prepped for a spay surgery only to find no ovaries or uteri in the abdomen. This usually occurs when the owner states the sex of their pet cat but no one checked! Cats are difficult to determine because the genitalia for both sexes are presented caudally just under the tail. The anus is located on both sexes just below the tail and is round. The **vulva** on females will be almost directly below the anus and is a straight slit opening; it looks almost like a semi-colon (Figure 6.22). This is called the anal–genital distance and is used on many animals to determine sex. The male's **prepuce** will appear as a rounded opening with a longer anal–genital distance away from the anus, approximately ½ inch in kittens and a full inch in adults. Think of a rather spread out colon. You should be able to make

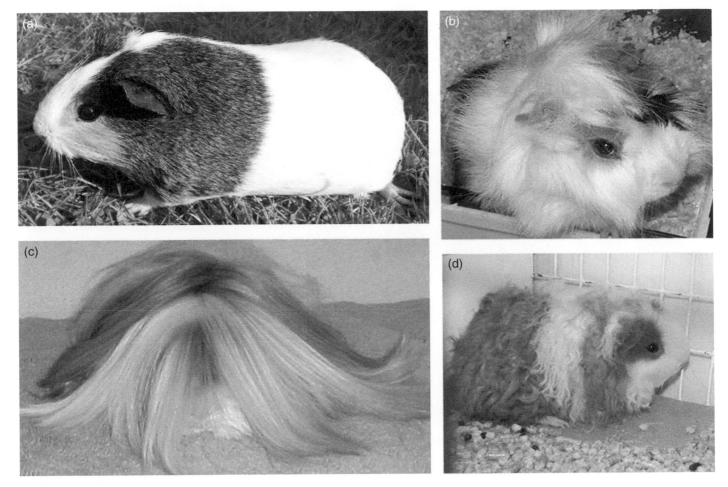

FIGURE 6.19 Guinea pigs: (a) English, (b) Abyssinian, (c) Peruvian, and (d) Texel. Source: Wikimedia Commons; Used under CC BY-SA 3.0, https://commons.wikimedia.org/wiki/File:Hausmeerschweinchen.JPG; https://commons.wikimedia.org/wiki/File:Rene_the_long-haired_Satin_Peruvian_Guinea_pig.jpg; https://commons.wikimedia.org/wiki/File:Swinka_morska.jpg; https://commons.wikimedia.org/wiki/File:Texel_guinea_pig.jpg.

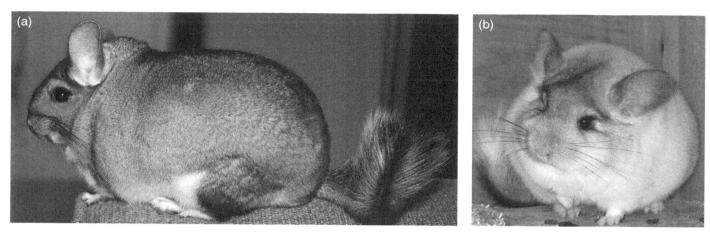

FIGURE 6.20 Chinchilla: (a) natural grey and (b) silver. Source: Wikimedia Commons. Used under CC BY-SA 3.0, https://commons.wikimedia. org/wiki/File:Chinchilla-Soelvmarmorert.jpg, https://commons.wikimedia.org/wiki/File:Chinchilla_lanigera1.jpg.

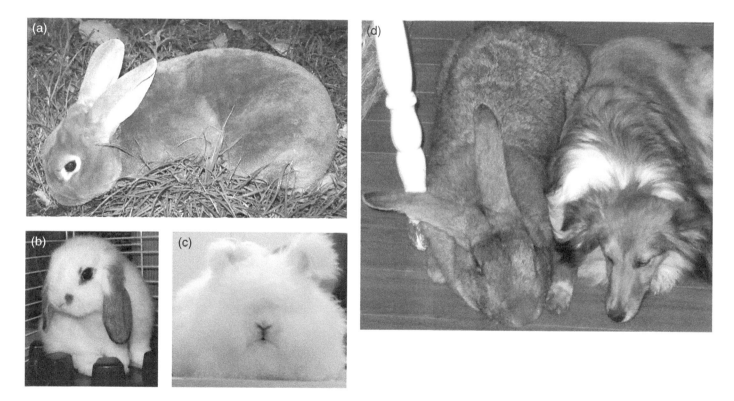

FIGURE 6.21 Rabbit breeds: (a) Rex, (b) Mini Lop, (c) English Angora, and (d) Flemish Giant next to Shetland Sheepdog. Source: Wikimedia Commons. Used under CC BY 2.0, https://commons.wikimedia.org/wiki/File:So_shy_Mini_Lop.jpg; https://commons.wikimedia.org/wiki/File:Runt_and_Paxie.jpg; https://commons.wikimedia.org/wiki/Category:English_Angora_rabbits#/media/File:Englishangora.jpg; https://commons.wikimedia.org/wiki/File:Gelbrex.jpg.

the penis protrude with gentle backward pull on the prepuce (Figure 6.23). The penis is cone-shaped and will have backward facing penile spines at the base. Of course, at maturity the males will have testicles that are situated above the prepuce but if the cat is neutered they will not be apparent!

Rabbits are sometimes difficult to sex because their genitals are similarly located and are tucked into the anal crevice so they are barely visible. To determine the difference, scissor the tail between your index and middle fingers and then place the thumb just below the anus. Pull the tail back, towards the spine gently but firmly and simultaneously press down with the thumb. This digital pressure will make the genitalia protrude. Males will have a tubular penis with a definite opening on the tip. Females will show a vertical slit and very little protrusion even if more pressure is applied with the thumb (Figure 6.24). See https://www.raising-rabbits.com/sexing-rabbits.html for a great website with photos on sexing rabbits.

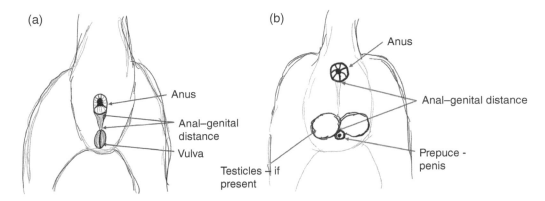

FIGURE 6.22 (a) Female and (b) male cat genitalia. Note the anal–genital distance.

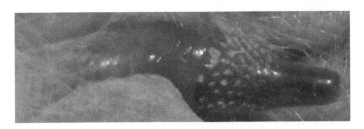

FIGURE 6.23 Cat's penis. Source: Wikimedia Commons. Used under CC-BY-SA 3.0, https://commons.wikimedia.org/wiki/File:Penis-cat.jpg.

Male hamsters, gerbils, mice, and rats are fairly easy to determine if you hold them around the shoulders and let their back legs hang. The testicles will drop into the scrotal sack and be visible. Female rats and mice will have visible nipples at 10 days of age. Plus, by using the **anogenital** distance, you will be able to judge male from female quite reliably. Figures 6.25 and 6.26 are photos of pocket pet genitalia.

Guinea pigs are a bit different anatomically. The female's vulva is shaped like a Y, whereas the male's prepuce is a round dot surrounded by the testicles (Figure 6.27).

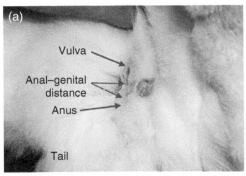

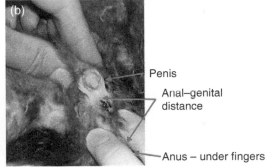

FIGURE 6.24 (a) Female and (b) male rabbit genitalia.

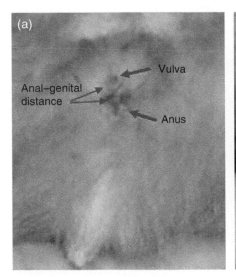

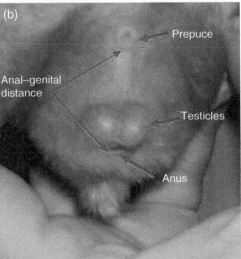

FIGURE 6.25 (a) Female and (b) male hamster genitalia.

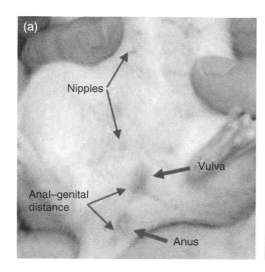
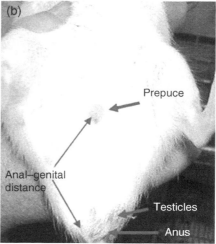

FIGURE 6.26 (a) Female and (b) male rat genitalia.

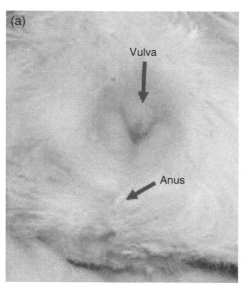
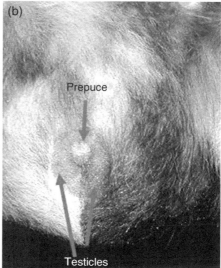

FIGURE 6.27 (a) Female and (b) male guinea pig genitalia.

Learning Exercise

While on your trip to the pet store ask the salesperson if you could possibly practice identifying male and female pocket pets. Ask if it is OK to take a photograph for your scrapbook.

Chapter Reflection

Write about what you learned in this chapter. How did learning about the different breeds of companion animals shape your thoughts about the different breeds? Did humans do justice to them all? Should designer breeding be encouraged? Can you reliably tell males from females?

CHAPTER 7

Feeds and Feeding

LEARNING OBJECTIVES

- Explain an animal's diet as related to its ecological niche
- Recall the differences in caloric content per gram of fats, proteins, and carbohydrates
- Calculate an animal's basic energy requirements (BER)
- Calculate the amount to feed an animal based upon information on the food label
- Utilize the information from food labels to feed prescription diets
- Feed hospitalized patients to ensure adequate nutrition
- Discuss the care required for tube-fed patients
- Discuss the feed options for livestock
- Determine the quality of baled products

NAVTA ESSENTIAL SKILLS COVERED IN THIS CHAPTER

IV. Examination Room Procedures

B. Basic procedures
   7. Be familiar with small animal nutritional requirements, therapeutic diets, pet food labeling standards, dry matter basis calculations, and the differences between pet food products

V. Small Animal Nursing

B. Animal care
   10. Prepare food and prescription diets – be aware of any special dietary needs

Tasks for the Veterinary Assistant, Fourth Edition. Teresa F. Sonsthagen.
© 2020 John Wiley & Sons, Inc. Published 2020 by John Wiley & Sons, Inc.
Companion website: www.wiley.com/go/sonsthagen/tasks

Appropriate nutrition for any animal is composed of the essential components that make up a healthy diet. The availability and demand for these nutrients depends on three factors: the **ecological niche** of the animal, the animal's metabolism, and the amount of stress the animal is undergoing at any one time.

The ecological niche is determined by the forage and feed available and the anatomic and physiologic adaptations of the animal to utilize the food as well as the resources and competitors in the environment. For example, **herbivores** or grazing animals like cattle, sheep, and goats have adapted their digestive systems to deal with the low nutritional value of grass on which they feed. **Ruminants** have four-compartment stomachs. Horses have large **cecums** where the breakdown of the cellulose in plants occurs making them herbivores too. Other animals have adapted monogastric stomachs and the dental formations to handle the types of foods to which they have access. For example, **carnivores** like cats, dogs, and ferrets have large canine teeth with which to tear meat from bones. Pigs and chickens are adapted to gaining their nutrition from both plants and meat; they are **omnivores**.

Metabolism is the process by which an animal processes food into energy to run the cellular processes, the conversion of nutrition into building blocks such as proteins, fats, acids, and carbohydrates, and the elimination of waste. In the animal world, the smaller the body the higher the metabolic rate. Metabolism in all animals changes as the animal ages. Younger animals have higher metabolic rates and different nutritional requirements from adults. As they mature, adults will require different nutrition to compensate for a slowing down of their metabolism.

Stress will also change the nutritional requirements of an animal. This includes work performed, environment in which it is performed, lactation, growth, changes in environment, and states of health. For example, a horse that does endurance racing will need more water, carbohydrates, and proteins to fuel its body than a horse that stands in a pen and is only ridden on the occasional weekend. An animal that is ill has different nutritional needs from a healthy animal.

Essential Nutrients – The Basics

Nutrients are absorbed from the food an animal ingests in the gastrointestinal tract. Enzymes and bacteria break down large molecules of food into simple molecules so that these can be absorbed through the intestinal wall. The simple molecules are water, carbohydrates, proteins, fats, minerals, and vitamins. These molecules are picked up by the capillaries in the intestinal wall and are carried through the body to maintain body functions.

While all these nutrients are required, they are not required in equal amounts. Water is required in the greatest quantity. An animal can go without eating for 2 weeks without serious damage to the body but it can only live for 3 days without water. Water is essential for transporting the molecules, is a component in most chemical reactions in the body, and acts as a solvent for other molecules. Absence of adequate water in the body is called **dehydration**. Without water the kidneys do not filter well and toxins build up creating damage to other organs. Eventually, the kidneys will shut down entirely and it is just a matter of hours before full organ failure follows.

Learning Exercise

Utilize the internet to find the daily water requirements for dogs, cats, horses, cows, sheep, goats, pigs, rabbits, and the pocket pets. Draw up a table to keep as a reference point.

Energy production requires three sources of nutrients; carbohydrates, proteins, and fats. These are measured in **calories**. Calories from food provide energy in the form of heat so the bodily functions can be carried out. Carbohydrates and proteins produce 4 kilocalories per of energy per gram. Fat produces 9 kilocalories per gram. Even though carbohydrates and proteins are equal in kilocalories, they are not equal in metabolism. Carbohydrates are quickly digested and absorbed, creating almost instant energy. If the body doesn't need that energy right away it is converted to fat and stored in fat cells and as glycogen that is stored in the liver and muscle. Carbohydrates come from anything that grows in the ground: grass, vegetables, grains (corn, wheat, millet, oats), rice, and trees. If carbohydrates are not available, the body will use protein and fat for energy.

Protein takes longer to be broken down and absorbed but will provide energy for 2–4 hours; it is used until gone. This is the difference between the instant energy carbohydrates provides and the long-term energy protein provides. Protein is essential in the diet because the body is virtually made of protein. Protein makes enzymes that power the chemical reactions in the body such as hemoglobin which carries oxygen in the blood. Protein comes from 20 amino acids, not all of which are essential to every species. One such amino acid is taurine which is essential for cats and is only available from meat. L-carnitine is produced from the amino acids lysine and methionine, and has a role in the production of energy by transporting fatty acids into cell mitochondria. This burns these fats within the cell to create usable energy.

Bodies do not store amino acids and so they must be consumed for use. Proteins are found in meat; beef, lamb, and goat have the highest percentage of protein, followed by pork and poultry. Eggs, nuts, soy, fish, rice, bean/lentils, corn, and wheat follow with lower amounts of protein. Meat by-products or meal are the internal organs, bones, and connective tissue that are ground up, cooked, and dried. The Association of American Feed Control Officials (AAFCO 2012a,b,c) states, meat by-products and meat meal are "the rendered product from mammal tissues, including bone, *exclusive* of blood, hair, hoof, horn, hide trimmings, manure, stomach and rumen contents, except in such amounts as may occur unavoidably in good processing practices"(AAFCO 2012b). Reputable pet food manufacturers only buy their meal from US Department of Agriculture (USDA) inspected facilities. This is a perfectly logical use of the parts of animals humans don't want to consume. Put it this way, if you give your dog a bone, hoof, or rawhide (meat by-products) as a treat it is no different from the meat by-products or meat meal on the label. These provide a good source of protein and the animal being used for food is used almost in its entirety.

Fats are used for energy and to provide nutrients for hair, skin and nails, or hooves. Fat helps the absorption of the **fat-soluble vitamins** A, D, E, and K. Fat fills fat cells which provide insulation. Fats are broken down in the body by bile that is formed in the liver, stored in the gallbladder, and released into the duodenum when fat is present. The enzyme lipase is also released by the gallbladder when fat is detected. These two break down fats into essential fatty acids called linoleic, linolenic, gamma linoleic, and arachidonic acids. They are essential because they are required for brain development, blood clotting, and controlling inflammation. Fats are found in the subcutaneous tissues of animals, eggs, milk, and plants including peanuts, soy, beans, seeds, and whole grains.

Minerals are required in varying amounts depending on the stage of growth. They are required to serve as **catalysts** in the body and function as transporting molecules that are required for body function. For example, calcium (Ca) is a vital mineral for the growth and maintenance of bone among other things. Macrominerals are those that are required in larger amounts. Microminerals or trace mineral are needed in much smaller amounts but are still required. Table 7.1 shows the macrominerals required, their use in the body, problems created when missing or deficient in the diet, and the source of the mineral.

Microminerals, also known as **trace minerals,** serve as catalysts in the body and transport molecules. These minerals need to be supplemented in small amounts. They are boron (B), cobalt (Co), copper (Cu), chromium (Cr), fluorine (F), iodine (I), iron (Fe), manganese (Mn), molybdenum (Mo), selenium (Se), and zinc (Ze).

Vitamins are essential, do not produce energy but they act as **coenzymes** and catalysts. Enzymes and coenzymes bind to proteins which facilitates the biologic activity of specific proteins in the body. There are two types of vitamins: water-soluble and fat-soluble. Water-soluble vitamins are B complex, choline, and C. They are not stored in the body and excess is flushed by the kidneys. The fat-soluble vitamins are A, D, E, and K and these are stored in the **adipose** tissues.

Understanding Pet Food Labels

There are a multitude of pet foods available. Some are glitzy and look great but are they really? Proper nutrition for hospitalized pets plays an important part in their recovery. We want to feed them the proper amounts but also make sure that amount has the proper nutrients. What is the protein, fat, carbohydrate, mineral, and vitamin content of these food choices? There are two organizations that regulate and sets guidelines for pet food labels. Remember the Food and Drug Administration (FDA) from Chapter 2? It is the governmental organization that makes sure imported foods are safe, produced under safe conditions and labeled truthfully. The AAFCO evaluates labels on a voluntary basis, and rate food manufacturers, develops and implements uniform and equitable standards that regulate the manufacturing and labeling of pet food. It also provides education on reading pet food labels and utilizes good research to make decisions about pet food choices.

Learning to Read Labels

Each label must contain certain information in a standardized format so that consumers can make good choices. The **Guaranteed Analysis** of ingredients is carried out by independent regulators to check for compliance with the nutrient requirements and label claims. All labels must have:

- Minimum statement of weight of contents – how much food is in the bag, can, or pouch.
- List of ingredients in descending order based on weight: the nutrients, protein, fat, fiber (carbohydrate), moisture content, minerals, and vitamins. If the label claims health benefits from a certain ingredient that must also be included in the analysis.
- Use of the food; if it is for young, adult, or geriatric animals, or certain disease conditions.
- Nutritional adequacy statement.
- Feeding guidelines with kilocalorie/cup.
- Name and address of the manufacturer or distributor.

TABLE 7.1			
Macrominerals			
Mineral – chemical symbol	Action or need in body	Problems caused	Source
Calcium (Ca)	Together with P gives structural strength to bones and teeth. Transfers information between cells, plays a part in nerve impulses, blood coagulation, and muscular contraction	Skeletal abnormalities, especially during growth and/or lactation Hypercalcemia or too much calcium can result in renal failure and mineralization of the kidney	Milk Ground egg shell Bonemeal
Sodium Na **NaCl** Chloride Cl	Together with Na it regulates blood pressure and volume. Regulates osmotic pressure and body pH or the acid–base balance	Low blood pressure Caused by vomiting, diarrhea, dehydration	Part of the salt molecule (NaCl)
Magnesium (Mg)	Important enzymes for muscle and nerve function, regulation of blood sugar levels and blood pressure. Used in the production of protein, bone, and DNA	Symptoms of extremely low levels include loss of appetite, vomiting, fatigue, weakness Can cause numbness, tingling, muscle cramps, abnormal heart rhythm, and seizures	Legumes, nuts, seeds, grains, milk
Phosphorus (P)	Along with Ca it maintains rigidity of bones and teeth. Important in cell membrane structure, provides energy at the cellular level, and is an important structural component of DNA and RNA	P can speed up kidney failure	Added as an additive to feed and is found in plants
Potassium (K)	Maintains water and acid–base balance, and osmotic pressure. Metabolizes carbohydrates and proteins. Regulates neuromuscular activity and heartbeat	In the young, slow growth, muscular weakness, stiffness, reduced heart rate, acidosis, nervous disorders, and death if totally deficient	K is found in the Earth's crust and is mined for supplements, it is also absorbed by grasses fed for livestock
Sulfur (S)	Essential component of enzymes and antioxidants that strengthen skin, hair, fur, and feathers. Important in cartilage health and the structure of proteins. Also importantin the pH balance of blood	Slow growth, reduced;milk production, and feed efficiency Severe deficiencies: anorexia, weight loss, dullness, and slow movement Excess sulfates in water can cause polioencephalomalacia (PEM) in cattle. May cause blindness, muscle tremors, difficulty walking, convulsions, and death	Forages, water, corn, gluten feed, distiller's grain

List of Ingredients

The list of ingredients is in order of quantity based on weight. Protein sources like meat are often listed first because of high water content they weighs more than meal, which has been cooked down to a powder. If the first ingredient on the label is chicken and the second is chicken meal, the FDA and AAFCO point out that if you could compare first and second ingredients on a dry matter basis, we would see that the chicken meal would have more animal protein than the first product listed had from meat. More about dry matter basis later in this chapter.

Adequacy Statement

Nutritional adequacy statement is used to help you match the pet's nutritional needs with a product. For example, Hill's™ Pet Nutrition W/D is a weight management diet formulated to help pets lose weight or

> **TABLE 7.2**
>
> **Comparison of Foods on a Dry Matter Basis**

	Purina – Dry Lamb and Rice		Purina – Canned Classic Ground Lamb and Long Grain Rice		Hill's Pet Nutrition – Advanced Fitness Lamb Meal and Rice
Crude protein (%)	26	29[a]	8	36[a]	24[a]
Crude fat (%)	16	18[a]	7	31[a]	16.5[a]
Crude fiber (%)	3	3[a]	1.5	7[a]	1.8[a]
Moisture (%)	12		78		0

[a]Dry matter (%).

as a dietary formula for diabetic dogs. The statement of nutritional levels established by AAFCO must be met for Hill's to label it as such. FDA notes that "Products labeled as premium or gourmet are not required to contain any different or higher quality ingredients, nor are they held up to any higher nutritional standards than any other complete and balanced products" (FDA 2019).

Feeding Guidelines

Feeding directions are required on pet food labels. They are set to show amounts in cups per the animal's weight. However, this is only a guide and it is recommended that you base the amount of food fed by the number of kilocalories required for that animal. Each label will include kilocalories/cup. Kilocalories are the same as calories used in human nutrition and we will use calories through the rest of this chapter, but first let's explore dry matter basis.

Dry Matter Basis

Dry matter basis is the percentage of protein, fat, and fiber once the moisture has been removed. By converting the feed basis percentage to a dry matter basis we can make an equitable comparison of food with variable moisture contents. Not only dry versus wet but also dry to dry foods. Why is this important? Pet foods with high moisture contents (canned) often show a protein percentage below 10% while its dry food counterpart is often listed at 15% or higher. Does this mean dry food has more protein than wet food? Not necessarily. If the wet food were to be condensed (removing the moisture), we would see an increase in protein because the food is less diluted. This analysis can be done with the protein, fat, and fiber in the diet. The formula for determining dry matter basis is:

Quantity/100 − moisture × 100 = ____ % in *dry* matter basis.

Let's compare three foods, two dry and one canned, two from Purina™, one dry from Hill's Pet Nutrition™, and all three with lamb and rice ingredients (Table 7.2). Note that there is more protein, fat, and fiber in the

canned product on a dry matter basis than shown on the label because of the moisture content. When we compare the two dry formulas from their lists of ingredients in the dry matter basis, they are close. Note that Hill's Pet Nutrition lists the percentages of the nutrients already in a dry matter basis, so you don't have do the conversion.

Application of Basic Nutrition

Calorie Requirements

One application of basic nutrition is to determine the **basic energy requirements (BER)** or caloric needs of an individual healthy pet. There are two rules:

1. Animals over 5kg: BER = (30 × BW in kg) + 70
2. Animal 5kg or less: BER − (60 × BW in kg) + 70

Example: The pet weighs 14lb. To fit the formula, we must determine if that is under or over 5kg. We remember from Chapter 1 how to convert pounds into kilograms so we take 14lb and divide by 2.2kg/lb = 6.36kg. Our pet weighs over 5kg, so we use rule 1. We put the patient's BW into the formula: (30 × 6.36kg) + 70 = 260.8 calories. Mark the patient's file as BER 261 calories.

If the pet is ill, injured, or has had surgery the caloric needs are usually higher to promote healing. The following are adjustments to the BER according to what is going on with the animal:

Boarding/cage rest: BER × 1.2 = ____ calories

Example: Pet from example was 261 BER × 1.2 = 313 calories

Surgery/trauma: BER × 1.3 = ____ calories
Cancer/sepsis: BER × 1.7 = ____ calories
Burns: BER × 2 = ____ calories

Learning Exercise

The patient is a 10-week-old Rottweiler puppy recovering from parvovirus. He weighs 23 lb. Determine his BER and then the additional amount he needs to recover.

Sometimes we must move the calories in the opposite direction to help a pet lose weight. The formula for that is:

Obesity: BER − 10–15%

Example: We have a cat that weighs 24 lb. To maintain that 24 lb the cat's BER would be:

$$24 lb / 2.2 kg / lb = 10.9 \text{ or } 11 kg (30 \times 11 kg) + 70$$
$$= 400 \text{ calories.}$$

To lose weight the cat needs fewer calories, so we need to subtract 10% or 15% of the calories the cat is consuming now. The first step is to convert the 10% to a decimal by dividing: 10/100 = 0.10 or 15/100 = 0.15, then multiply the current calories by the decimal point. Formula is: 100 calories × 0.10 = 40 calories. The 40 calories are subtracted from the current 400 calories to get our new BER: 400 − 40 = 360 calories.

Learning Exercise

If we want to reduce the diet by 15% how many calories would we end up with for this cat?

These formulas are something to keep in a small notebook until you have them memorized. This is good information to use on your own pets to keep them from becoming obese or getting too thin which is almost as bad.

How Much to Feed

The next thing we need to determine is how much to feed. Pet foods must have a label on the package that recommends an amount of food per pound of body weight (Figure 7.1). As you can see, the label shown in Figure 7.1 is for kitten food and has two amounts: one for kittens under 4 months of age and one for 4–6 months of age. Note that this is a daily feeding and it is recommended that you split this amount into 2–3 servings.

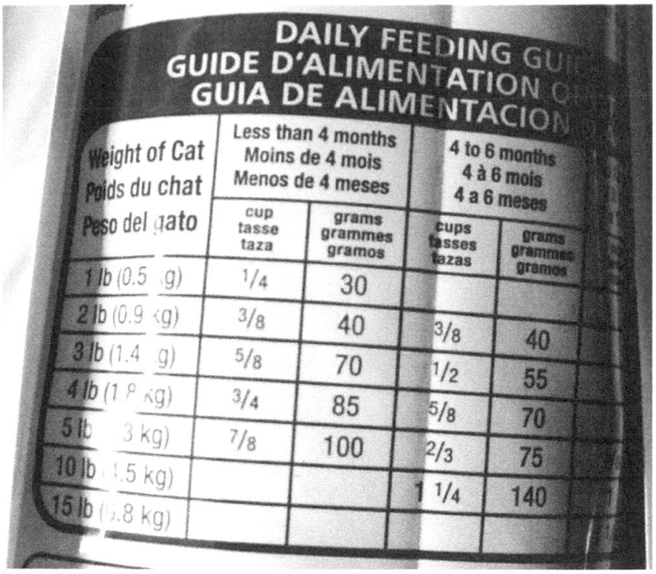

Weight of Cat Poids du chat Peso del gato	Less than 4 months Moins de 4 mois Menos de 4 meses		4 to 6 months 4 à 6 mois 4 a 6 meses	
	cup tasse taza	grams grammes gramos	cups tasses tazas	grams grammes gramos
1 lb (0.5 g)	1/4	30		
2 lb (0.9 kg)	3/8	40	3/8	40
3 lb (1.4 g)	5/8	70	1/2	55
4 lb (1.8 kg)	3/4	85	5/8	70
5 lb (3 kg)	7/8	100	2/3	75
10 lb (.5 kg)			1 1/4	140
15 lb (.8 kg)				

FIGURE 7.1 Bag label – growth formula for kittens.

Learning Exercise

- Why would there be two different amounts for a kitten that is under 4 months of age versus one that is 6 months of age?
- What are the two feeding amounts listed on the label for the following kittens: 3-month-old kitten that weighs 4 lb gets _____ cup and a 6-month-old kitten that weighs 4 lb gets _____ cup.
- To split this into two meals it would be ____ cup for the first kitten per serving and ____ cup for the second kitten per serving.

TIP BOX 7.1

To halve fractions, double the denominator and leave the numerator alone. For example, half of 1/2 cup is 1/4th.

Now let's look at the kitten food label again. See where there is a huge jump from 5 lb to 10 lb and from 10 lb to 15 lb? What happens if the kitten you are weighing is 8 lb and 5 months of age? No need to panic or guess, we can use math to help us figure it out. Let's look at the label again, we notice that a 2 lb cat at 4–6 months is to get 3/8th of a cup. We can divide the 3/8th cup in half which is 3/16th and multiply it by 8. Here is the formula (Figure 7.2).

$$\frac{8}{1} \times \frac{3}{16} = \frac{24}{16} = 24/16 = 1.5 \text{ cups}$$

1.5 cups / 2 = 0.75 or ¾ cup per serving

FIGURE 7.2 Multiplying a whole number with a fraction.

Learning Exercise

Utilize the internet to go to the Hill's Pet Nutrition, Inc website at this URL: https://www.hillspet.com/dog-food/ib-canine-natural-chicken-and-brown-rice-recipe-mature-adult-dry

Scroll down and select Average Nutrient and Calorie Content. You will see a table listing the ingredients and calories/cup. Figure out the BER for a 40 lb, 7-year-old, English Springer Spaniel and the amount in cups of food the dog should be fed daily. Then scroll up and click on Feeding Guide and check your work.

Ideal Weight of Dog Poids idéal du chien Peso ideal del perro		Weight Management Gestion du poids Manejo del peso		Maintenance Maintien du poids Mantenimiento del peso	
lb	kg	cups tasses tazas	grams grammes gramos	cups tasses tazas	grams grammes gramos
5	2.3	3/4	60		
10	4.5	1 1/4	105	7/8	70
15	6.8	1 3/4	145	1 1/2	125
20	9.1	2 1/4	185	2	165
30	14	3	245	2 1/2	205
40	18	3 2/3	300	3 1/3	275
50	23	4 1/4	350	4	330
60	27	4 3/4	390	4 3/4	390
70	32	5 1/2	450	5 1/2	450
80	36	6	495	6 1/4	515
100	45	7 1/4	595	7	575
120	54	8 1/4	680	8 1/4	680
				9 1/3	765

At Hill's, we believe that great nutrition can transform the lives of pets, and the pet parents and vets that

FIGURE 7.3 W/D dry dog food label.

Prescription Diets

There are many specialty diets referred to as prescription diets produced by various manufacturers. As the name implies, these are only available through veterinary prescription. These diets meet the special needs of individuals with different diseases or conditions. For example, low sodium diets to reduce fluid retention in patients with cardiac failure, low protein diets for kidney failure, urinary diets to reduce crystal production, and hypoallergenic diets for pets with skin or food allergies. There are diets for obese pets to lose weight, one for gastric upsets, and one for anorexic animals, and so on. These diets are usually available in dry or canned food options. They have the same information on the labels as discussed earlier and must ensure their claims of helping with these various diseases. Let's look at Hill's Pet Nutrition's W/D or Weight Management Diet. Utilize the internet to look at this diet (https://www.hillspet.com/dog-food/pd-wd-canine-dry) or see Figure 7.3.

Note that the label includes an amount for weight management meaning to lose weight, and weight control for maintenance of weight, or this diet can also be used for management of diabetes in dogs. The crude fiber, or indigestible fiber, makes the dog feel full and the protein and higher fat contents maintain a more stable blood glucose level throughout the day.

Learning Exercise

Figure out the amount of food to feed a diabetic American Cocker Spaniel that is 21 lb. Look at the recommended feeding chart and then figure out the caloric needs based upon his BER.

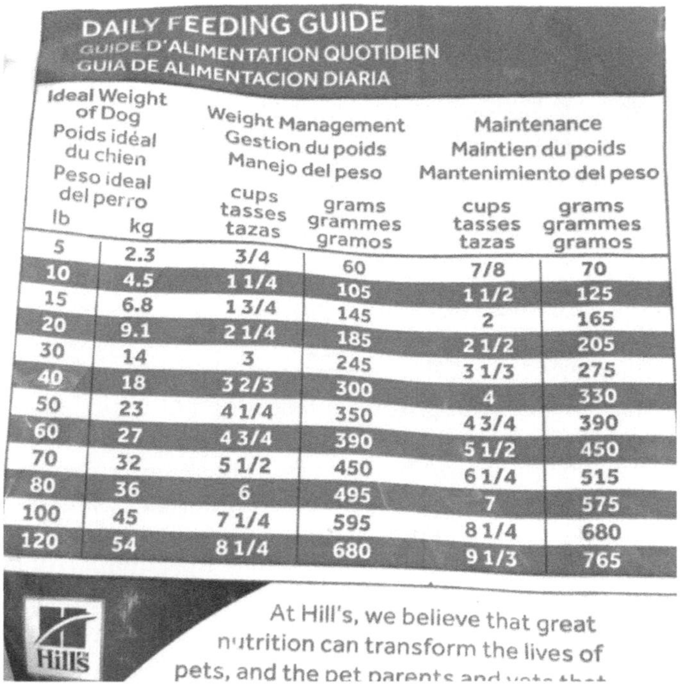

Feeding the Hospitalized Patient

There are five factors influencing patient feeding and appetite in the veterinary hospital that work against maintaining the patient's well-being:

1. Age of the patient
2. Additional nutritional requirements brought on by illness or injury: BER + calories
3. Patient's potential decreased appetite due to the illness, injury, or condition
4. Specific challenges an illness imposes on a patient
5. Unfamiliarity of the food and the environment in which it is offered

No one formulation meets the needs of all age groups. The nutritional requirements are not the same for a kitten as they are for a geriatric cat. Kittens and puppy food are fed for up to 1 year of age for most breeds. Some of the larger breed cats and large breed dogs mature later, with some taking up to 2 years to fully mature and so require kitten or puppy food for longer. From puppy and kitten food they should be transitioned to adult formulas. For dogs, the switch from adult to senior diets depends on the size of the dog. Little dogs tend to live into their teens and some make it into their twenties. Switching them to a senior diet usually takes place at 10–12 years of age. Medium-sized breeds it is usually around 7–8 years old and for large breeds 5–6 years of age. Cats should be switched from an adult to a senior food at the age of 7.

If it is your job to feed the hospitalized or boarding pets, check the record and the cage card for any specific directions on feeding the pet while in the hospital. If there isn't anything marked for food selection it is important to ask the veterinarian in case a prescription diet was intended or that food was to be withheld for a diagnostic test or surgery. Remember when figuring out how much to feed an ill or injured patient you need to find the basic BER and then add in the extra calories depending upon their illness or injury. For boarding pets, a quick check of the record will tell you its age and you can go from there for food selection. Sometimes owners will bring their own food in for a boarding pet, especially if they are on a particular diet.

Anorexic patients are the most challenging because not eating isn't an option! It slows down healing and it is especially detrimental if cats don't eat. Cats cannot go without eating for more than a few days. When they refuse to eat or cannot eat, they may develop a potentially fatal condition known as **hepatic lipidosis**. Alert the veterinarian about a cat that refuses to eat at the first refused meal, then keep a careful eye on the patient. You may apply the following techniques to both dogs and cats if they are not eating well or not eating at all.

First look at the circumstances the pet is in. Is it feeling threatened by others? Try hanging a towel over the cage door when feeding. Try using pheromone sprays that induce calm, or try setting it next to a good eater which may stimulate the reluctant pet to eat for fear of losing its portion. Check for other environmental issues. Some cats will not eat next to a litter box, especially one that has been used. Clean the box and try again or let the cat eat in an empty kennel, then return it to its assigned cage and clean the dining kennel. Sometimes the pet just simply misses home. Having an article of clothing worn by their owner or their favorite blanket in the kennel will make them feel less anxious.

A second thing to try is to increase the **palatability** of the food. Heating food slightly increases its aroma and flavor. Be mindful of using the microwave as too hot will turn them away and may cause a painful burn. Mixing a small amount of water and heating a patient's food sometimes increases acceptance. Blending it in a food processor or blender until smoothie consistency may also tempt some to eat. Cats smell their food more than taste it so offering some "stinky fish food" may do the trick. Placing a small dab of food on their paws or tip of the nose may get them to taste the food and stimulate them to eat. Be aware that if there is nasal congestion, they may not be able to smell the food. Clean the **nares** with a warm wash cloth, and maybe a few drops of saline into the nostrils will help clear the mucus. If thick, a nasal bulb syringe can be used to **aspirate** the discharge. Always check with the veterinarian before doing this.

A third attempt is force feeding. This sounds like you jam a bunch of food down the throat, but it really needs to be extremely gentle and slow. Place the food at eye level with the pet. Some patients will begin to eat on their own after the first few mouthfuls of being fed. Dip your finger into the food and gently open the patient's mouth and rub the food against the roof the mouth. Allow the patient time to process what just happened and the food itself, if it decides to swallow, offer the dish, if it doesn't try to eat try another dab on the hard pallet. If using food from the refrigerator warming it slightly before offering it or force feeding it will help the process. Warm food is digested easier as well.

Another technique is to use a food that is designed to be given by syringe or to liquify the diet in a blender. Steps to syringe or force feeding a patient are:

- Fill a syringe with the food
- Place the tip in the corner of the mouth adjacent to the back teeth
- Push the corner of the mouth forward to make a pouch
- Tip the nose up slightly and squirt the food slowly into the pouch
- Allow the patient to swallow before continuing with more food

This can be extremely taxing to the patient, so it is a good idea to break the feedings into smaller amounts and feed throughout the day. Stressing the patient out can cause them to continue to refuse food. Be patient; always feed slowly to prevent **aspiration** of the food. Make careful notations in the patient's records on amounts and times of feeding. Never fight with an animal over food, it wears them out and they may develop a learned aversion to food. Alert the veterinarian if the animal puts up a fight as there are other alternatives to force feeding with a syringe.

If all feeding efforts fail the veterinarian may decide to insert a **nasogastric** or **pharyngostomy tube**. This is a tube that is inserted into the nares or through a small incision in the neck, and down the esophagus until the tip enters the stomach. The tube is secured over the top of the patient's head or neck with sutures and a bandage. Liquefied food is injected through the tube as needed allowing for easier feeding. The nasogastric tube is used for short periods of time and the pharyngostomy tube is for long-term feeding.

Both tube placements require maintenance so they do not plug up from the diet being injected. Before and after feeding they should be flushed with a small amount of water. You can discuss how much per flush with the veterinarian because a cat will not need as much as a Great Dane! Clean the tip off with warm water and a paper towel. Make sure the cap on the end of tube is on securely. Clean any drips from the bandage material to keep it from becoming foul smelling.

Remember the amount of food to be fed should be calculated based upon the patient's BER + illness, injury, or condition. It is important to keep careful records of how much was eaten and when in the patient's record. Monitoring urine and fecal output is also important. What goes in must come out and sometimes there is a problem with that process and if missed can create another whole set of problems. Alert the veterinarian if the patient is not eliminating properly.

Open food cans should be labeled with the open date, whom it is for, and your initials, then placed in the refrigerator for storage. This is not only to make sure the patient is fed properly, or food is wasted, but also for billing reasons. It is important to recoup the expense of feeding a special diet. Another reason is if sending the diet home with the patient they get their can or if the patient has gone home the diet can be thrown.

Water Availability and Consumption

Water is not considered a nutrient but is essential to life. Without water a patient becomes **dehydrated** quickly and if severe enough can lead to death. The smaller the patient the quicker the level of dehydration. Water must always be accessible and in adequate volume unless otherwise specified. Check water frequently throughout the day, refill before it is gone. Access should be easy for all patients. Small puppies and kittens might not be able to reach into a standard water bowl so select one that is shallow enough, so they can reach. If the water dishes are held in place by a bracket, the screws holding it in place can be loosened and the bracket lowered to allow easier access for shorter adult patients. Pocket pets drink out of sippy tubes attached to bottles. These tend to go empty quickly or if they leak the animal can be without water quickly. Check and if bottles are empty figure out if it is from a leak before refilling; you may have to replace it with a new cork or bottle.

Spilling of water is a huge issue for two reasons: (i) the animal doesn't have access to water; and (ii) it makes the kennel wet. Both are uncomfortable situations that no pet should be exposed to for any great length of time. Checking the kennels throughout the day will catch these mishaps and correcting them immediately is important. If the water is spilled utilizing standard water bowls, perhaps it could be changed out for a heavy crock type bowl or a dish or pail that can be attached to the kennel door. Sometimes you must get creative if there aren't the options describe above. A appropriately sized rock scrubbed clean may weigh down a bowl enough to keep it from tipping. Make sure it isn't so big that it displaces too much water and big enough that it can't be swallowed! Whatever the choice, ensure the patient has enough water for a 12-hour period.

If the patient isn't drinking alert the veterinarian of this development. He/she may decide to administer fluids either orally or by subcutaneous or IV infusion. Water is given orally by syringe and utilizes the same technique described for liquid food. Subcutaneous fluids are given under the skin with a needle attached to an IV drip set which is attached to an IV bag of fluids. Approximately 25–50 mL per subcutaneous location can be given depending on the size of the patient. The location is usually along the side, where there is excess skin. IV fluids require a catheter to be placed into a vein, often the cephalic vein. Careful monitoring is required to make sure the catheter is not pulled out or dislodged. Careful monitoring and speed of the amount of IV fluids is very important. If given too fast the fluids are not absorbed and may migrate to the lungs causing fluid overload symptoms.

Fluids are usually calculated upon the animal's weight and depth of dehydration. The daily amount of fluid is administered throughout the day in evenly divided amounts. Marking the IV bag with a sharpie pen or a piece of adhesive tape that includes amounts, times for infusion, and rates helps to ensure that the fluid amounts are administered correctly.

Feeding Livestock and Poultry

The same rules apply to feeding livestock and poultry as to all other animals. A clean, fresh source of water available always is just as important to them as it is to companion animals. When it is hot outside check more often as animals will consume more water than usual. When it is cold outside make sure the water hasn't frozen. If it is freezing a heater designed to keep the water warm can be added to the bucket or tank.

Livestock require the same nutrients, although in differing amounts, as carnivores. Livestock gain their nutrients from plants, grains, and supplements. The mixture of forages, grains silage, and supplements is called a ration which is balanced carefully to provide nutrition for the animal. Forage, also known as roughage, makes up the bulk of their diet and can be the main source of nutrition. Forage is grass and grain plants that are often baled as hay and fed in racks or the animal is turned out in pastures where it grazes on its own. Grains, including oats, wheat, and corn are also used to supplement livestock rations and provide a boost in protein, especially poultry. Silage is another form of food fed to livestock and consists of the entire corn plant ground up and stored in a pit. Supplements are often fed in the form of blocks that are set out with access ad lib or they are mixed into the grain ration. The blocks can be pure salt or a mixture of minerals. This book cannot cover even the basics in balancing a ration for livestock. If interested check to see if any local colleges have a livestock feeding course or see if there is one available online. Many county extension agencies have information for balancing rations as well.

Your job as a veterinary assistant may include feeding the livestock. Checking the quality of the feed before feeding is important. Forage in the form of hay should smell of green meadows freshly mowed. It should appear dry and leafy without excess thistles, other weeds, or woody stems. Moldy feed, excessive weeds, and dust can be detrimental to the animal's health. Mold appears as a dark, powdery substance or as white, wet slime on the forage and will have a "moldy" smell. Moldy food and excessively weedy forage will often be rejected, thus putting the animal at risk for not getting enough nutrition. If it is eaten it can cause digestive issues. Dust can be inhaled and cause wheezing and coughing. Alert the inventory manager of the issues so that clean food can be ordered.

Visiting a livestock food store is an educational experience. Reading labels to determine contents of the feed, looking at baled products for content and smell are both ways to learn about feeding livestock and poultry.

Feeding Other Species

Pocket pets are usually easy to care for by simply feeding them the foods developed specifically for their species. These can be purchased from any wholesale distributor, so your inventory manager will have a good source to go to for ordering food. A word about guinea pigs, they are unable to synthesize vitamin C and so must get it as a supplement either in vitamin C drops or in their food. If purchasing food with vitamin C added, make sure it is fresh as the vitamin C does have a short expiration date. It is often better to purchase vitamin C treats or feed foods high in vitamin C if a guinea pig is hospitalized. Ferrets are full on carnivores and like cats require high

quantities of proteins and fats. Feeding a quality cat food to these animals is acceptable.

Chapter Reflection

Process the information from this chapter and describe what you learned, what surprised you, or what made you think.

References

Association of American Feed Control Officials (AAFCO). 2012a. How to understand a dog or cat food label. 2012a. https://talkspetfood. aafco.org/readinglabels (accessed June 29, 2019).

Association of American Feed Control Officials (AAFCO). 2012b. What are byproducts? https://talkspetfood.aafco.org/byproducts (accessed June 29, 2019).

Association of American Feed Control Officials (AAFCO). 2012c. What's in the ingredients list? https://talkspetfood.aafco.org/ whatisinpetfood (accessed June 29, 2019).

Food and Drug Administration. 2019. Animal health literacy, pet food labels – general. https://www.fda.gov/animal-veterinary/animal-health-literacy/pet-food-labels-general#Claims (accessed July 12, 2019).

Suggested Reading

Anon. Choosing the right food for your senior dog. *MedicAnimal.* https://www.medicanimal.com/Choosing-the-right-food-for-your-senior-dog/a/ART111515 (accessed June 29, 2019).

Anon. Dry matter basis calculator for pet food. *Paw Diet* 2018. https:// www.pawdiet.com/articles/dry-matter-basis-calculator-for-pet-food/ (accessed June 29, 2019).

Anon. How to reading a pet food label. *Hill.'s Pet* 2019. https://www. hillspet.com/dog-care/nutrition-feeding/how-to-read-dog-food-labels (accessed June 29, 2019).

Anon. Unwholesome ingredients in your dog's food? *Tufts Your Dog* 2017. http://news.vet.tufts.edu/2017/02/unwholesome-ingredients-in-your-dogs-food/ (accessed June 29, 2019).

Danks L. The role of calcium and phosphorus. *Veterinary Practice* 2014. https://veterinary-practice.com/article/the-roles-of-calcium-and-phosphorus (accessed June 29, 2019).

Mandal A. What is metabolism? *News Medical Life Sciences* 2019. https:// www.news-medical.net/life-sciences/What-is-Metabolism.aspx (accessed June 29, 2019).

Martin LJ. Dietary fats explained. *Medline Plus* 2018. https:// medlineplus.gov/ency/patientinstructions/000104.htm (accessed June 29, 2019).

CHAPTER 8

Restraint of Animals

LEARNING OBJECTIVES

- Assess the species for behavior and safely approach
- Utilize fear free techniques for exams and procedures
- Safely move patients from one location to another
- Apply appropriate restraint per procedure being performed while utilizing appropriate restraint equipment as needed and adapting restraint techniques as per patient's reaction

NAVTA ESSENTIAL SKILLS COVERED IN THIS CHAPTER

IV. Examination Room Procedures
A. Restrain patients
   1. Small animals
      a. place and remove small animals from cages
      b. place and restrain small animals on tables and floor
      c. apply dog and cat safety muzzle
      d. apply Elizabethan collar
      e. apply restraint pole
      f. demonstrate standing, sitting, lateral, sternal, and dorsal restraint positions
      g. recognize when to alter normal restraint for compromised patients in the exam room (i.e. ringworm, contagious diseases, ectoparasite infestation) and describe appropriate action or personnel to notify
   2. Restrain birds, rabbits, pocket pets, reptiles, and other exotics (optional)
   3. Large animals (optional)
      a. halter, tie, and lead horses
      b. restrain cattle and horses

Tasks for the Veterinary Assistant, Fourth Edition. Teresa F. Sonsthagen.
© 2020 John Wiley & Sons, Inc. Published 2020 by John Wiley & Sons, Inc.
Companion website: www.wiley.com/go/sonsthagen/tasks

Physical restraint increases the competency of the veterinarian and technicians. If used effectively it reduces patient stress and prevents harm to all. A calm, confident attitude by a patient's handlers reassures an animal and elicits cooperation. Loss of temper, yelling, or hitting can result in injury to staff or patient and is never appropriate. Skilled handlers always control their emotions and treat animals kindly but firmly and patiently.

Although this chapter covers some of the major methods of physical restraint for dogs, cats, pocket pets, livestock, and horses, the reader is directed to texts, websites, and videotapes devoted in their entirety to animal restraint. Supplementary resources are listed at the end of the chapter.

Restraint is much like ballroom dancing – it is a coordinated effort. The veterinarian or technician takes the lead; the assistant follows. In following, the assistant must anticipate the actions of the other staff member and respond so smoothly that the movements of the two are seamless. For example, as a patient is lifted to the exam table the restraint (*dance*) begins and must be maintained until the examination is complete and the animal is returned to the floor (*music ends*).

There are some basic rules to observe while you are in charge of restraint:

1. Never take your hands or eyes off the patient. Watch and listen to the patient for cues to it becoming upset.
2. Be aware of what the other personnel are doing; watch, listen, and anticipate their next moves.
3. Pay attention to the patient's body language. Make modifications in restraint techniques to respond to changes in the patient's attitude.
4. Modify the restraint technique to present the body part that needs to be examined. This means you will be constantly changing the position of the patient and the restraint technique used.
5. Use your whole body when restraining, not just your hands.
6. If you are losing control, let people know; "I'm losing it, or it is slipping out of my hand!" Never just let go as that is how people get hurt. Try to hang on as long as you can and perhaps that may be all the time needed to complete the procedure.
7. *Always use minimum amounts of restraint first.* Distraction techniques, easy handling from the beginning of the procedure, and advancing only as needed.

Reflection

Think of how a patient would feel if handled roughly and without compassion. How would they react? How would they feel? Then think of how you can alleviate those reactions and feelings as you learn restraint and then as you practice it throughout your career. How will you best learn "the dance" when it comes time to restrain a patient for a procedure?

Restraint of Companion Animals

Restraint in the veterinary clinic has under gone a revolution of sorts. Gone are the days were we immediately placed a companion animal into a restraint hold the moment their feet hit the exam table. Research has shown this made pets and owners extremely anxious, to the point where both dreaded going to the veterinary office. The current trend is to make the visits as stress and fear free as possible.

This doesn't mean that you never hold a leg or head, it just means that we are going to be more mindful of how soon and how long those holds will last. It also means we will be more mindful when an animal struggles. We used to think "never give up, never surrender" when we restrained a patient, but now we release a patient after a certain length of struggle time and after several tries. Instead, we try different holds, some restraint equipment and, if those fail, chemical restraint may be needed such as sedatives, tranquilizers, or general anesthesia. These drugs are safe to use on just about all patients and many of them have reversal agents that clear the effects from the patient, so they go home without feeling groggy or semi-conscious.

Patient Defenses

Before we go further, we need to discuss the arsenal of natural weapons animals bring to the table. Cats and ferrets have sharp canines (Figure 8.1) and claws that create deep punctures that often become infected. Both tend to bite numerous times and rake with their claws when fighting. Ferrets will often bite and not let go – you may have to put them under running water or dunk them into water to make them let go!

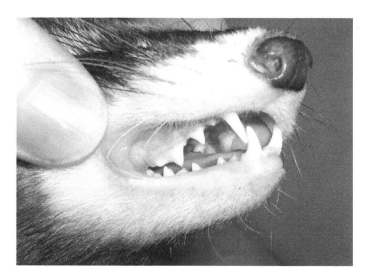

FIGURE 8.1 Ferret dentition. Source: https://commons.wikimedia.org/wiki/File:Buffy_teeth.jpg. Public Domain.

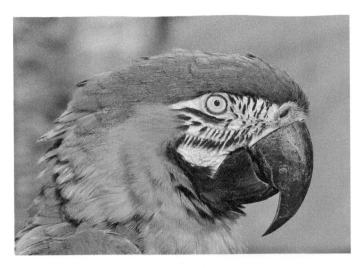

FIGURE 8.2 Parrot beak. Source: Wikimedia Commons. Used under CC-BY-SA 3.0, https://commons.wikimedia.org/wiki/File:Ara_ararauna_qtl3.jpg.

Assessing Behavior and Safely Approaching Companion Animals

As we first deal with a patient we want to keep three things in mind to ensure the safety of the people involved and the safety and well-being of the patient. These are not in any order; they are all equally important:; field of vision, body language, and species characteristics of prey versus predator behavior.

There are two types of animals; those that are **prey animals** and those that are **predators**. Each have different behaviors that have evolved to keep them from dying, prey animals from being eaten by predators and predators from starving! All animals have the "fight or flight" response to danger, meaning they will try to get away but if cornered will fight. Figure 8.3 shows both responses in action; the dog is in flight and the cat is in fight response.

Dogs have large canine teeth that cause deep punctures, and molars that crush tissue causing bruises. Plus, they tend to hang on and shake their heads while biting which causes rips and more damage to the underlying tissues. Birds will use their beaks; some, like the large parrots, are so strong they can amputate fingers (Figure 8.2). Some birds have pointy beaks that can pluck an eyeball out. Rodents have large, long front teeth and will often bite when handled, which is painful but not life-threatening. Horses and cattle are accurate with their feet and will kick or stomp on you. Cattle, sheep, and goats all use their heads as battering rams.

This information is not to scare you into giving up your dream of working with animals, it is simply to bring awareness that we, in comparison, are puny and weak! We need to use our heads and all our senses including our intuition for self-preservation when approaching animals to feed, care for, or perform a procedure! Fortunately, we have big brains and if you are smarter than the animal and can utilize the following knowledge you may survive without being hurt or getting others hurt. Never underestimate an animal or believe that they couldn't possibly hurt you, they may not set out to do so but careless handlers can cause the animal to become fearful or aggressive.

Reflection

What animal defenses have you the most nervous or scared? How do you see yourself overcoming these fears?

Reflection

Can you think of other patients seen by veterinary clinics that can be classified as prey or predators?

However, not all will respond in the same manner. Prey animals tend to respond to danger at a greater distance than predators, moving away from perceived danger quickly before they must defend themselves. We can use this characteristic when we need to move prey animals from one point to another. We also keep this in mind when working with predators so that we don't inadvertently corner them, thus causing a fight.

Approach an animal within its field of vision to avoid causing them to startle. All animals will startle if a person suddenly appears from their blind spot. Speak up to let them know you are there before coming into range, touch gently and with confidence after you have announced your presence.

Prey companion animals are rodents, rabbits, and birds (although some are predators, these are usually not kept as pets). Their eyes are placed at each side of the skull providing a wide **peripheral** field of vision such that their visual field extends far out to the sides of the body with only a small blind spot directly in front of their face and directly behind their rear end. This wide range of vision allows them to see something approaching from the side without moving their head (Figure 8.4). For example, the rabbit, as a prey animal, has a wide range of vision to each side that narrows straight ahead of its face. Rabbits will use both eyes to view what is directly in front of them. However, there is a blind spot directly in the middle of their face and directly along their back which extends behind their rear end.

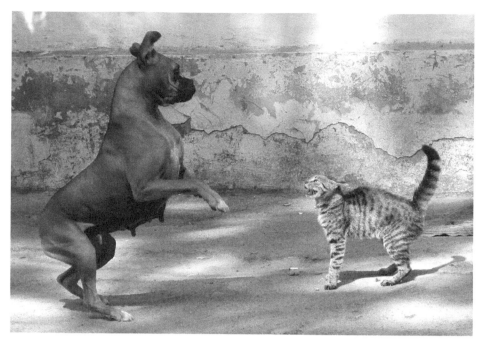

FIGURE 8.3 Flight and fight response. Source: Wikimedia Commons. Used under CC-BY-SA 2.0, https://commons.wikimedia.org/wiki/File:This_was_a_timely_capture_(3926001309).jpg.

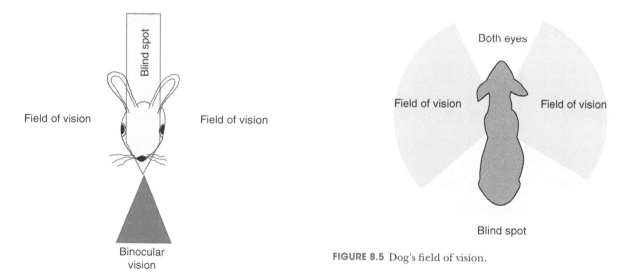

FIGURE 8.4 Rabbit's field of vision.

FIGURE 8.5 Dog's field of vision.

Dogs, cats, and ferrets are carnivores and so their eyes are more forward on their faces. This gives them slightly less peripheral vision than the prey animals (Figure 8.5). Their blind spot is also bigger. They cannot see much past their shoulder when looking straight ahead but use both eyes to see right in front of them, thus not having much of a blind spot to the front. Knowing the field of vision of animals allows a handler to approach safely.

As the handler approaches an animal it is important to assess their behavior. Animals use body language to communicate with each other and by learning what that body language is saying we can assess behavior and approach the animal safely. Let's discuss dogs and cats separately.

Most of the dogs we deal with are friendly towards people and are easy enough to approach without too much concern. However, if you don't know the dog it is best to consider them to be potentially aggressive and approach with caution. We can use our body language to avoid stimulating aggressive dogs and to calm nervous dogs when approaching. We will want to use what the fear free initiative calls the "considerate approach" such as kneeling on one knee and offering a treat for all friendly, nervous, or scared dogs. Speak kindly, avoid direct eye contact, and reach under their chin to give a bit of a gentle scratch as the other hand is offering a treat. If the contact is accepted in a friendly manner proceed to either picking the animal up or moving it into position on the floor.

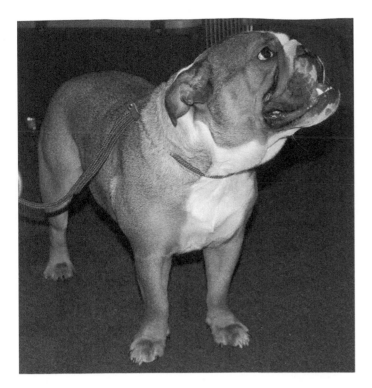

FIGURE 8.6 Friendly dog. Source: Wikimedia Commons. Used under CC-BY-SA 3.0, https://commons.wikimedia.org/wiki/File:Buldog_angielsi_671.jpg.

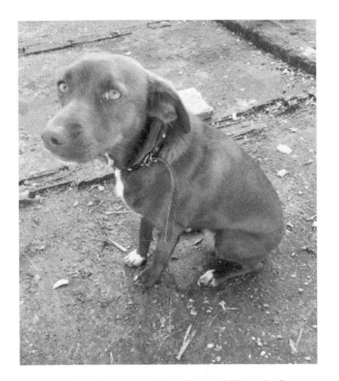

FIGURE 8.7 Submissive or scared dog. Source: Wikimedia Commons. Used under CC-BY-SA 3.0, https://commons.wikimedia.org/wiki/File:Alertita.jpg.

If we approach a dog with our bodies turned full frontal to them and make direct eye contact, this is dog speak for "I'm the dominant one here and let me show

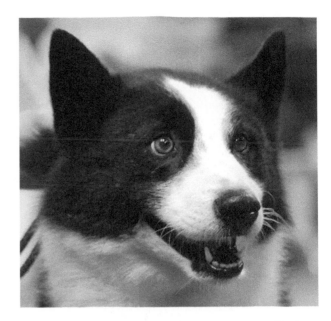

FIGURE 8.8 Nervous dog. Source: Wikimedia Commons. Used under CC-BY-SA 2.5, https://commons.wikimedia.org/wiki/File:Karelski_pies_na_nied%C5%BAwiedzie_LM.jpg.

you why." It is a flat-out challenge and the dog can either accept the challenge or feel threatened by it, both resulting in a defensive response! It is very important to determine the dog's personality before you approach. For this we use their body language.

The body language between friendly, submissive, nervous or scared, and aggressive dogs is good to learn and once you get the signals down it gets easier to discern. Of course, the friendly dog will greet you with tail wagging, an open mouth, and a happy expression on their face (Figure 8.6). Submissive dogs may approach you with their whole body tucked, shoulders hunched, tail held tightly between their back legs almost curling themselves in as if to protect their rear ends (which they are), ears lowered, and a sideways body position to your body (Figure 8.7). Submissive dogs may whimper and roll on their backs at your feet. A nervous or scared dog will be jumpy, with ears flicking from up to plastered to the side of their heads. They may be panting and shivering, the **sclera** clearly visible around their eyes which they dart around the room trying to watch everything at once (Figure 8.8). With these dogs, it is easier to push them

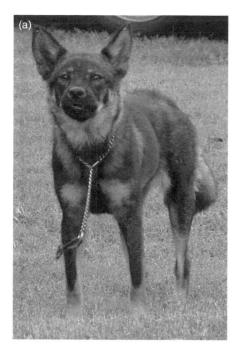
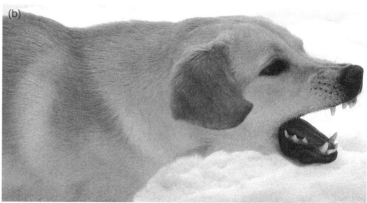

FIGURE 8.9 Aggressive dog body language: (a) showing mild aggression, with mouth open, eyes and ears directed forward, tail straight out from body, and front legs spread wide; (b) hackles raised, head even with shoulders, mouth snarling, eyes and ears directed at antagonist. Source: Wikimedia Common. Used under CC BY-SA 2.0, https://commons.wikimedia.org/wiki/File:Labrador_Growl.jpg; https://commons.wikimedia.org/wiki/File:2003-09-08_Dog_showing_aggression.jpg.

into flight or fight. Let them approach you first, offer treats and kind words, move slowly and confidently.

Aggressive dogs will often try to engage your eyesight, be aware of this and avert your gaze either at their feet or over the top of their heads. Use your peripheral vision to look at them. Aggressive body language includes the head lowered even with the shoulders, ruff standing on end, and often their tails are straight out from their bodies (Figure 8.9). Eyes and ears will be pointed at you and their tail may or may not be wagging.

It is to be hoped that the aggressive dog will be identified and come with a muzzle already in place. However, any dog can be pushed into biting and so listen to your instincts. If you feel like the dog is potentially a biter or may bite because of the procedure, a muzzle can be placed on the dog in a fear free manner, which is discussed a bit later in the chapter.

Approaching cats can be very easy or it can be very hard. The fear free method is to allow the cat to acclimatize itself to the room by roaming around and exploring for a bit. This often puts a cat at ease and, being a cat, it will often end up on the exam table by its own volition. This is the time to slip in and offer a treat. A cat that has been brought into the clinic in a carrier should not be unceremoniously dumped out onto the table, nor do you reach in and pull it out. It is recommended that the entire lid be removed and then an assessment of its behavior can be made. If the cat choses to walk out on its own it is allowed to go exploring as just discussed. Otherwise the ensconced cat is examined and treated

TIP BOX 8.1

When allowing a cat to explore the exam room make sure all the doors are shut and the staff side door should have an indicator about a cat being loose in the room.

while hunkered down in its "safe place," in this case the carrier.

It is important to read a cat's body language and if the cat is scared, nervous, excited, or aggressive prepare other ways of handling the cat, which are discussed later. For now, Figures 8.10–8.13 provide a description and visualization of body language that can help you know what the cat is feeling. Remember that cats vocalize in several ways so listen as well as observe!

A relaxed cat may or may not be purring, irises will be at normal dilation, whiskers lowered, often laying on its side with feet extended (Figure 8.10). Vocalization will often be a purr. This not a worried cat.

Cats show annoyance by hooding or closing their eyelids to slits, they often move to a **sternal** position, as if to be ready to jump up and move (Figure 8.11). Whiskers will be up but not straight out at this point. Ears may move from flat to erect. However, it will not take much to push this cat into becoming angry. A soft coaxing voice, an offered treat, and very gentle handling may bring them around to relaxing. Vocalization may be a low grumble.

Figure 8.12 is a montage of pictures showing the various reactions of cats to unsettling experiences. The cat

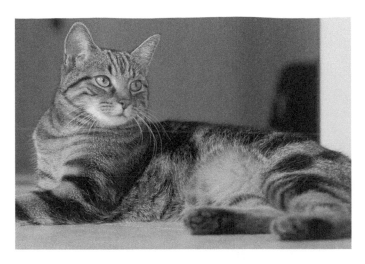

FIGURE 8.10 Relaxed cat. Source: https://commons.wikimedia.org/wiki/File:European_shorthair_procumbent_Quincy.jpg. Public Domain.

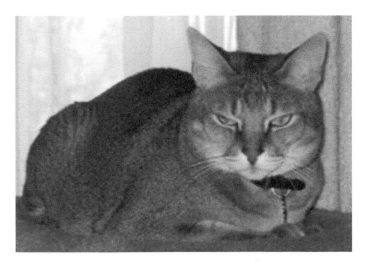

FIGURE 8.11 Annoyed cat. Source: Wikimedia Commons. Used under CC-BY-SA 3.0, https://commons.wikimedia.org/wiki/File:Chausiecatexample.jpg.

in Figure 8.12a has a startled appearance; whiskers straight out, body positioned to escape, irises narrowed to a slit. The kitten in Figure 8.12b is nervous or scared, body position is hunched in order to move quickly, whiskers are straight out and its vocalizing. Both may or may not be exhibiting the hair standing on end along its back, like the photo in Figure 8.12c. This can indicate anxious, scared, nervous, excitement, or anger; you must take it in context of the situation. The cat in Figure 8.12d is a bit harder to determine, is it stupefied, resigned to its fate, or ready to explode? The context of the picture is that it is being examined at a cat show by a judge. The fully dilated eyes and whiskers pulled down may indicate nerves, excitement, or maybe even enjoyment. This picture demonstrates that we don't always know what the cat is feeling and so a person needs to be ready for anything when dealing with not only cats but all animals.

Look and listen; a low-pitched growl that seems to be coming from deep within may be your first warning of impending cat explosion. Stop what you are doing to avoid escalating into a very angry cat. The cat in Figure 8.13 is very obviously upset and angry. Back arched, hair standing on end, hissing or screaming vocalization, whiskers straight out and up, foot poised to strike. No one wins at this point, it is better to let the cat calm down and perhaps discuss sedation options with the veterinarian.

Learning Exercise

As you go through your daily life, pay attention to body language. Dogs, cats, and people! What does their body language tell you? Are they friendly, scared, nervous, aggressive?

Ferrets are gregarious and curious about their surroundings. However, they may be scared if not used to car rides or strangers. Allow them to walk out of the carrier and explore a bit. Be aware, however, that they can fit themselves into tiny spaces and will be extremely difficult to remove if they feel cornered. Once on the exam table, a smear of peanut butter on the ventral abdomen will keep them busy for general exams and often subcutaneous injections.

Aggressive behavior can be aroused by fear, pain, territorial instincts, dominance behavior, sex drive, and maternal protection of young. These stresses lower tolerance limits, so selection of restraint techniques based upon these behaviors is highly recommended in order not to push an animal into aggressive behaviors.

Fear and pain will cause all animals to lash out. They do not always understand that you are trying to help. Extreme care must be taken to ensure not only the animal's safety, but also that of the personnel doing the work. Sedation or tranquilizers are usually the only choice at this point to handle the animal safely.

Territorial instincts in both dogs and cats are often forgotten about. Cats establish their territory very quickly and a calm cat put into a kennel may turn into a very angry cat because you are infringing on its territory (i.e., the kennel). This may also be the reason why cats refuse to come out of carriers and get quite upset when the carrier is "invaded." Dogs will also establish territory and become "cage aggressive." They may lunge, barking and growling at other dogs as they pass by. A towel or blanket placed over the door of the kennel is one way to keep the peace. That and placing these dogs at the very end of the room so passers-by are limited will help. Dogs and birds are also hierarchical. This is where a top animal leads and everyone else falls in line. The point is when introducing a new animal into the pack or flock it is

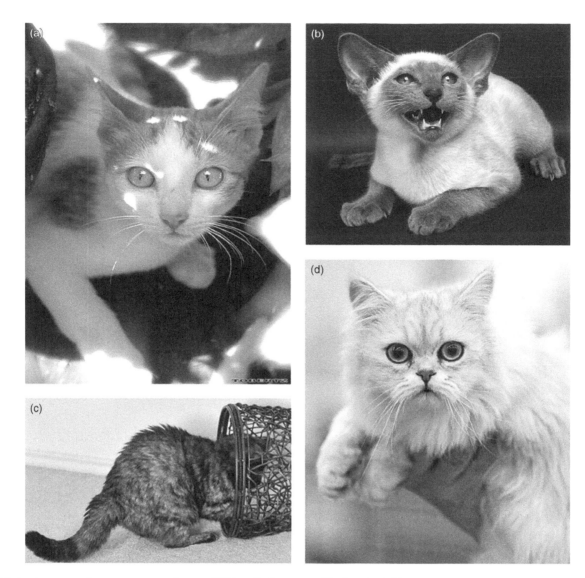

FIGURE 8.12 Anxious, scared, or nervous cats. Source: Wikimedia Commons. Used under CC BY-SA 3.0, https://en.wikipedia.org/wiki/Cat_communication#/media/File:Siam_blue_point.jpg; https://commons.wikimedia.org/wiki/File:Surprised_cat.jpg; https://commons.wikimedia.org/wiki/File:Abby_playing_in_basket.jpg; https://en.wikipedia.org/wiki/List_of_cat_breeds#/media/File:Tiffanie_at_cat_show.jpg.

important to know that a fight may erupt, and you don't want to be caught in the middle of a rumble! This is avoided or reduced by introducing animals with cages close enough for the animals to smell and look at each other but not to have physical contact with each other.

Sex drive in males can be an overpowering urge that can turn normally very docile animals into very aggressive animals if you are the one keeping them from their target. Maternal instinct also has a very strong effect on behavior, again even the most docile animal will become aggressive if their offspring is being "attacked." From a human's perspective this may be just a wish to pet the youngster! Dogs, cats, and ferrets bear young that spend the first few weeks of life blind, deaf and helpless, totally dependent on their mother for survival. Mothers can be defensive of their young and often get quite agitated when their young vocalize. If procedures such as tail docking or dewclaw removal is to be carried out it is best to take puppies to a back room, so the mother can't hear them. Excessive handling of newborn kittens can sometimes cause the mother to eat her young. Again, this is a defense mechanism, although we may think it is horrible. It is best to leave the family alone until the newborns open their eyes and ears and are becoming mobile.

Reflection

Think about all of the instinctual behaviors patients have: maternal instincts, territorial instincts, and sex drive. Why do these make such an impact on how a patient may behave?

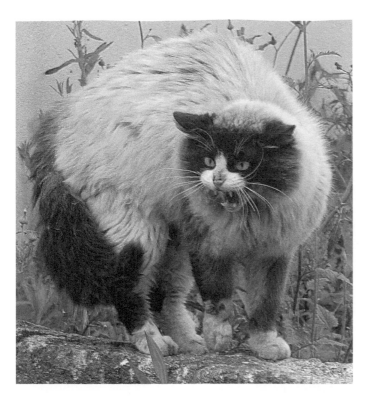

FIGURE 8.13 Very angry cat. Source: Wikimedia Commons. Used under CC-BY 2.0, https://commons.wikimedia.org/wiki/File:Gato_enervado_pola_presencia_dun_can.jpg.

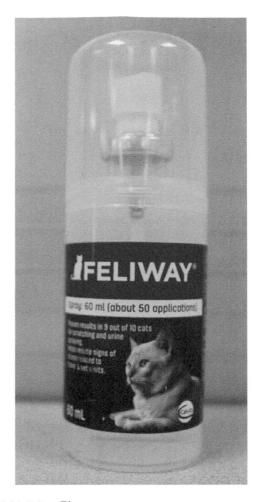

FIGURE 8.14 Feliway™ spray.

Restraint procedures need to be modified if patients are contagious in any manner. All personnel should be made aware of the possible contagion so that proper clothing items can be adorned before coming into contact with these animals. A lab coat over scrubs or coveralls and gloves are the usual PPE required. After the patient has been seen, proper disinfecting of the room is an absolute must. If the patient had fleas, an insecticide formulated to kill fleas should be used.

Utilize Fear Free Techniques

The fear free approach was initiated by Dr. Marty Becker with the mission to: "prevent and alleviate fear, anxiety and stress in pets, by inspiring and educating the people who care for them" (https://fearfreepets.com). This program brought together experts from across the field of veterinary medicine, animal trainers, shelter personnel, animal boarding and daycare owners, groomers, and pet owners to develop programs for fear free veterinary clinics, fear free homes, and fear free trainers and other pet professionals. The programs award a certification after completion.

The goal is to provide care to animals that may be sick or injured without causing undo stress from being handled aggressively, which in many cases induces fear, stress, and anxiety, not only in the pets but the owners as well. This movement is catching on across the country and by enrolling in the online courses you increase your value as a veterinary assistant.

We have already mentioned how to greet a dog or cat using fear free techniques, but it really starts before the animal walks into the room. All traces of the animal before it should be erased. This means wiping down all the surfaces in the exam room, including the chair, with a disinfectant or deodorant spray and paper towels and sweeping the floor free of hair and other debris, then using a pheromone spray to induce calm such as Feliway™ for cats or Adaptil™ for dogs (Figure 8.14). Spritz the room after each visit and your clothing once or twice a day. If using a towel for the exam table, which is recommended, spritz that with the spray as well.

Dogs are greeted while they are still on the floor. The assistant kneels into a considerate position and offers a "low end" treat. These are usually hard biscuits broken into a few pieces. While being offered with one hand the other is reaching under the neck to offer up a little gentle scratch. If accepted, the dog can be lifted to the table with another treat offered as soon as its feet touch the table. If the hard biscuit isn't accepted, then a soft chewy treat is offered and if that is not accepted then perhaps Kong™ filling or cheese spray on an applicator

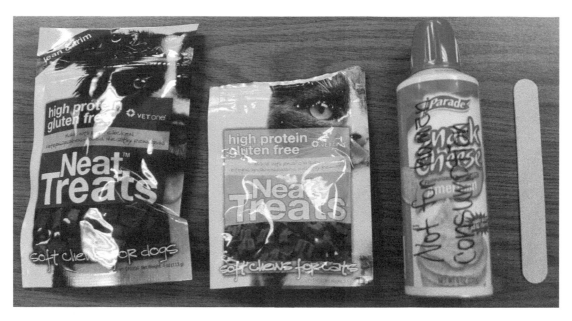

FIGURE 8.15 Range of treats.

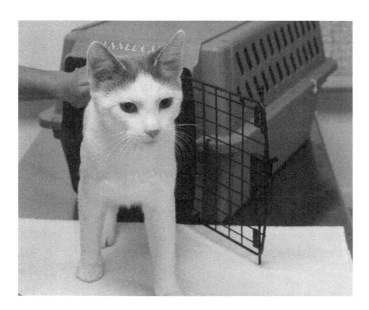

FIGURE 8.16 Cat leaving carrier.

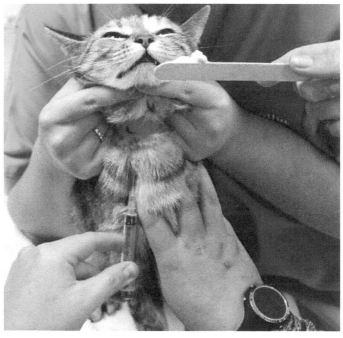

FIGURE 8.17 Using treats and blowing to distract from a procedure.

stick is offered (Figure 8.15). It is to be hoped that one of those three treats will be accepted. If not, lift the animal to the table and try again. Not all patients will take the treat and so extra gentle handling and speaking to the pet is important.

Cats are allowed to leave the carrier and explore the exam room (Figure 8.16). Their treat selection starts with the soft chewy treat, then the spray cheese, and the final offering is some great smelly canned food. Move them to the table, find the cat's itchy spot, either behind the ears, base of tail, or under the chin, while continuing to offer up a treat now and then. The treats or blowing into the face are used as a distraction when a procedure is started tand while the procedure is being carried out (Figure 8.17).

Maintain a hand on the pet at all times while they are on the table. To put it into perspective for pets on a table, think of yourself being on a mountain ledge with a lengthy drop right beside you. **Vertigo** or anxiety usually affect us as negatively as it does the pet standing on an exam table.

And that is the start! We won't go any farther because this book cannot nor should not try to reproduce an already established program. Instead, we would encourage you to invest in yourself by registering to become a certified fear free practitioner! What the rest

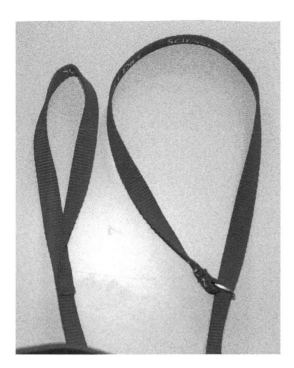

FIGURE 8.18 Slip leash.

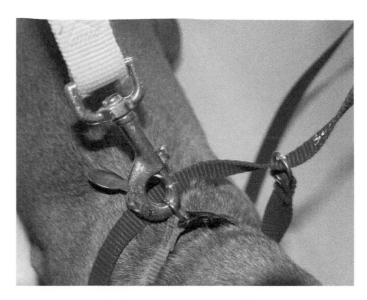

FIGURE 8.19 Double leash technique.

of this chapter discusses is the proper use of restraint techniques and equipment available for those not yet utilizing fear free techniques.

Learning Exercise

Research fear and stress free handling. The Fear Free Pets website (https://fearfreepets.com/) will provide proper training which would make you an extra valuable employee!

Safely Moving Patients from One Location to Another

The veterinary assistant is often called upon to help move an animal from one place to another inside the hospital. Knowing how to secure a pet for transport will increase the safety of the people and animals involved.

Dogs are often brought to the clinic on a leash. It is often the clinic's policy to send the owner's leash home with them, so it isn't lost. This makes a transfer of leashes in order. Always carry a leash in your pocket. This is often a slip leash (Figure 8.18) that opens easily to accommodate any sized head. The slip leash is placed over the dog's head and tightened gently so as not to choke the dog. The owner or you can unhook the owner's leash. Some clinics will insist on double leashing dogs. This is where you would put a second 6 ft leash with a clip onto the collar loop (Figure 8.19). The handle loop on one leash is passed over your

hand and onto your wrist and the other loop is held in your hand. This may seem like overkill but if you've ever had a dog escape from you, that extra length to grab can be a life saver. Even small dogs that are being held and passed to you should be leashed. At some point you may have to set them down in order to open a door or to set up a kennel. Having them leashed allows you to accomplish those tasks without fear of having them escape.

Placing a dog into a kennel is often very easy if you toss a couple of treats in before them. Allow them to move into the kennel or place them in the kennel if holding them and close the door a bit so your body and the door are blocking any escape. Remove the leashes and place the cage card and ID collar on the kennel and dog, respectively.

Reflection

Why is it so important to identify patients and the kennel they are assigned to stay in while at the practice?

Cats and ferrets are often brought into the clinic in a carrier. If that is the case, inform the owner that you will be right back with their carrier to take home with them. Transport the patient to the kennel, open the door to the kennel, and then hold the carrier just inside the kennel. Open the door to the carrier and see if the cat or ferret will walk out on its own. You can also try tossing a couple of chewy treats into the kennel before the cat or ferret. If the patient starts to walk out, allow it to get at least half way out before starting to slide the carrier back out of the kennel, be ready to close the door if the cat should try to escape.

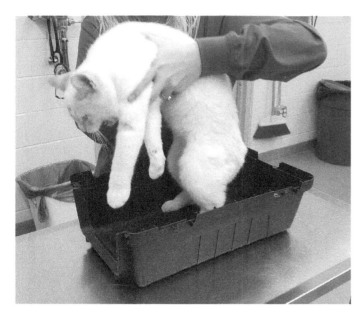

FIGURE 8.20 Cat in carrier transfer by lift to kennel.

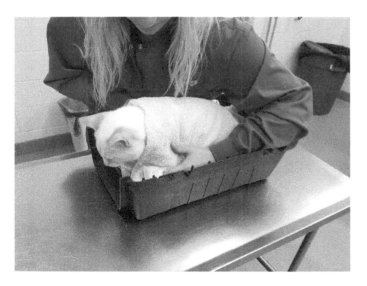

FIGURE 8.21 Cat in carrier transfer with towel to kennel.

If the cat or ferret won't step out, take the lid off the carrier and lift with both hands one over each shoulder and quickly move it into the kennel (Figure 8.20). If the patient should be upset, use a large, thick towel to cover it completely and then scoop it up as if it is the contents of an upside-down taco and into the kennel (Figure 8.21). Offering a few chewy treats after such egregious handling may be appreciated. Replace the lid to the carrier and return it to the owner. Then return promptly to the patient to place cage card and ID collar on the patient, respectively. Remember to snip off the excess ID collar after it is fitted around the neck.

If a cat, ferret, or small dog is carried into the clinic you will most likely be handing the pet. It doesn't hurt to put the slip leash around the animal' neck. It is another security step if the animal should leap from your arms.

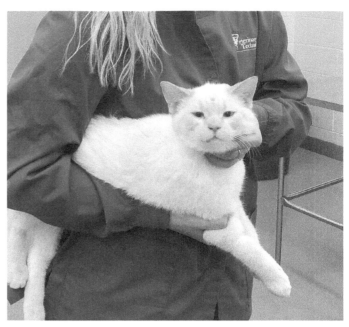

FIGURE 8.22 Carrying cat or small dog properly.

To carry a small patient properly, slide your non-dominant hand under its chest coming out between the front legs using your fingers to grasp the front legs (Figure 8.22).

> ### Reflection
>
> Can you think of other ways that cats and ferrets could be removed from a carrier? What treats or tricks could you come up with?

Use an elbow to pin their body against your side. The other hand slips the leash over the head and, holding onto the loop, cradle the head under the jaw with that hand. This allows you to let go of the head to open doors but hang onto the leash in case the animal should try to escape. Toss a treat into the kennel and place the animal into the kennel, facing the treat, then remove the leash. Put an ID collar on the pet and cage card on the kennel. Give them water, unless told not to because of an upcoming procedure, which in that case the cage card is marked to reflect that procedure. If the first treat was accepted, another treat can be offered to take the sting out of being placed into a kennel, if not leave it in case the patient is a shy eater. Adding a towel or blanket from home or a piece of the owner's clothing will also help the patient settle down. Double check that the kennel or run door is securely latched.

Medium-sized dogs are placed in the floor level kennels and large dogs are put in runs. Avoid lifting these sized dogs if possible. Walk the dog up to the door of the kennel, toss in a couple treats and tell them to "kennel."

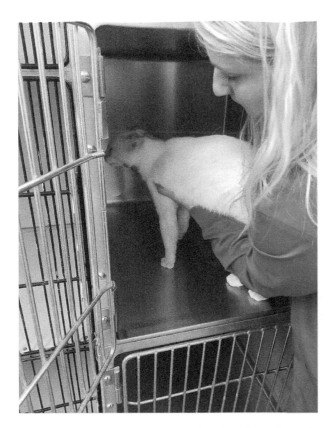

FIGURE 8.23 First step in removing a small patient from a kennel.

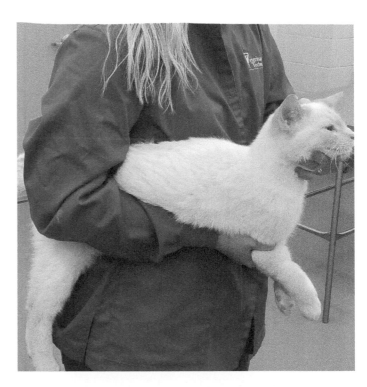

FIGURE 8.24 Removing a small patient from a kennel.

It is to be hoped that they know this command and will walk in on their own or perhaps the treat will entice them to go into the kennel or run. If not, open the door, use the leash to point its head into the kennel, then squat down and give them a little boost in that direction with a hand across their rear end. Do it gently and not so forcibly that its head hits the back wall of the kennel. Let them eat the treat if they desire, then gently pull their head with the leashes so you can remove them. Repeat with ID collar, cage card, comfort item, and water dish. Double check that the kennel or run door is securely latched.

When it is time to do the procedure or for the animal to go home, approach the kennel calling out the animal's name. It is to be hoped that they are at the door waiting, because they associate you with all those treats! Carefully open the door and offer a treat. As the patient is munching on it, slip the leash around the neck and if there is a collar attach a second leash. Snip the ID collar off with your scissors and leave it in the kennel for now. If the patient is small, position the pet so its head is going in the same direction as your non-dominant hand (Figure 8.23). Reach over the back and slide your hand under the chest so that its body is laying on your forearm and that hand can clasp the front legs. Lift the patient up and pin its body with your elbow against your side, all done gently of course (Figure 8.24). Transport to exam table or to the owner in the reception area. If the patient

has left the hospital, return to the kennel and clean as described in Chapter 4.

Medium and large dogs are retrieved from kennels similarly. Again, offer a treat to get them to come to the front of the kennel or run. Open the door slightly, using your body or knee to block them from escaping and apply the leashes (Figure 8.25). Follow the same procedure as described for removing the patient from the kennel or run.

General Restraint Techniques for Dogs and Cats

Many procedures like physical exams, **aural**, **oral** and **ophthalmic** examinations and medications, vaccinations, anal gland evacuation, and toenail trims can be accomplished with minimal restraint and virtually the same techniques for both dogs and cats. Some will object to a procedure, especially if sore or injured, so modifications will be needed. This could be a change in the hold, the use of restraint equipment, or the use of a sedative.

Reflection

Think about the differences in small, medium, and large patients. Think of ways to get them into and out of kennels and runs. Can you come up with any treats or tricks to do so gently?

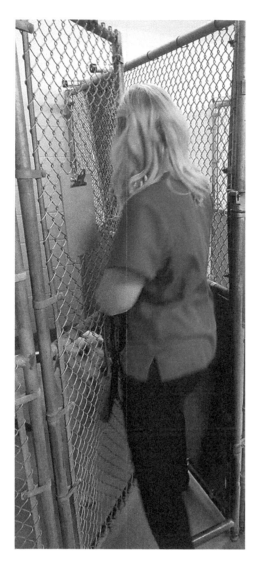

FIGURE 8.25 Blocking the door to the kennel.

Restraint for Examinations, Medications, and Procedures

Exam tables are used to elevate smaller patients to perform physical exams, draw samples, or give medications. Tables are slippery and can cause anxiety in the patient. Prevent this by placing a towel or cushion covered with a towel on the table before putting a patient on it. Almost all sized patients can be examined on a table; however, dogs over 50 lb are usually examined on the floor. The exam table rarely accommodates their size and if it wobbles because of their weight it is even more nerve-racking for the patient.

While on the table your main job is to keep the patient from falling off, but not clamping them down to the table for the entire length of the examination. Let the patient stand or sit as they see fit while the veterinarian is listening to heart, lungs, and gastrointestinal sounds (Figure 8.26). Note the hand positions in Figure 8.26, gentle without clamping hard onto any one part of the body. If a patient should fall off the exam table they can sustain substantial injuries. This would be an example of an **iatrogenic injury** and can be the basis for a malpractice suit!

While the patient is sitting on the table you may be asked to provide access to examine the eyes, ears, or mouth. The patient can either be in sitting position or in a sternal position. Snuggle the patient's body up to your body. Reach one arm over the patient's body and using that forearm to gently pin the patient's body against yours. Use both hands to steady the head for whatever body part the veterinarian needs to examine. Figure 8.27 shows holding the head for an examination of eyes, but a slight adjustment can be made for an ear exam. This usually involves flipping the pinna over the head and

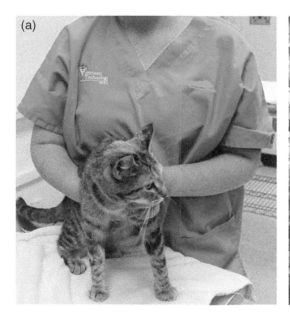

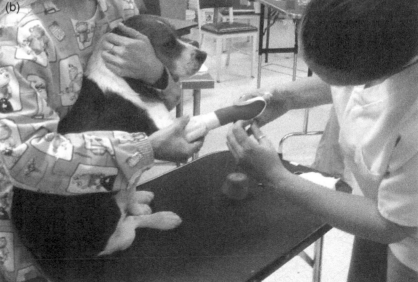

FIGURE 8.26 Sitting table restraint for general examination and procedures.

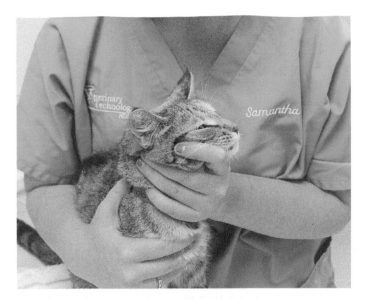

FIGURE 8.27 Head restraint for eye exam.

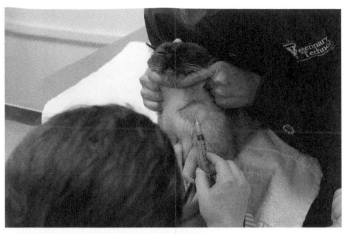

FIGURE 8.29 Restraining for jugular venipuncture.

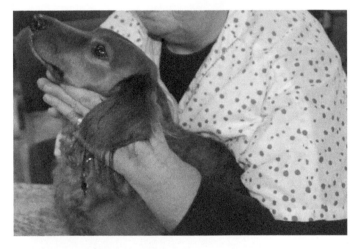

FIGURE 8.28 Holding the head for oral examination.

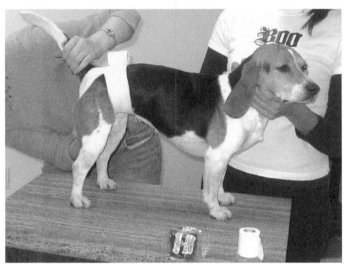

FIGURE 8.30 Standing restraint for abdominal and perianal exams.

using your thumb to hold it in place. If the patient requires its oral cavity to be examined, hands placed to either side of the head with fingers resting against the mandibles allows the veterinarian to open the mouth for an examination (Figure 8.28).

Jugular venipuncture is often used when a large amount of blood is needed for tests. The initial body placement is the same, note how the restrainer in Figure 8.29 uses her body to "corral" the cat. Place index fingers along each side of the mandible and gently raise the head (Figure 8.29). It is to be hoped that someone is available to offer treats on a stick to help distract the patient.

The veterinarian will ask you to have the pet stand for abdominal palpation (Figure 8.30) and to examine the anus and genitals. The patient in Figure 8.30 is a calm dog and is tolerating the examination well; however, if the area is sore or the veterinarian needs to express the anal glands a more restrictive hold would be prudent.

You would gather the animal's body close to yours and place one arm over the back and around the neck while the other supports the abdomen to keep the patient from sitting down. This works well for small and large dogs. For cats you may need to pick them up and pin them to your side as if you were carrying them, see Figure 8.24.

If working with a small dog or cat that doesn't like being handled, wrapping them in a towel is an easy way to control their bodies without exerting a lot of pressure and causing anxiety. Start with the length of the towel laid cross-wise to the table. Set the patient just shy of the middle of the towel's length. Cover the front paws with one side of the towel and then the rear end (Figure 8.31a). Bring the shorter end over the body and tuck it snugly under the legs (Figure 8.31b). Bring the longer end of the towel over the body wrapping snugly (Figure 8.31c). Then keep wrapping the towel until it is completely around the patient (Figure 8.31d). Grasp the towel where all the ends meet just behind or to the

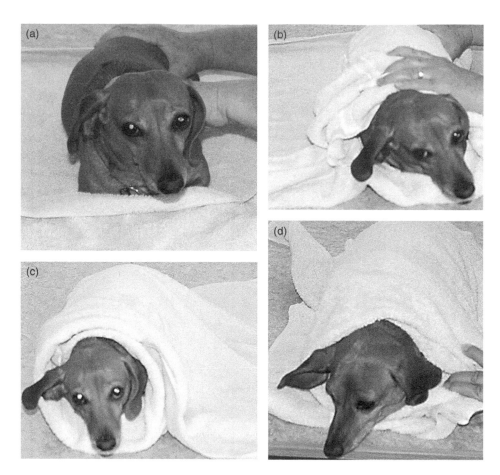

FIGURE 8.31 Towel wrap.

side of the patient's head. If you need to you can grasp the patient around the neck or the scruff if the patient is going to try to bite. It can be a bit tricky doing that with the towel in your grasp as well, but if the other hand is free you could reach around the patient's body to control the head. The veterinarian can come up through the back of the towel for the auscultation and palpation. A front leg or rear leg can be extruded for an injection or blood draw from the cephalic, saphenous or femoral veins (Figure 8.32).

To examine the head, the front legs are covered so they can't swipe at the veterinarian when looking at the structures on the head. You or the veterinarian can grasp the head with one or both hands and maneuver it in whatever way is necessary for the exam or treatment (Figure 8.33).

Sometimes, an animal needs to be laid onto their side, this is called lateral recumbency. This hold is used for examinations of the side, abdomen, and prepuce of the patient, for administering subcutaneous fluids or injections, **cystocentesis** and IV injections, or blood draws from the lateral saphenous vein of dogs and cats or the femoral vein of cats. This hold is also used to take a lateral or medial view of a front or back leg or a lateral view of thorax or abdomen. This can be done by one person on any patient smaller than 45 lb. For larger patients it

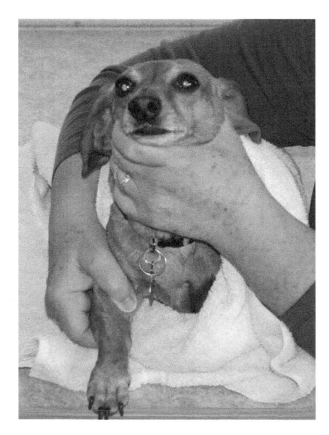

FIGURE 8.32 Extruded front leg for injection.

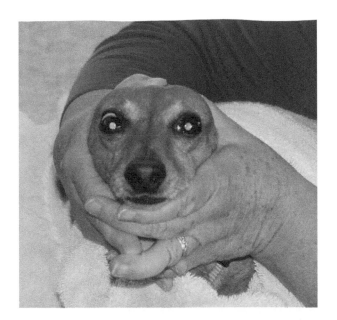

FIGURE 8.33 Examining the head using a towel.

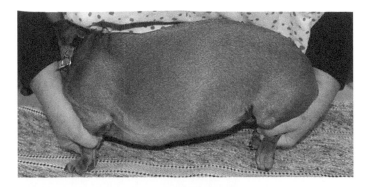

FIGURE 8.35 Arm's reaching over the top and grasping legs.

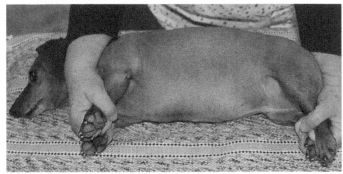

FIGURE 8.36 Holding the patient down with wrist and arm.

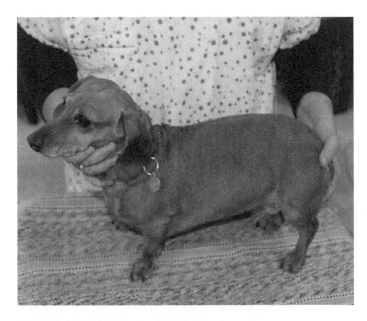

FIGURE 8.34 Positioning for lateral recumbency.

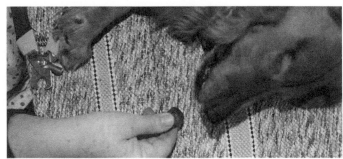

FIGURE 8.37 Offering treats while in lateral recumbency.

takes two people working in tandem with the legs. Once in position the person on the front end will take over holding the animal in position.

For lateral recumbency, start by positioning the body of the patient length-wise on the table and perpendicular to your body (Figure 8.34). Reach both arms over the patient's back and grasp both front legs with one hand and both back legs with the other hand (Figure 8.35). Lift and move the legs away from your body, allowing the patient's back to slide down your chest. Keep hold of the legs, position the wrist holding the front legs over the neck and the arm holding the back legs over the flank or along the rear end (Figure 8.36).

Only apply a light pressure in these areas to keep the animal in the down position.

If the animal should struggle, lift the legs up slightly towards the ceiling and apply a bit more pressure to the neck and flank. The *instant* the patient stops struggling, release the pressure and lower the legs back to the table. This is a reward for lying still. Another technique is to use treats while the patient is lying down to keep them occupied. Cheese on a stick or the soft chewy treats work very well with both dogs and cats (Figure 8.37). If this hold is being done for an IV injection or blood draw, the hand holding the back legs releases both, while the hand holding the front leg raises them towards the ceiling just a bit, so the patient is resting on its shoulder blade. Keep the wrist of the hand holding the front legs on the neck.

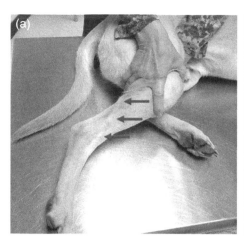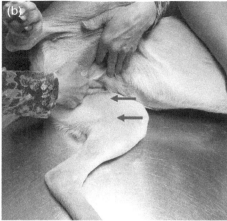

FIGURE 8.38 Restraining and occluding for IV: (a) saphenous and (b) femoral veins.

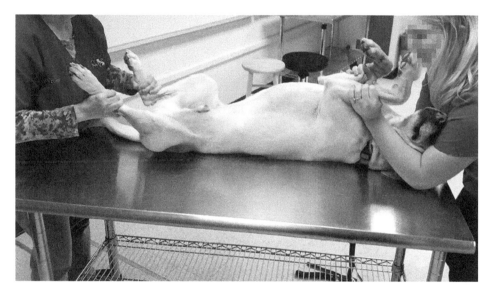

FIGURE 8.39 Dorsal recumbency.

Then the free hand can occlude for the saphenous or femoral veins (Figure 8.38).

Dorsal recumbency is just one more step to the lateral recumbency technique. After they are in lateral recumbency, you simply roll them onto their backs. Often, you will need a second person to keep them in that position. One person takes the front legs, one in each hand, and arms are positioned on either side of the head. The other person holds the back legs, one in each hand (Figure 8.39). If a third is available, ply the patient with treats. This hold is used for examinations, cystocentesis, and ventrodorsal radiographs.

Sternal recumbency is when the dog or cat is held upright on their sternum. This is a good hold for eye, ear, and oral cavity examinations as well as for IV cephalic and jugular vein access. It can also be used for radiographing a front leg or paw. Set the patient on the exam table or floor as if you were going to perform a lateral recumbency. Place one hand under the chin and the other hand on top of the hips or rump. At the same time

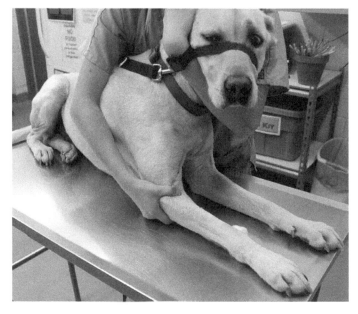

FIGURE 8.40 Occluding the cephalic vein in sternal recumbency.

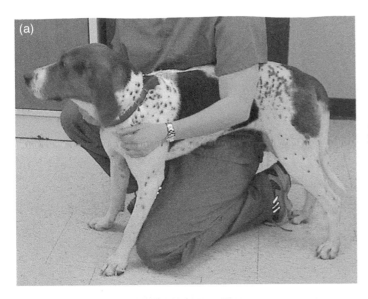

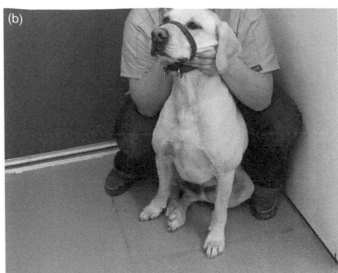

FIGURE 8.41 Large dog floor restraint.

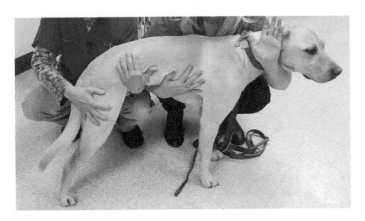

FIGURE 8.42 Lifting a large dog.

push down on the hips as you lift on the chin, if it's a dog say, "sit!" Once the patient is sitting, slide one arm over the shoulders and in tandem with the other hand slide the front feet forward. Keeping the one arm over the shoulder, reach up to grasp the chin in tandem with the other hand to steady the head. Or with the arm over the shoulder encircle the neck with that arm and use the other to occlude the cephalic vein (Figure 8.40). Be able to switch hands to hold the other leg as needed.

Working with large dogs often requires you to either squat down or to kneel with one knee and fold or sit on the other leg (Figure 8.41). In Figure 8.41 note how the student is squatting over the dog and she is in the corner not the dog. This prevents the dog from feeling trapped.

Lifting large dogs should be a team effort. It is important to note that years of lifting dogs over 45 lb, especially by yourself, will take its toll on your back. Extend your work life by asking for help when lifting and always use your legs to lift, *not* your back! To lift a large dog as a duo, stand shoulder to shoulder with the dog placed perpendicular to your legs. Squat down beside the dog, one

person uses her arms to encircle the neck and thorax, the other encircles the abdomen and goes around the back end of the dog (Figure 8.42). On the count of three, lift simultaneously and place the dog on the table (Figure 8.43). The person in charge of the front end of the dog resumes full control of the dog on the table.

Learning Exercise

Practice! The only way to become proficient at the restraint techniques listed is to practice. If you have pets at home they are now your practice aids! If you have a stuffed animal practice on that. Have your roommate or family member move it about and bark or growl! If school will allow it book practice times. If you volunteer at a rescue ask if you could practice there. Record how things went, how did the different animals respond to being held in the various holds? Did you learn anything new while practicing?

Restraint Equipment

On occasion, a patient may be too naughty to get close to it, but whether it is scared, territorial, or aggressive, a restraint devise that can be used is the capture pole (Figure 8.44). The capture pole has a loop that can be closed by pulling back on the end of the pole. It is designed so that you cannot choke an animal but will hold the body away from the handlers. Use the capture pole to secure the head while another person can give a sedative (Figure 8.45).

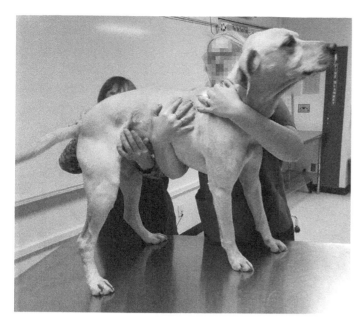

FIGURE 8.43 Assuming control of large dog on table.

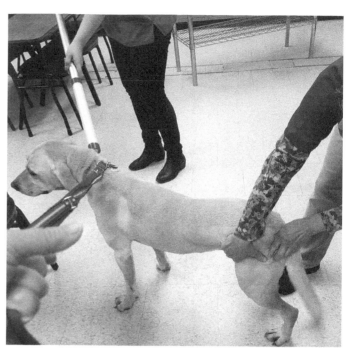

FIGURE 8.45 Using capture pole to give a sedative.

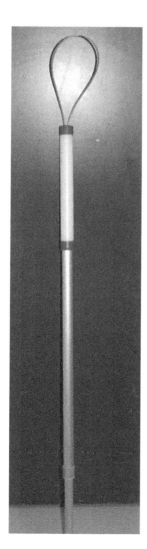

FIGURE 8.44 Capture pole.

If the owners think their dog may bite, applying a muzzle is in order. There are several muzzles available as seen in Figure 8.46. Muzzles A, B, and D are used on dogs and muzzle C is the cone muzzle recommended for cats. The first two are easy to slip on over the dog's muzzle with the straps being fastened around the ears. The trick is to select the appropriate size to fit around the muzzle. Muzzle D is a cage or basket muzzle and is the one recommended as a fear free device. This muzzle can be put on without a lot of struggle. Offer the dog a taste of spray cheese on an applicator stick so they associate the smell with something good. Then spray the front of the muzzle with the cheese. Hold it up to the dog and allow it to stick his face into the basket to get the cheese. Quickly buckle the muzzle straps behind the ears (Figure 8.47). If using muzzles A and B, one restrainer will have to steady the head with hands on either side of the neck and back of the head. The other person holds the straps open widely, one in each hand, and slides the muzzle onto the patient and quickly clasps the straps behind the ears.

Cats too may need to be muzzled and the plastic cone muzzle is the best one to use as it has a wide enough opening for them to breath normally and it covers their eyes which is also a distraction technique. Wrap the cat up in a thick blanket or towel as previously described (Figure 8.48). Another person unwraps just the head and slides the muzzle over the face and secures the ties behind the ears (Figure 8.49). Often this will calm an angry cat because they can't see what is going on, so they often give up. However, whatever the procedure is may spark their anger

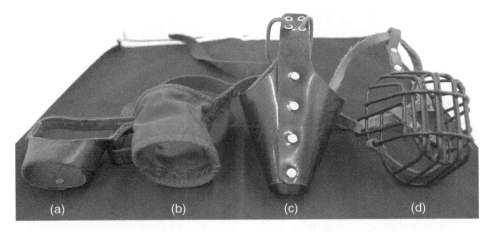

FIGURE 8.46 Types of muzzle. Source: Joshua Sherurcij, Wikimedia Commons. https://commons.wikimedia.org/wiki/File:German_Shepherd_with_Muzzle.JPG

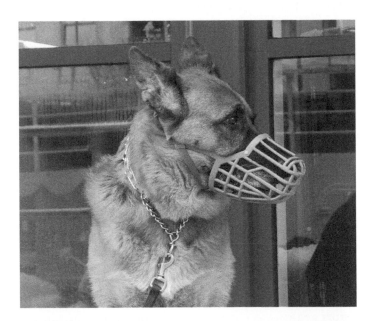

FIGURE 8.47 Applied muzzle.

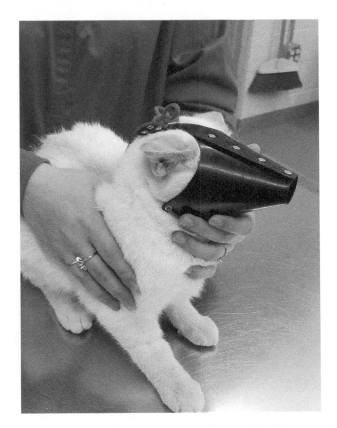

FIGURE 8.49 Cone muzzle on cat. Source: Sheldon, Sonsthagen, and Topel, 2017. Reproduced with permission of Elsevier.

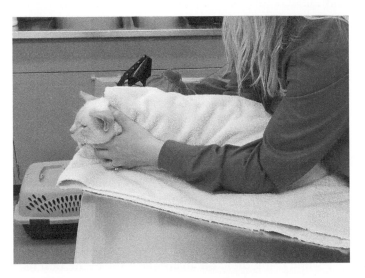

FIGURE 8.48 Cat folded in blanket. Source: Sheldon, Sonsthagen, and Topel, 2017. Reproduced with permission of Elsevier.

again, if possible, sedatives could be used in addition to the muzzle.

An Elizabethan collar is designed to keep dogs and cats from chewing on wounds or surgical incisions. The collar must be longer than the patient's nose otherwise they may still be able to reach. The patient's collar is usually attached to the Elizabethan collar using the loops along the inside edge (A in Figure 8.50). Then both are placed around the patient's head and the long strap is used to secure the cone closed. Adjust the patient's collar

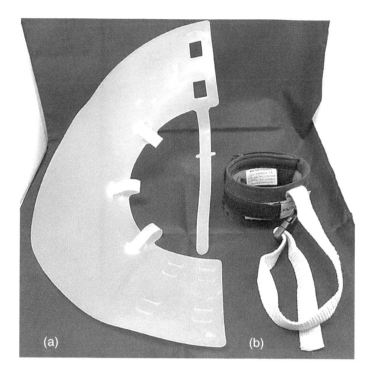

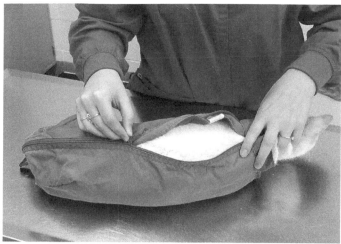

FIGURE 8.52 Cat being zipped into bag. Source: Sheldon, Sonsthagen, and Topel, 2017. Reproduced with permission of Elsevier.

FIGURE 8.50 Elizabethan collar (a); and no-bite neck brace (b).

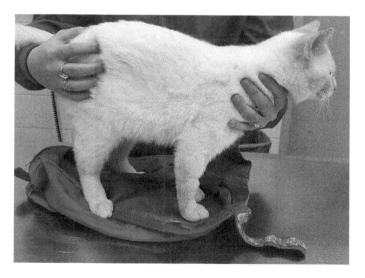

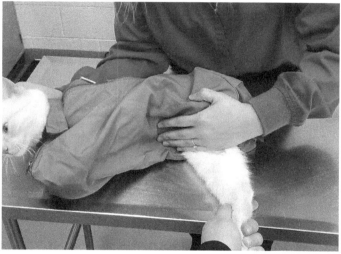

FIGURE 8.53 Cat with back leg exposed. Source: Sheldon, Sonsthagen, and Topel, 2017. Reproduced with permission of Elsevier.

FIGURE 8.51 Cat set down on top of cat bag. Source: Sheldon, Sonsthagen, and Topel, 2017. Reproduced with permission of Elsevier.

to make it snug around the neck, just so it can't be pulled off, you should be able to slip two fingers between the collar and neck. Because the collar is longer than the nose, the food and water dishes must be elevated so they can still drink.

Another type of anti-mutilation device is the No-Bite Neck Brace (B in Figure 8.50). This is a hard-plastic brace that encircles the neck and is attached to the animal with a strap that encircles the chest. It is a little bit less restrictive than the Elizabethan collar. However, some patients are contortionists and will get at their wounds when this collar is used.

Cat bags or feline restraint bags are also used when a cat is squirrelly or a bit naughty. The bag is opened wide and the cat is set down on top of the bag (Figure 8.51). The neck strap is placed around the neck and the zipper is pulled to enclose them in the bag (Figure 8.52). Front and back legs are accessible through the zippered openings (Figure 8.53). Never leave a cat unattended in a cat bag on a table. They can still roll and if they roll off the table they can get hurt.

Gauntlets are heavy leather gloves used when dealing with an animal that wants to bite or scratch (Figure 8.54). They don't protect you from bites as teeth can go through the leather, but it does tend to slow them down so you can get your fingers out of the way. Gauntlets reduce your tactile sensation, so it is important to modify your grip when using them on an animal. One of the best uses of them is as a distraction technique, put your fingers only in half way and while the animal is biting on the

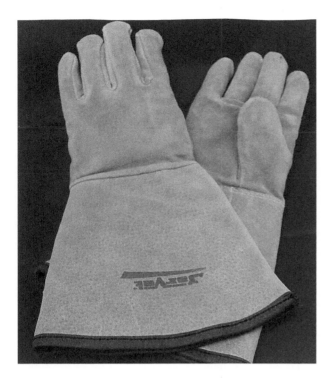

FIGURE 8.54 Gauntlets.

empty finger holes the other hand can reach around and grasp the animal long enough to slip the other glove all the way on and assist with a hold around the neck and grasp the feet. Another person should be standing ready to give a sedative and/or muzzle.

Learning Exercise

Schedule a time to look over the instruments discussed at school. If they don't have them or you are studying remotely stop by a veterinary practice and explain that you are going to school and ask if they would let you see their restraint equipment. Perhaps they will allow you to either watch while they are using the equipment or take a photo of the instruments.

Restraint of Pocket Pets

Rabbits and ferrets are becoming increasingly popular house pets. Rabbits are never carried or held by their ears. To carry them, their head is tucked into the crook of your elbow and their bodies are supported along your forearm and snugged against your body, lay your other hand on top of the shoulders. Rabbits rarely bite but their back feet can be used to rake your arms and body. They are very sharp and can cause quite severe gashes. When putting rabbits down on a table or inside a kennel

they tend to hop forward quickly to get away from you. This could mean they hop off the table or hop into the back wall of the cage. Don't let go of them immediately when their feet hit the surface, they will do their little hop and you can still control their forward motion. Rabbits can hurt their backs by kicking out with their back legs. It is important to keep the rabbit in sternal recumbency or if going into lateral recumbency wrap them tightly in a towel, as described for the cat. Rabbits do not appreciate slippery surfaces, so a cushion and towel are both needed to make them feel more at ease on the table.

Ferrets, guinea pigs, and rats are picked up by grasping them over the shoulder and then quickly supporting their rear ends until they can be cradled in your arms. Hamsters are often asleep during the day so make sure you wake them up with a knock on their cage. Give them a moment before reaching in for them or you will see a very frightened and angry hamster chatter its teeth! Which in turn is very frightening for us! A gentle way to pick up hamsters and gerbils is to scoop them up. Cup both hands and lower them down on each side of the patient, bring them together in a scooping motion and bring your hands together so the patient is encircled by your hands. If you are worried about bites, a pair of light cotton gardening gloves will slow them down a bit.

In the suggested reading section at the end of this chapter there is a list of websites that should have more information on handling techniques for blood draws and injections done on pocket pets.

Reflection

Think of a pocket pet coming to a veterinary practice. Will they be scared and nervous or calm and collected? What could you do to help them calm down?

Restraint of Pet Birds

When a bird is brought to the veterinary clinic it is usually a very sick bird. The goal is to not stress the bird further so, if possible, the bird is "examined" inside the cage without touching it at all. If you must hold the bird, one thing you have to remember is bird's breathe using a "bellows" like system. So, any constriction of the thorax can suffocate the bird. The goal is to hold the bird without injuring them and not being injured by the bird. Their bullet-shaped body and wings makes it difficult to hang on to them and if they are **psittacine** birds their beaks can cause damage to fingers, even amputation! Some people recommend using a small wash cloth or towel to reach into the cage to grasp the bird from behind. Position the index finger and thumb on either side of the head just below the eyes. Very gently hold the bird with the rest of the fingers in a "cage" like hold rather than touching the bird. This will help prevent the possibility of suffocating the bird. Once out of the cage, resting the bird on a folded towel will help make them comfortable and you can grasp their feet at that time. If you can cover their head that will calm them as well. Others suggest allowing the bird to step off a perch and onto your hand or arm. Bring the bird close to your chest with its breast facing yours. Reach up from behind with the other hand and grasp the bird around the head in the same manner as described previously. Again, cage your fingers around the thorax. If the bird is small, like a parakeet or cockatiel, you can pin their feet with your little finger. If the bird is larger, like an amazon or cockatoo, you will need to use the other hand to control the feet. Once they are caught you can extend a wing for flight feather or toenail trims.

Learning Exercise

Utilize the internet to find videos on bird handling. Review at least two or three that show the capture and holding techniques described. What did you observe? Did you pick up any tips or techniques?

Restraint of Livestock

Defense strategies of livestock as prey animals is to flee first. For all but the pig, their eyes are placed at each side of the skull such that their visual field extends far out to the sides of the body with only a small blind spot directly in front of their face and directly behind their rear end.

As you can see from Figure 8.55, the horse, like cattle, sheep, and goats, will use one eye at a time to view what is directly in front of them and to each side. This wide range of vision allows them to see something approaching from the side without moving their heads. Note the side vision is anchored at the point of its shoulder. This will be important when we talk about moving prey animals without use of force.

Pigs have more forward-facing eyes and so their field of vision is limited like a predator's vision. However, those large ears hear the tiniest of noises and their sense of smell is like a dog's (Figure 8.56). If the animals cannot flee or they feel threatened, they – like dogs and cats – have an arsenal of weapons with which to defend themselves or their offspring.

Cattle will use their head as a battering ram to knock you down and then will kneel and to use their head to pulverize you into pulp. They can also kick with their

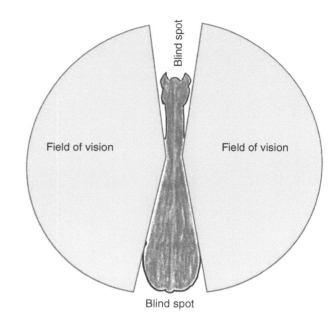

FIGURE 8.55 Horse's field of vision.

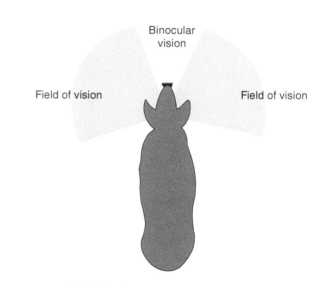

FIGURE 8.56 Pig's field of vision.

back feet in an arc pattern, out to the side then backward. They are very accurate and can kill a person if caught at the full extent of the leg. Some cattle have horns that can gore an unwary handler. Horses can strike out with their front feet or paw at you or they can rear up and come down on you. Hind feet can kick with either one leg or both legs at the same time. Horses also bite and if they do it is difficult to make them let go, and the process to escape their bite often leads to more severe damage to tissues. To walk behind a horse or cow you should either pass 7–8 feet behind them or as close to the rump as possible. This will reduce the amount of damage a kick will cause. However, both can give a short pop with their back feet that can cause severe bruising to your leg or if it happens to be your head it can kill you! Sheep and goats will ram you with their heads, which can knock the

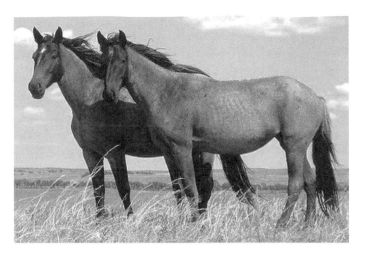

FIGURE 8.57 Alert horse. Source: Wikimedia Common. Used under CC-BY-SA 2.5, https://commons.wikimedia.org/wiki/File:Nokota_Horses_cropped.jpg.

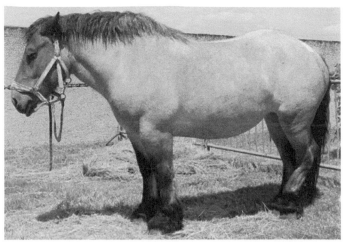

FIGURE 8.58 Sleeping horse. Source: https://commons.wikimedia.org/wiki/File:Cheval_ardennais_expo.jpg. Public Domain.

wind from your lungs. This is very uncomfortable but not usually life-threatening, unless they happen to ram into your head. That can cause severe damage to the skull, brain, and neck. Boars have tusks they use to slash and a powerful bullet-shaped body to knock you down. They have been known to eviscerate their foes. Sows will knock you down and trample you. They too can bite and have canine teeth that can cause severe damage. With all that being said, livestock and horses are not aggressive most of the time. The only time they are is when you are messing with their offspring or it is mating season.

Assessing Behavior and Safely Approaching Livestock

Horses are always approached on the left side of the body. This is in part due to custom and training, as both sides have equal fields of vision. As you approach look at the body language, is the horse aware of your presence? Alert body language is head up, with ears and eyes pointed toward you (Figure 8.57). Sleeping body language is head hanging down, standing on three legs with an overall slumped appearance (Figure 8.58). Each need to be approached cautiously but in different ways. The alert horse is approached slowly and offered a treat of some kind, either a small pail of grain or treat nuggets; allow a small mouthful or one nugget. Speak to the horse and reach up slowly to pet the horse either on the side of the face or along the neck. If the horse is sleeping, especially in a box stall with its rear end facing the gate, the handler needs to speak to the horse to wake it up. Never step into a stall without announcing yourself as this will startle them, and you may end up getting kicked, squished, or stomped. Never try to chase horses, unless you are on a horse, even then it is tricky, and they will leave you in the dust!

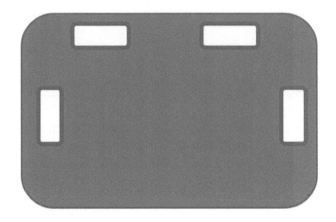

FIGURE 8.59 Pig hurdle.

Cattle, sheep, and goats are usually moved as a group into a smaller enclosure. The direction of approach is at or behind the point of shoulder depending on which way you wish to move them. Approaching at the point of shoulder will move them in the opposite direction from you and behind the point of shoulder will move them forward and away from you. To move them straight away from you walk at 5–6 feet just to the right or left of the blind spot directly behind them. Cattle and sheep usually move as a herd or flock as there is safety in numbers. Sheep have an extremely strong **flocking** instinct and if you can get one to go in the right direction the entire flock will follow. Goats, however, will often scatter in every direction. It is better to entice them into a pen with grain or treats.

Pigs are a bit more contrary and will often turn and look at you as you approach. The use of a hurdle (Figure 8.59) can seem like a solid wall to them and they will move away from it coming up to their position. The hurdle can also be used to direct them right or left. Plastic paddles are also used to gently swat them on the rear to move them forward or on the left or right shoulder to move them in the opposite direction.

You should never beat on any of the livestock to get them to move. Using the point of shoulder and a cheerful shout of "git up" or "move" is often all you need. Remember the fight or flight response, give the animals time to sort themselves out at gates or going into enclosures. If pushed too hard they will try to get away which either results in them scattering, or turning back upon you, with heads lowered to move past, around, or over you.

Reflection

Now that you have learned a bit about livestock and horses, is there anything that makes you nervous or scared about working with them? How will you combat those feelings so that you may handle them safely?

Maternal Behavior

Maternal instinct has a very strong effect on behavior, even the most docile animal will become aggressive if their offspring is being "attacked." Which from a human's perspective may be just a wish to pet the youngster! Livestock mothers can be quite dangerous if they feel threatened. Calves, lambs, kids, and foals can be worked on in front of the mothers; however, you must keep a watchful eye on them as they may come to their defense if the youngsters vocalize in distress. Cows are extremely dangerous when working on or around their calves (Figure 8.60). Handlers often need to place ear tags and treat the umbilical cord, this handling is done

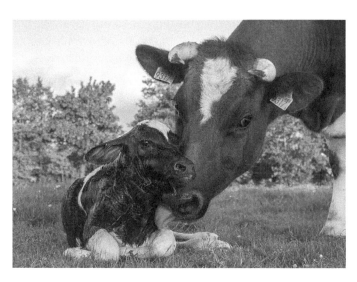

FIGURE 8.60 Cow with newborn calf. Source: Wikimedia Commons. Used under CC-BY-SA 3.0, https://commons.wikimedia.org/wiki/File:New_born_Frisian_red_white_calf.jpg.

as soon as possible after birth and this may cause the cow to feel the newborn is being threatened. If they perceive a threat their response was described previously, and they will stand guard; if you move, they will take after you again. Foals must be worked on with mothers' present, otherwise the mares tend to go crazy with fear and worry and will try to get to the foal even if it must hurt itself to do so. Never remove a newborn lamb from their mother's sight as they often reject them when returned. Piglets must be removed from the mother's sight and hearing before being worked upon. They get very upset when they hear their piglets squeal and have been known to climb out of pens to get to their offspring.

Territory

Horses are not so much territorial as they are hierarchical. This is when there is a top animal that leads and everyone else falls in line. The point to remember is when introducing a new animal into the herd it is important to know that a fight may erupt, and you don't want to be caught in the middle of a rumble! This is avoided or reduced by introducing animals with fencing situated close enough for the animals to smell and look at each other but not to have physical contact with each other.

Sex drive in males can be an overpowering urge that can turn normally very docile animals into very aggressive animals if you are the one keeping them from their target. Be very cautious and follow all the safety rules when dealing with these animals, especially with dairy bulls and stallions. The sheer size and weight of these animal can cause severe damage to a human.

Learning Exercise

Research the reasons for maternal, territorial, hierarchical, and sex drive behaviors in livestock and horses. Why have these developed and how can we use them to our advantage when working with these patients?

Restraint Techniques for Horses and Livestock

Horses are led and "controlled" by a halter. The reason for the quotes around controlled is that even if the person is 200 lb on the end of a lead rope attached to a halter, if that horse wants to get away it is going to get away! For that reason, there is one rule to keep in mind when working with a horse. *Never trust a horse!* This may sound harsh, but they are prey animals and will try to flee if startled or frightened. If they can't get away, they will fight or run over you to escape. You must be

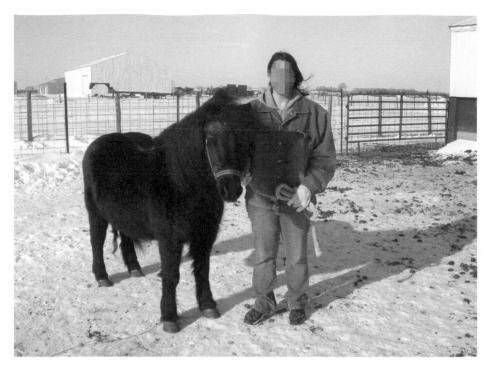

FIGURE 8.61 Placing a halter on a horse. Source: Sheldon, Sonsthagen, and Topel, 2006. Reproduced with permission of Elsevier.

hypervigilant when working with horses, not only towards the horse but to what is happening in the environment. It is to be hoped that you will be somewhere that people can't suddenly appear, slam a door, or make a loud noise. All of these may frighten the horse to the point of fight or flight.

When removing a horse from a stall first make sure the horse hears you approaching, call out its name or knock on the stall door. Most horses will turn and look at you, if they don't step close to the back end and lay a hand on their rump *but* only if they are awake and aware of your presence. If they are asleep call out their name again.

Move confidently toward the head and offer a pat and/or a treat, many horses appreciate treats. Apple and carrot treats are available and having some of both in your pocket will often win over a horse. Some will have a preference liking one over another, and some won't like them at all. A pocket full of pellets or handful of grain will sometimes be the ticket as a distraction. After making friends, tie the lead rope with an over hand knot around the neck. Shake out the halter to get it into position and slip it over the nose. Then reach across the poll to grasp the neck strap and bring it over the neck. Buckle the neck strap making sure the metal rings are not riding on any bony parts of the face and that the nose piece is high enough to not block the nasal passages. Hook the lead rope to the center ring under the chin. Then grasp the lead rope with your right hand just below the halter rope clip and coil the rope in your left hand.

Stand to the side of the horse (Figure 8.61). If it is still facing away from the door, step toward the horse and pull the lead rope to the right making them turn around away from your body. If you step back and pull them toward you, they could knock you down as they swing their rear ends.

If moving a horse out of a stall, pen, or barn you "send" the horse through the doorway first. Point the horse's head toward the door and give a forward tug on the lead rope. A command like "getup" or "forward" is given with the forward tug. Allow the coils to unwind in your hand to give them enough slack to proceed through the door. This protects you from being run over if the horse should be startled from behind. There would be nowhere to go but over you as you walk through the door. As their rear end clears give a gentle tug on the lead rope and the command "whoa" to let them know they need to turn and face you as you walk through the door.

To lead the horse, gather the lead rope coils in your left hand, give a gentle tug forward on the lead rope with your right and step forward. Walk along side of the horse, parallel to the front leg. This prevents the horse from stepping on you from behind.

When working with a veterinarian it is important to work on the same side as the veterinarian. This is to prevent the horse from moving over the person offering the least path of resistance (Figure 8.62). As an example, if you are standing on one side, big and tall, and the vet is squatted down on the other side looking at a leg, the vet is the path of least resistance. If something should startle the horse it will move away from both of you when

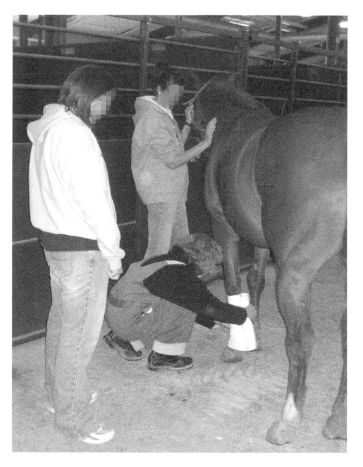

FIGURE 8.62 Proper positions while working on a horse.

standing on the same side. If not, then the vet could be seriously injured.

Horses respond well to distraction techniques. Treats or grain are almost always welcomed. Patting them and talking to them works to keep their attention on you, cupping an eye with your palm, or rolling up loose skin on their necks and wiggling it works as well. Another method is to use a small diameter nylon rope with a clip on one end. The clip is attached to one side of the halter ring and the end is run through the opposite ring over the nose. The rope is then placed under the horse's lip and gently tightened to make them really pay attention to that thing under their lip. It should not be jerked as this can cause pain and make them jump away. The use of twitches may still be used in some practices but with the advent of good and safe sedatives they do not need to be used.

Stocks are a great device to use for procedures on horses (Figure 8.63). It is designed with two gates between four stout posts, connected by horizontal rails. The horse is led towards the gate and sent in as the handler walks on the outside of the stock. Just before the horse moves through the other end the gates are closed. The horse can be cross-tied to the end posts by attaching another lead rope to the halter.

Picking up feet on horses can be a bit dangerous and it takes strength and a sound back. The horse should be tied to a vertical post or have someone hold the horse and apply distraction techniques. To pick up the front

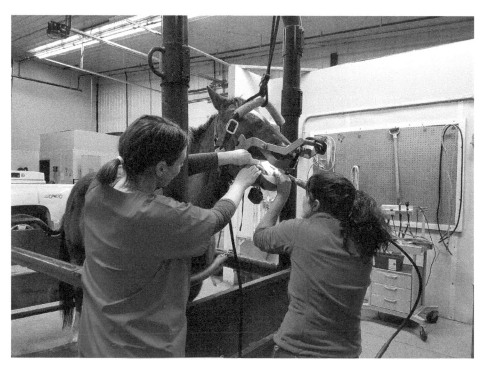

FIGURE 8.63 Horse in stocks for dental work.

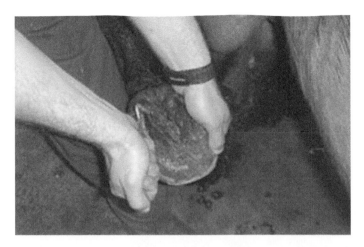

FIGURE 8.64 Picking up front foot. Source: Sheldon, Sonsthagen, and Topel, 2017. Reproduced with permission of Elsevier.

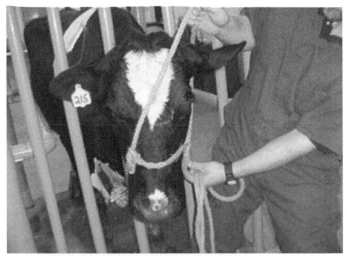

FIGURE 8.66 Stanchion head gate – cow being haltered. Source: Sheldon, Sonsthagen, and Topel, 2017. Reproduced with permission of Elsevier.

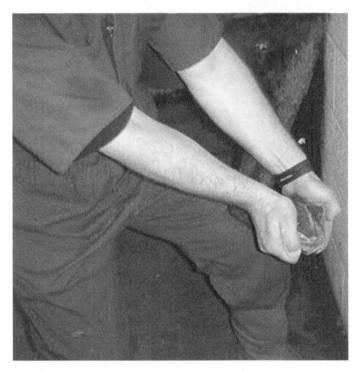

FIGURE 8.65 Holding back foot on knee. Source: Sheldon, Sonsthagen, and Topel, 2017. Reproduced with permission of Elsevier.

leg face the rear end of the horse. Slide your hand down the leg to the fetlock, encircle and lift up, giving the command "lift" or "give." If the horse doesn't pick up its foot, lean into it and that will usually make it either shift its weight or pick up the foot (Figure 8.64).

Hold the foot on a bended knee or while holding the foot slip your inside leg around the horse's leg and hold the foot between your legs. This frees up the hands to hold and clean the hoof. The rear leg is picked up in a similar manner, but never put it between your legs! Once the foot is picked up stretch the leg out behind the horse and rest it on your knee. Again, this frees the hands to

clean the hoof. (Figure 8.65).When finished with a foot, do not just drop the leg, set it down gently.

To return a horse to its stall send them through the door as previously explained. This time you stay outside of the stall, give a gentle tug to turn them around and remove the halter. Step up to the left side of the head, unbuckle the neck strap and lower the halter off the nose. A treat and a pat are always appreciated, step back and close the door to the stall.

Learning Exercise

Practice! If possible, try to get more practice on horse restraint. List the techniques described and then schedule an appointment with your school to have access to a horse. If that isn't possible, do you know someone that has a horse that would be appropriate for you to practice with? Is there a stable near you that would allow you to practice on one of their horses? Keep track of how the horse reacted to each technique. Did you learn any tricks or techniques?

Beef cattle are worked upon in a chute. This YouTube video (https://www.youtube.com/watch?v=UjWsNOls5_M) is an excellent demonstration of how that piece of equipment is used. If the head needs to be worked on, a halter is place on the head and tied to the side of the chute. Dairy cattle are usually haltered and worked on in a stanchion. This is like a horse stock with a head gate at one end that prevents forward and backward motion, and solid posts with horizontal bars to prevent side to side movement (Figure 8.66).

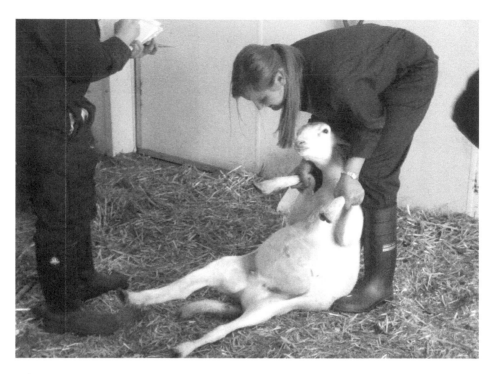

FIGURE 8.67 Setting up a sheep.

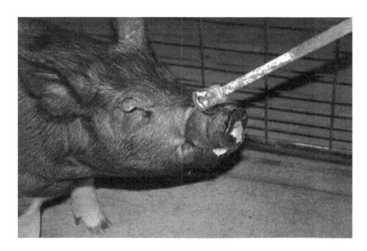

FIGURE 8.68 Hog snare. Source: Sheldon, Sonsthagen, and Topel, 2017. Reproduced with permission of Elsevier.

The website http://www.sheep101.info/201/handling. html is an introduction to working sheep. The only thing they don't show is setting a sheep up on its rump. This is a multi-step process that takes some practice but even the most diminutive person can do it with minimal trouble. The sheep's body is placed perpendicular to your legs, with its shoulder against one of your legs. Reach over the top to the opposite side of the sheep and grasp the flank with one hand and the chin with the other hand. Turn the neck into the "off" shoulder, lift up on the flank until the rear leg is lifted off the ground. Using the leg against its shoulder as a pivot point, step back with the other leg and pull the sheep off balance. This lays them on their sides

and a quick shift of hands to the front legs can put them on their rump (Figure 8.67). Then you can let go and balance the sheep's body between your legs in order to shear, draw blood, or trim hooves.

Goats are handled much like tiny horses. Haltering and picking up legs are very similar, they are just a more manageable size and don't require as much care in not being trampled.

Pigs are either worked in a group pen or as individuals. To separate them out or to move them you would use a device called a hurdle (Figure 8.59). It is made of plastic or wood and is solid with thoughtfully placed hand holes. When placed in front of pigs they will stop and if placed on the right side of them they will go left and vice versa. Plastic paddles are also used to move a group, one should never use them to beat on a pig just a gentle whap will get them to move. Individuals are worked upon by either picking them up or applying a hog snare. Piglets are picked up by a back leg and quickly moved to be cradled in your arms against your abdomen. This avoids the screeches they emit when caught. A 30–40 lb pig is also captured by a back leg, and the other leg is grasped as soon as possible. They are held upside down until the procedure is over. Pigs weighing 45–80 lb can be held the same way with two people, holding a leg apiece. Any pig over 80 lb should be captured with a hog snare (Figure 8.68). The loop is held in front of the pig; their natural curiosity will cause them to nibble on the loop when they do pull the handle back capturing the top jaw. The pig will pull backwards, and you pull backwards as well, at this point you are at a stalemate which is good because the pig will stand there for ever! Blood draws and simple procedures can be done with the hog snare in place. However, ear protection must be worn as they squeal and shriek their displeasure. The snare is only effective for about 30 minutes, after that the snout can lose feeling and they may rush forward. To remove the snare, pop the handle forward to release the loop and pull it out of the pig's mouth quickly. Otherwise it could get hung up and caught on their canine teeth or tusks and will become a flying projectile as it shakes its head.

Chapter Reflection

After working through this chapter, learning the techniques, and practicing at school, what impact did it have on you when restraining patients? Were you able to keep your cool and not get upset? Were you confident or scared? Did the patients feel safe in your hands or were they nervous and scared? If the latter what can you do to keep them calm and safe?

Reference

Sheldon CC, Sonsthagen T, Topel JA. *Animal Restraint for Veterinary Professionals*. St. Louis, MO: Mosby Elsevier, 2017.

Suggested Reading

Restraint and Behavior of Dogs and Cats

https://www.pennfoster.edu/~/media/Files/PDF/SampleLessons/396-Veterinary%20Technician%20Associate%20Degree.ashx

https://www.slideshare.net/TahmeenaHassan/physical-restraining-methods-of-dogs-and-cats-52536008

https://www.slideshare.net/MarthaImperato/cats-i-behavior-and-restraint-of-cats?next_slideshow=2

Restraint of Cattle

https://www.gla.ac.uk/t4/~vet/files/teaching/clinicalexam/preexam/restraint.html

Restraint of Horses – application of twitch and chain shank

http://cal.vet.upenn.edu/projects/fieldservice/Equine/eqrestr/eqrestr.htm

Restraint of Sheep

http://www.sheep101.info/201/handling.html

Restraint of Rabbits and Pocket Pets

Veterinary Key – Rabbits https://veteriankey.com/rabbits-4/

Assessing the Health and Welfare of Laboratory Animals

http://www.ahwla.org.uk/site/tutorials/BVA/BVA08-Rabbit/Rabbit.html

http://www.ahwla.org.uk/site/tutorials/BVA/BVA06-Rat/Rat.html

http://www.ahwla.org.uk/site/tutorials/BVA/BVA03-Gerbil/Gerbil.html

http://www.ahwla.org.uk/site/tutorials/BVA/BVA05-Mouse/Mouse.html

http://www.ahwla.org.uk/site/tutorials/BVA/BVA09-Ferret/Ferret.html

Knots and Ropes

Texts on animal restraint rightfully begin with the use of ropes and knots. Although this may seem unusual, without this knowledge an assistant will be unable to provide effective animal restraint. A length of rope can quickly become a leash, halter, hobbles, or security with the quick application of the following knots. This can mean the difference between a patient injuring itself, clients, co-workers, or you!

Knot Tying Terminology

Knot tying uses a specific terminology in order to follow directions on how to tie the different knots.

Knots: the intertwining of parts of a rope or two ropes together.

Hitch: the intertwining of loops arranged so the **standing part** pushes against the **end**, securing the rope to an animal or object.

End: the end of the rope that can be freely moved and manipulated (Figure 9.1).

Standing part: the "other" end of the rope that is either the long end, secured to the animal or inanimate object or held still while the **end** is passed around it to make a knot or hitch.

Bight: a sharp bend in the rope. This is can be made with either the **end** or the **standing part**. To use shoe tying as an example, when you make a "bow," you are making a bight!

Throw: when the **end** is wrapped around another end or the standing part of the rope being used (Figure 9.2). When tying your shoes it is the first tie. As you wrap one shoestring (**end**) around the other (**end**), you have made a throw! (Figure 9.2).

Loop: a complete circle made to start a knot or hitch. It can be made in the **standing part** or **end**. Depending on the knot, the end is passed under or over the standing part, as Figure 9.3 shows. It is important to

Tasks for the Veterinary Assistant, Fourth Edition. Teresa F. Sonsthagen.
© 2020 John Wiley & Sons, Inc. Published 2020 by John Wiley & Sons, Inc.
Companion website: www.wiley.com/go/sonsthagen/tasks

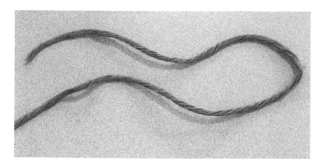

FIGURE 9.1 End, standing part, and bight.

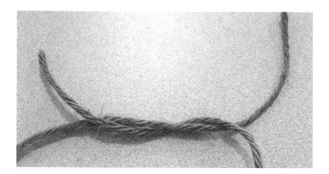

FIGURE 9.2 Throw.

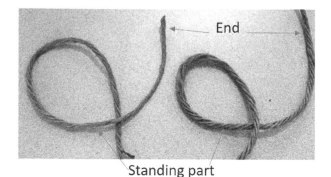

FIGURE 9.3 Loops – left end under the standing part, right end over the standing part.

make the **loop** in the right direction so the knot is tied correctly.

Overhand knot: a quick and easy way to secure the **end** of a rope from fraying or to produce a loop to make a fixed bight (Figure 9.4).

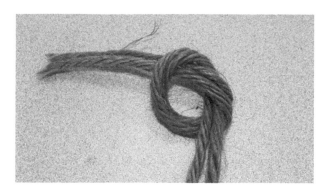

FIGURE 9.4 Overhand knot.

Types of Ropes

The choice of material and flexibility depends on the rope's purpose. Ropes are made of many types of materials and are of varying thicknesses (Figure 9.5). The diameter is expressed in fractions of an inch, such as ⅝, ½, or ¼ inch. Strength varies by material and diameter. Ropes are flaccid to stiff depending on the material used to construct the rope. A cotton rope with a small diameter and good flexibility is suitable for positioning a small, anesthetized animal during surgery or radiography. A stronger nylon rope with some stiffness is more suitable for maintaining a loop while slipping it over a kenneled dog's head. A thistle or hemp rope is rough to the touch. Flexibility should be such that knot retention is secure. The surface must be smooth enough to be comfortable for both the patient and the handler. A thick, stiff rope characteristic of the lariat used for large animals is harsh to the touch but doesn't damage the tough hide of a calf or cow. A soft cotton or nylon rope of medium diameter and approximately 6 ft long can be used to make horse halters.

Prevent Fraying

Rope is purchased from hardware and feed stores in requested lengths. When purchasing rope in this manner, it becomes necessary to treat the ends with some technique to prevent fraying or unraveling. Nylon or synthetic ropes will fray quickly if the ends are not secured. There are several ways to secure the ends of rope. One is to apply tape around each end, leaving ¼–½ inches of rope sticking out; a quick pass through a candle or disposable lighter flame will melt the ends together and prevent fraying (Figure 9.6). The tape can be removed after the ends are melted to facilitate it being passed through a ring or loop. A temporary fix is wrapping the ends tightly with tape; however, tape becomes brittle over time and often slips off. A simple overhand knot tied at the end of the rope will also prevent unraveling (Figure 9.6). Unfortunately, the thickness of the tape and the overhand knot may prevent the insertion of it through small loops while tying a knot.

A third technique of securing an end is to **whip** it with smaller cords. This is called whipping (Figure 9.7).

Whipping is wrapping a small diameter cord around the ends of cotton rope to prevent fraying. A thick kitchen string or lightweight nylon cord about 12–24 inches long is needed in order to give you a deep enough whip.

1. Start on one end of the rope with unfinished ends. Make a bight in the center of the whipping cord. Place it on alongside the rope with the **bight** adjacent to the end of the rope.
2. Use long **end** of the whipping cord to begin tightly encircling the rope and the bight of the whipping cord about 2 inches from the end of the rope (Figure 9.8). Place each wrap adjacent to each other, without a space between the wraps or wrinkles or twists in the cord. Wrap toward the end of the rope until you have all but ½ inch of the rope covered with the whipping cord. You should be close to the bight. Stop wrapping and put the end of the whipping cord through the bight at the end of the rope.
3. Pull the other end of the whipping cord left free at the beginning of the wraps until the bight and the wrapping end of the cord are pulled under the wraps, about half the length of the wrapped cord (Figure 9.9).
4. Trim the end of the cord used to pull the bight under the wraps close to the first wrap, then trim the rope within ¼ inch of the end (Figure 9.10).

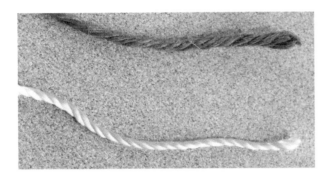

FIGURE 9.5 Examples of types of ropes.

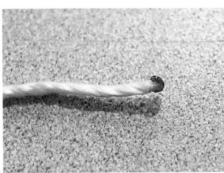

FIGURE 9.6 Melted and tied ends of nylon rope.

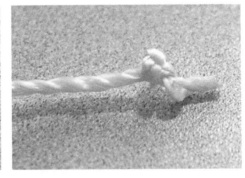

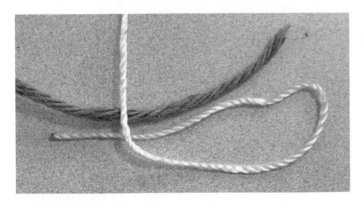

FIGURE 9.7 Start of whipping.

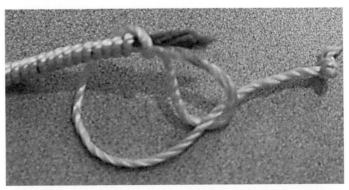

FIGURE 9.8 Wrapping the whipping cord.

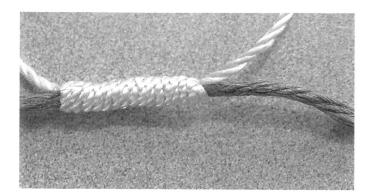

FIGURE 9.9 Ends tucked under the wraps.

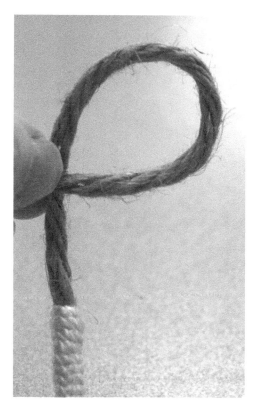

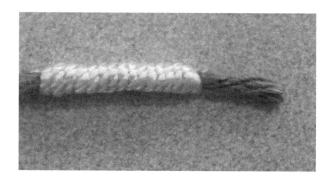

FIGURE 9.10 Completed whipping with ends trimmed.

FIGURE 9.11 Starting loop for hanking.

Hanking a Rope

Hanking is a method of shortening long ropes or extension cords for storage. It provides a quick release of a rope's length without tangling or knotting. This technique works well on extension cords as well.

1. Form a **loop** that with the **end** passing under the **standing part** and hold it together with your non-dominant hand (Figure 9.11).
2. Reach through the **loop**, grasp the **standing part** and bring **bight** through the **loop**. This makes a second loop in which the next loop will be brought through. Repeat the process of forming the loops to form a continuous chain (Figure 9.12).
3. When no more loops can be made, bring the **end** through the last loop and tighten. To untie the rope, pull the **end** out of the last loop. This will start the "unlooping" process. If it does not, you may have selected the wrong end! Try again at the opposite end (Figure 9.13).

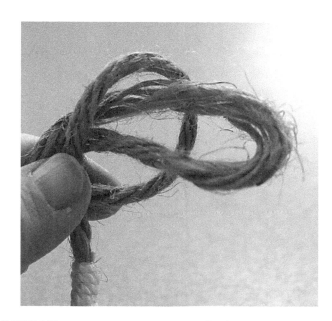

FIGURE 9.12 Making loops within loops or hanking.

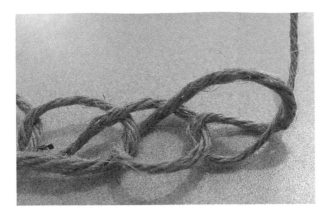

FIGURE 9.13 Finishing and untying the hanked roped.

Types of Knots and Hitches

In veterinary practice, there are seven frequently used knots: the halter tie, square knot with its variants such as the reefer's knot, sheet bend, bowline, and the bowline on a bight. The half hitch and clove hitch are also used to secure patients for various reason in the veterinary practice.

When securing a conscious patient to an object, the knot must meet two requirements: (i) quick release by the handler and (ii) the knot does not tighten on the patient if the end is pulled or the patient struggles. This may not be achieved with a single knot, but several knots used in tandem will meet these requirements.

There are three important rules to remember when tying any animal to an immovable object:

1. Always tie a patient with a quick-release knot. The halter tie meets this rule because if the patient gets into trouble it can be quickly released.
2. A patient must be tied in such a way that it does not become tangled. This may result in frightening a patient and causing an injury to either itself or the person trying to untangle it.
3. A rope is never tied around a patient using a knot that continues to tighten if tension is placed on the end or standing part. Circulation or airways can be compromised if such a knot is used, causing injury or death.

Types of Knots

The following are instructions for tying knots. Practice all of these knots with not just a strand of rope but hook something to one end! It is a different experience not being able to manipulate both ends of a rope. It will make you a better and safer knot tier and you will use them throughout your lifetime.

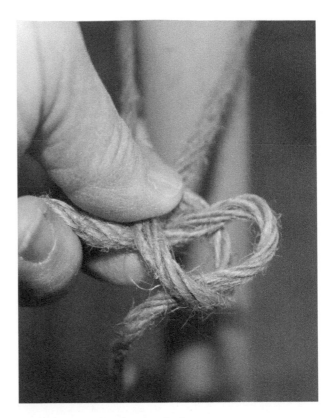

FIGURE 9.14 Halter tie – forming the loop.

Halter Tie

Livestock are often secured to inanimate objects like fence posts or rings attached to walls. The halter tie is used to tie a patient to these objects. If the patient gets tangled up or is in some other predicament, the knot can be quickly untied by pulling on the end. The halter tie will always release even if the patient pulls on the standing part and tightens it around the object. This is the only knot that should be used to tie a patient to a fixed object.

1. Start with at least a 6 ft leash or halter rope with the clip end attached to a collar or halter, respectively. Pass the **end** of the rope from left to right around a vertical post. Hold the **standing part** in your left hand and the **end** in your right, the two should be parallel to each other. Form a **loop** in the **end**, so it passes over the standing part of the loop. Place it on top of the **standing part** in your left hand, as close to the post as possible. Pinch the loop and **standing part** together with your left index finger and thumb (Figure 9.14).
2. With your right hand reach through the **loop** from the top and grasp the **end** just far enough down to make a **bight** by folding the rope between your index finger and thumb. Making sure the end is under the **standing part,** pull the bight up through the loop.
3. Tighten the knot by pulling on the **bight** and pushing the loop close to the post (Figure 9.15).

4. Some patients have figured out that if they pull on the end, the halter tie comes untied. To prevent this, place the end loosely through the bight. To untie the

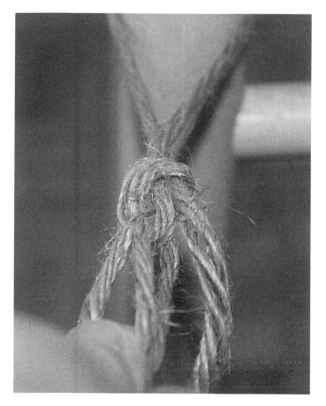

FIGURE 9.15 Tightening the knot by pulling on the bight.

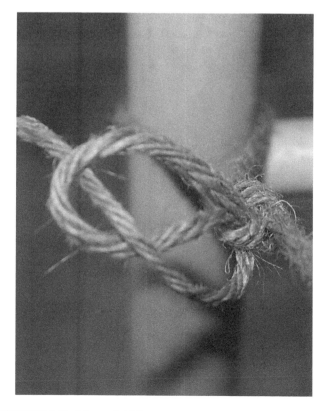

FIGURE 9.16 End through bight.

rope, remember to remove the end from the bight. Give the end of the rope a firm tug and the knot should untie quickly and easily (Figure 9.16).

A vertical post is stronger than a horizontal post for securing livestock and horses. A post can actually be pulled out of the ground. This can cause a whole new issue as the resulting breach in the fence could release the patient from captivity and the resulting drag of fencing material continues to scare the animal as it runs away. No matter how hard the animal pulls on this knot it should release quickly and easily even during this kind of scenario.

Practice makes perfect. If the knot does not untie easily, you have not tied it correctly. If the animal can back up and untie the knot by applying pressure to the standing part, then the knot was not tied correctly. Often it is because the loop was formed with the end under the standing part. It is important to be able to tie this knot quickly and accurately which requires practice.

Square Knot

The square knot is used whenever a knot must remain secure, without slipping even if tension is applied to one or both ends. The square knot is the foundation for the reefer's knot and all suture knots. This knot is unique because as tension increases, the knot becomes tighter, which prevents it from loosening. However, no matter how tight the knot becomes, it can be untied easily by pushing the ends and standing parts toward the knot (Figure 9.17).

When this knot is tied correctly, it never slips either tighter or looser. This is imperative for suture knots and when going around an animal's body part. The key to tying a perfect square knot every time is to remember the end that you start your throw with is the end that is used to make all the throws. The square knot uses both ends and the resulting loop is the standing part.

1. Hold an **end** in each hand, place the right **end** over the left **end** to make a X (Figure 9.18a). Make a throw with the right **end** which now becomes the left **end** (Figure 9.18b).

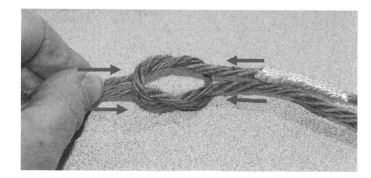

FIGURE 9.17 Untying a square knot.

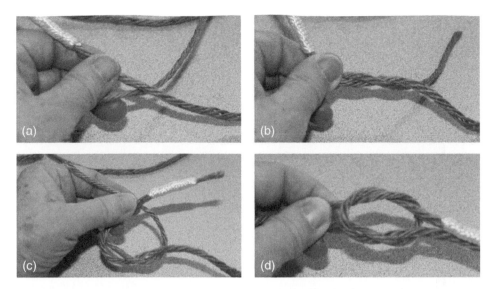

FIGURE 9.18 Tying a square knot first throw.

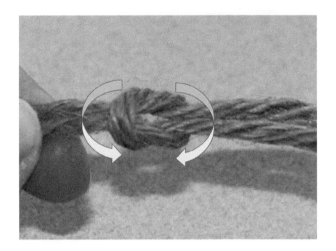

FIGURE 9.19 Properly tied square knot.

Remember: "right over left, left over right" or "left over right, right over left" when tying a square knot. The key is to remember which end was used to make the first throw and to continue to use that end to make the second throw!

2. Place the left **end** over the right end, forming another X and make another throw. This restores it as the right **end** again (Figure 9.18c). Pull the **ends** and **standing parts** tight (Figure 9.18d).

A non-slipping noose forms that does not tighten or loosen if tension is applied to the ends or standing parts.

To check that you have tied it correctly, grasp both ends and part of the loop closest to the knot and push them toward the knot. You should see two interconnected loops (Figure 9.19).

If you are tying this around a patient's body, make one end shorter than the other so that when you finish, you

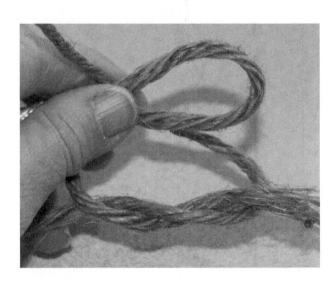

FIGURE 9.20 Reefer's knot – bring the bight through as the second throw.

have a length of rope that can be used to tie the body part to another to secure it out of the way. Never tie a body part to an inanimate object unless using a halter or collar.

Reefer's Knot

The reefer's knot is based on the square knot and is tied like a square knot but uses a bight made in one of the strands to provide a quick release. It would be similar to tying a shoelace with only one bow.

1. Make the first throw as described for the square knot. Before making the second throw, make a bight in the left **end** and wrap that around the right **end** (Figure 9.20).
2. Tighten the knot by pulling the bight one way and the end the other. This makes a one-loop bow. To untie the knot, pull on the end of the bow (Figure 9.21).

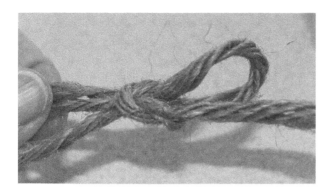

FIGURE 9.21 Reefer's knot – tightened knot.

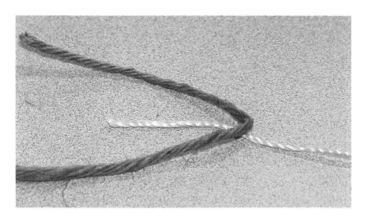

FIGURE 9.22 Sheet bend first step.

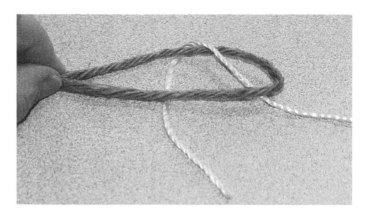

FIGURE 9.23 Sheet bend second step.

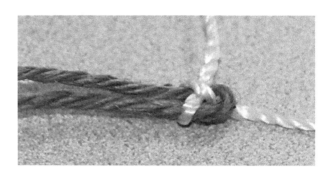

FIGURE 9.24 Sheet bend final step.

To make sure this knot will not tighten down, pull on the sides of the loop. If it moves, you have not made the throws correctly. This can be used to tie a fractured limb up to an IV pole for surgical preparation.

Sheet Bend Knot

If a long length of rope is needed but only short pieces are available, this knot will connect the ropes of different diameters and conformation securely.

1. Make a **bight** close to one **end** of the thickest rope so that you have an elongated U on one **end**. Both **ends** of this rope will be pointed in the same direction (Figure 9.22); one **end** should be substantially shorter than the other. Grasp the lighter rope at one **end** and bring the **end** up from underneath the **bight** in the thick rope right where it bends.
2. Pass the **end** underneath both of the thick ropes, bringing it over the top of those **ends** and then lift a portion of the lighter rope and pass it under itself (Figure 9.23).
3. Tighten the knot by pulling all four **ends** in opposite directions. As you pull it tight, you should see the **bight** in the thick rope and an X forming in the lighter rope. The lighter rope should have one **end** under the **bight** of the thick rope and one **end** over the **bight** (Figure 9.24).

The knot should not fall apart and it should *not* look like a square knot. If it does, you did not go under the lighter rope as described. Because this is a variation of the square knot, it will be easy to untie by pushing the ends toward the knot.

The sheet bend is also used as a tail tie in horses and cattle. The U is made with the hair on the tail bent at the tip of the vertebrae as the thick rope and then a ½ or ¼ inch rope or cord is used to as the lighter rope. This allows you to tie the tail to a front leg or neck using a halter tie.

> **TIP BOX 9.2**
>
> If a patient's tail needs to be tied out of the way, always tie it to the patient's body. That way, if the patient should happen to get away, the tail goes with!

Bowline

A bowline is a non-slipping knot that can be used to safely secure ropes around an animal's body part or a load to a trailer. This knot is sometimes difficult to master, but once you can tie it correctly, it is a great all-purpose knot. It is very easy to untie because of the way it is tied, no matter how tight the knot is pulled.

1. Pass the rope around a body part or object; leave the left end longer than the right. The left end now becomes the **standing part**. Make a loop with the left

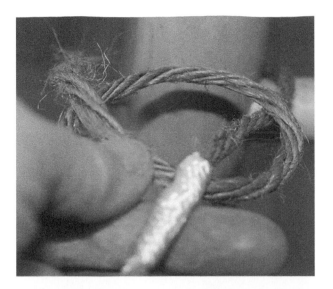

FIGURE 9.25 Bowline knot first steps.

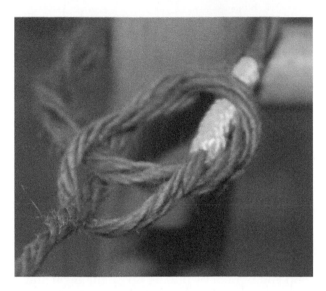

FIGURE 9.26 Bowline second step.

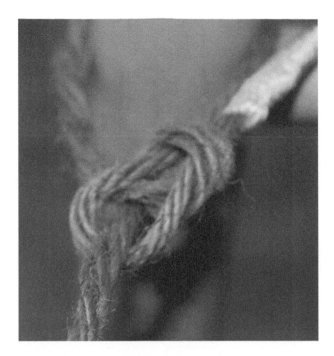

FIGURE 9.27 Bowline final step.

hand rope, with the **end** under the **standing part** (Figure 9.25).
2. Grasp the right hand rope and bring the **end** up through the loop, around the **standing part**, and back down through the loop (Figure 9.26).
3. Tighten the knot by pulling the **end** up and the **standing part** down. You should see two loops: the one made in the standing part and the one made by the end around the standing part (Figure 9.27).

If the knot slides, you have not tied it correctly and need to retie it so it does not cut off circulation or respiration if used around a leg or neck. Usually, the issue is from making the loop the wrong way.

To untie the knot, grasp and pull the loops in different directions, this will loosen it right up, no matter how tight it is.

Bowline on a Bight

The bowline on a bight creates a non-slip noose with equal length ends that can be tied to a fixed object or another part of the animal. This knot is particularly useful in equine and large animal practices when securing patients to prevent kicking or when tying limbs out of the way. The two long ends can be used to secure legs to the animal's own body.

1. Fold the rope in half, which makes a **bight** in the middle of the rope and gives you two long **ends**. Use the **bight** as an **end**, form a large circle by making a throw around the two strands of the rope. Make sure the resulting circle can pass over the head and around the neck, leg or other body part of the animal. Hold the large circle at the top with your left hand (as indicated by the red arrow); pass your right hand fingers through the bight and with your index finger and thumb, grasp the two strands of the throw, as indicated by the blue arrows (Figure 9.28).
2. Drop the top of the circle being held by your left hand and grasp the **bight** with your left hand, indicated by the green arrow. Pull the **bight** toward the two ends in the direction indicated by the green arrow. At the same time pull the two strands in your right fingers in the opposite direction as indicated by the red arrow (Figure 9.29).

TIP BOX 9.3

To remember how to tie the bowline, use this saying: "The rabbit comes out of the hole, goes around the tree, and back into the hole."

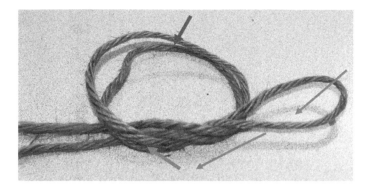

FIGURE 9.28 Bowline on a bight first steps.

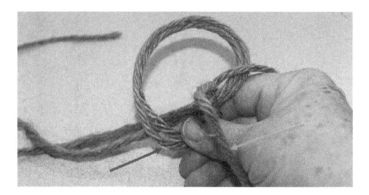

FIGURE 9.29 Bowline on a bight second step.

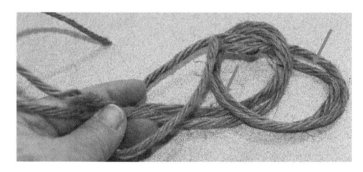

FIGURE 9.30 Bowline on a bight third step.

3. Switch your hold to the two strands coming from each side of the knot, as indicated by the blue arrows and pull in opposite directions to tighten the knot (Figure 9.30).
4. Note the **bight** indicated by the green arrow. This is what you would grab to loosen this knot. If you don't see this you made the knot wrong or you didn't pull the two strands indicated by the blue arrows in the right direction, as indicated also by the blue arrows (Figure 9.31).

The resulting non-slipping noose can be placed over the patient's head. You can use the two long ends to anchor the back legs to the neck to prevent kicking or to pull the legs in a certain direction to get them out of the way.

When tying the legs, use two half hitches around the leg followed by a halter tie to secure the rope.

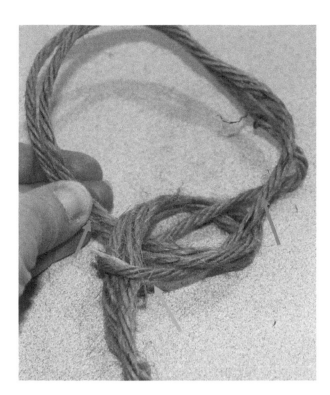

FIGURE 9.31 Bowline on a bight final step.

Overhand Knot

The overhand knot, can be used to make a loop leash that can be safely used around the neck as a leash or around a limb to secure it to a table.

1. Make a **bight** on one **end** of the rope. Make it as close to the **end** as possible (Figure 9.32).
2. Grasp the **bight** at the bend and fold both strands into a **loop**. Continue to move the **bight** through the **loop** and tighten by pulling up on the **bight** and down on the **ends** (Figure 9.33).
3. The result is a single strand loop secured by two strands of the knot. To make a leash, bring the long end through the loop. This creates a leash that will not stay tight when pressure is released. To make a handle, tie another over hand knot on the opposite end, only make it big enough to fit your hand (Figure 9.34).

Never use a slip knot to make a leash. If the resulting loop is made with the long end it may get placed around a neck or limb and it will tighten down and stay tight even after the ends are released.

Hitches

Hitches are used in the veterinary practice for a number of reasons. The half hitch is used to secure a rope to a leg, post, or cleat. Cleats are typically found on the sides of surgery and X-ray tables, cattle chutes, and horse stocks. Remember that hitches stay secure because the

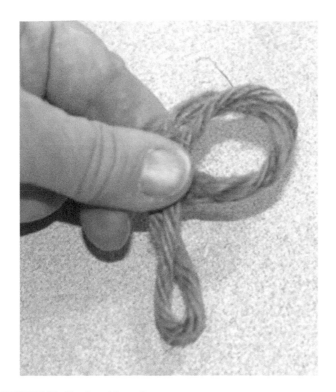

FIGURE 9.32 Overhand knot first step.

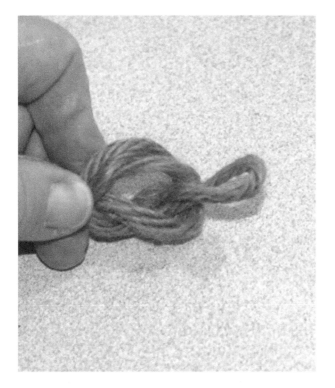

FIGURE 9.33 Overhand knot second step.

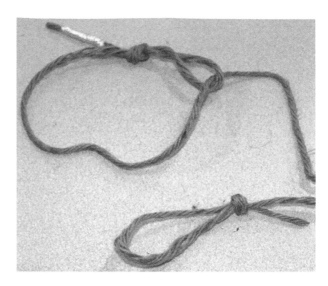

FIGURE 9.34 Overhand knot final step for making a loop leash.

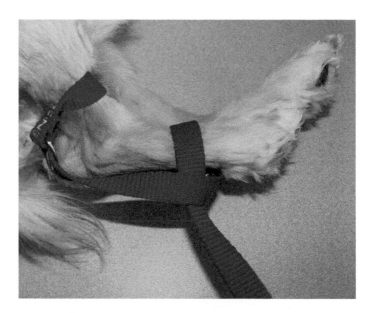

FIGURE 9.35 Loop and half hitch secured to a leg.

end presses the standing part against the leg, post, or cleat. Also note that hitches are actually loops made either by placing the end under or over the standing part and then stacked one upon another! It will matter a great deal which way the loop is made; if the rope stays in place you made it the right way!

Tying a limb to a surgical table is a commonly used technique utilizing hitches and a slip leash utilizing an overhand knot.

1. Start with a rope leash; bring the handle end through the loop or ring, creating a circle that opens and closes with tension when released or applied to the end. Slip the loop around the limb above the elbow or hock; pull the end to make it snug but not extremely tight. Make a hitch by forming a loop that opens away from you in the end and slip the loop around the leg, below the circle usually at midleg. Make the loop snug but not tight around the limb (Figure 9.35).

2. Use the end to secure the limb to the table by winding the end around the cleat once in a figure eight, then make a half hitch by making a loop with

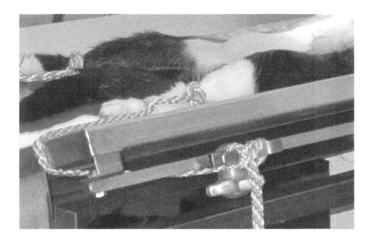

FIGURE 9.36 Leg secured to surgical table.

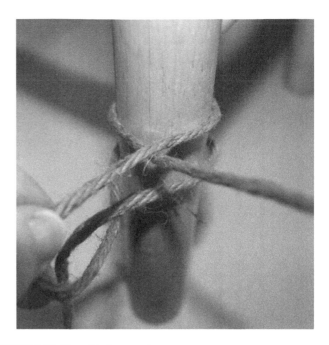

FIGURE 9.38 Clove hitch second step.

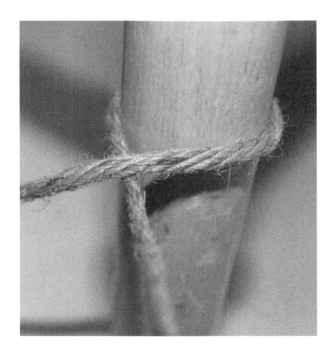

FIGURE 9.37 Clove hitch first step.

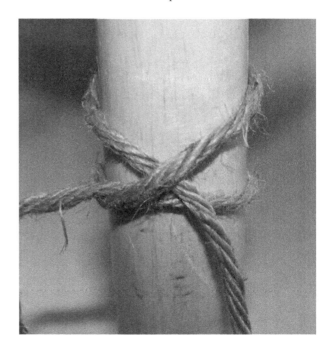

FIGURE 9.39 Clove hitch final step.

the **end** under the **standing part** and place it around one of the cleats; pull to tighten. To loosen, push up on the end; this will release the pressure applied to the standing part (Figure 9.36).

Clove Hitch

The clove hitch can be used to secure a rope to an object and leave two long ends available to tie something up to it or to secure a load on a trailer. The clove hitch is made with two half hitches, each made in opposite directions then stacked one on top of the other. This is great to secure loads to trailers as you can tighten one end of the rope over the load with one rope while the rope will not come loose because it is being kept in place by the first half hitch in the stack.

1. Pass one **end** of the rope around the object. You can make one **end** longer than the other or keep the rope **ends** even. Drape the right **end** over the left **end**. Drop the right **end** as the left will hold it close to the object. The left strand now becomes the **end** and the **standing part** (Figure 9.37).
2. Grasp the left rope as pictured with one hand making a **bight** and bring the **end** around the object with the other hand. Pass the end through the **bight** (Figure 9.38).
3. Grasp both ends, one in each hand and tighten. The result should be two loops around the object with an X forming the standing part (Figure 9.39).

If using ropes to tie a load down on a trailer, secure one end of the rope to the trailer with a bowline knot. Pass the rope over the load to the opposite side of the trailer. Apply a half hitch around a beam or ring, pull the rope tight. Cross over the load again, and use another half hitch. Continue this pattern until you get the load sufficiently secured, then finish off with a clove hitch to secure the rope to the trailer. The clove hitch will not come undone even if tension is applied to one strand or the other.

Chapter Reflection

Now that you have learned how to tie knots and how to use them on patients, think of times when a good knot would have come in handy, and share those experiences. How you will make sure that you have tied a knot properly.

Suggested Reading

Animated Knots by Grog. https://www.animatedknots.com/horse-farm-knots (accessed July 2, 2019).

CHAPTER 10

Management of Hospitalized and Boarding Pets

LEARNING OBJECTIVES

- Provide appropriate environment for hospitalized patients
- Care for recumbent patients, including administering enemas
- Provide appropriate exercise for hospitalized and boarding pets
- Execute appropriate socialization for hospitalized and boarding pets
- Follow veterinary prescribe treatment plans
- Understand how diseases enter the body
- Assist with in-hospital patient care including bathing and dipping
- Accurately obtain vital signs, body conditioning scores, and weights
- Determine the well-being of patients and recognize signs of pain
- Properly collect, label, and store voluntary urine and fecal samples
- Assist with euthanasia and recognize signs of grief in co-workers

NAVTA ESSENTIAL SKILLS COVERED IN THIS CHAPTER

V. Small Animal Nursing (Large Animal Nursing – Optional)
A. Safety concerns
   2. Utilize patient and personnel safety measures
B. Animal care
   1. Provide routine record-keeping, and observation of hospitalized patients, i.e. stress importance of notations made when cleaning and feeding
   2. Demonstrate a basic understanding of:
      b. common diseases
      c. common medical conditions
   6. Demonstrate understanding of a treatment plan

Tasks for the Veterinary Assistant, Fourth Edition. Teresa F. Sonsthagen.
© 2020 John Wiley & Sons, Inc. Published 2020 by John Wiley & Sons, Inc.
Companion website: www.wiley.com/go/sonsthagen/tasks

8. Perform therapeutic bathing, basic grooming, and dipping of small animals
12. Demonstrate an understanding of euthanasia and post mortem care
13. Capillary refill time and normal mucous membrane evaluation
VII. Laboratory Procedures
A. Assistance in the laboratory
    1. Collect voided urine samples
    5. Collect voided fecal samples for examination
    9. Handle disposal of deceased animals

Depending on your hospital or clinic you may be taking care of pets that are boarding, recovering from surgery, or are sick and may be contagious. Each one of these need a little bit of tender loving care and appropriately sized accommodations to their respective needs. Remember, these are beloved pets and they get lonely, spending a few minutes talking to them and giving them a few pats as you move through the room will be of comfort to them. Above all though, they need a clean, stress free environment in which to live and heal. A vital job for the assistant will be to ensure these requirements are met.

Housing Requirements – Kennel Set-up

Kennels and runs should always be ready to receive a patient. The basic set-up is clean newspapers on the bottom of the cage, an empty cage card, and ID collar inside the kennel. The newspaper is good for soaking up spills and containing debris. It is also good for dust collection for cages that may not be used very often because of size or position in the room. The newspaper can be folded up to capture the dust or debris from the pet and disposed of in the garbage. This would be appropriate for recycling.

When a patient is admitted to the hospital there are some considerations to take into account. The selection of a kennel or a run will depend on the size of the patient. It must be large enough for the patient to stand, move, and turn around easily. They should not have to negotiate around food and water dishes when shifting positions. Metal cages tend to be cold so a layer of newspaper covered with a towel or blanket is often required. Clean, soft, dry bedding large enough for an animal to stretch out on comfortably should be provided for each patient. Many will enjoy burrowing into the blanket for warmth and comfort. Instead of the newspaper some

clinics use a rubber mat with holes for drainage as the resting area. A towel can be laid over the mat but if the patient is **incontinent** or tears or chews at the bedding just the rubber mat is provided.

Water is the next priority and it should always be available, unless otherwise directed. Always place the water dish in a spot to avoid it being tipped over easily. Check on patients throughout the day to make sure they all have water and that none are sitting in a wet or soiled cage. If found, clean it out and resettle the patient immediately. A wet patient is a sad and potentially unhealthy patient.

Reflection

Determine how you will set up a kennel or run for a patient. What comfort measures can be taken to ensure a comfortable and sanitary kennel or run?

Water and Food Consumption – Elimination

The consumption of water can be tricky to determine unless you are paying attention to the amounts given. This is especially important with cats as they are not great drinkers in the first place and when stressed are even more apt to not drink. Measuring the water presented and when being replenished may be asked of you for some patients. Making note of the amount of water consumed in the record is very important with these patients. Be conscious of the amount of water available. If you arrive in the morning to an empty bowl, which has not been dumped, perhaps a bigger bowl is in order to last the night. Alert the veterinarian if water is being consumed in larger amounts than normal for that sized pet. There may be a medical issue that has not been investigated. Failure to consume all the offered food, especially if formulated to their daily caloric requirements, must be written in the patient's file. The veterinarian may choose to adjust the diet for the patient based on this information.

If elimination of urine and feces is not normal more notations are in order. Urine descriptions include yellow, straw-colored, or red. You may be asked to catch the urine to measure the output. This is important when there is a concern for kidney function. Feces descriptions include degree of firmness, from normal to watery, which can be indicated with plus signs. Normal is + and watery is ++++; also note if the feces contained blood or mucus. Normal elimination would indicate no straining for both; an indication of straining is important to note.

Reflection

How will you note or keep track of which animal is drinking and how much as well as elimination patterns? Devise a way to know exactly who is doing what under your care.

Environmental Considerations

Think of the patient's needs from the perspective of the individual. Environmental factors influence patient well-being. Factors such as temperature, humidity, and ventilation have an important role in patient comfort. Airflow into a kennel with solid walls is very limited making it warmer than the room. Obese and long-haired patients may get too warm and will often lay down close to the kennel door. Short-haired patients will either be just right or will retreat to the rear of the cage where it is warmer. Setting the water dish and the resting blanket or mat will be dictated by these behaviors. The overly warm patients will appreciate their water dish set to the back of the kennel and their blanket towards the front and vice versa for the warm patient.

Pay attention to the patient that is disturbing their bedding. It can be an indication of anxiety, pain, anger, or frustration. Anxiety can sometimes be calmed by placing a towel over the cage door and making sure the door is latched securely. This provides a quiet, dark place that often allows the patient to calm down and rest. When checking on this patient just a peek inside is enough. Depending on the patient, it may be better to not disturb them until it is time for treatments, potty breaks, or feeding. Their cage, unless soiled or wet, is often not cleaned until the animal has adjusted and is no longer emotional. If the patient will be in the clinic for a long

period of time an article of comfort from home is a good way to help them adjust. You may also use the pheromone spray to help calm them down.

Light–dark cycles are important for well-being. Body temperature and activity levels are influenced by exposure to light. The artificial environment of the hospital alters exposure to light and dark. Lights should be on during normal daylight hours and off during nighttime hours. Many wards will have timers for the lights, so a periodic check of these timers is important as sometimes they get turned off and either don't turn on or don't turn off. Often timers are regulated by small switches with pegs that are put in place by a screw. There is usually an on peg and an off peg that can be placed at 12-hour increments. The screws become loose as the timing wheel rotates, and they fall off, thus making the timer stay on or off until it reaches the next switch. Return the pegs to the correct times and hand tighten or gently tighten the screws with a screwdriver.

Noise and odors add a negative effect to the wards, not only for people but for the patients within. Strange noises in a veterinary clinic are frightening and distracting to patients. A constant barking dog should be assessed to see why it is barking. If from boredom, try giving it a busy toy with peanut butter or spray cheese. If from nervous energy, perhaps a romp in the exercise yard will help. If just plain nervous or anxious, placing a towel over the door may help. Odors can also be anxiety producing. Cats smelling dogs nearby, or rodents and birds smelling cats nearby can cause high anxiety. If possible, house like species together in one room or if that isn't available try to separate the species with an empty cage in between. Males smelling females in heat may become frustrated and aggressive towards the handler that is keeping him from his true love! Keeping these two as far apart as possible, even to the point of putting them in different rooms, will help.

While animals use their sense of smell more acutely to evaluate the world around them, they also use their vision as we do. The sight of a large dog may frighten a small dog or kitten housed across the room; likewise, a dog can become frustrated by the fact that it cannot get to the cat it would like to chase. By recognizing the possibility of this reaction and hanging a towel or piece of newspaper over the door to block one or the other's view is a smart idea.

Reflection

Think about ways that you can remember to check on the patient's well-being. How can you make a kennel or run a safe and fearless place for a hospitalized patient?

Socialization and Exercising Hospitalized Patients

Pets are accustomed to human–animal interaction. Therefore, it is important to provide positive interaction for each patient whenever it is handled. Offering treats during treatments and procedures if possible and when you start cleaning the kennel helps to keep the patient from becoming fearful of your approach. If the procedure doesn't allow treats, then talk in a gentle, soothing voice and stroke them calmly. Find their "itchy" spot, then a cuddle and praise after the procedure will go a long way in gaining cooperation and trust. These positive reinforcements put patients at ease which in turn will make it more likely that they will eat, rest, and respond to the treatments.

Exercise and play are important for the hospitalized and boarding patient. Hospitalized patients may be on restricted exercise so always check before taking them outside. Boarding pets will appreciate the opportunity to be out of their kennel for a walk or romp in the exercise yard. Adult dogs are most likely to be house-trained and will not soil their kennel or run. Twice daily at least 10-minute walks to stretch their legs and relieve themselves is very important to their mental health. If the hospital has a fenced in yard a longer break with other pets is appropriate. Let the pets meet each other while still on the leash. If there are no indications of aggressiveness, then they can romp together. Never leave the pets or patients unattended during these breaks, not only to make sure they don't get into a fight but to make sure they don't escape. Remember to double leash the dogs as you transport them from the ward to the exercise yard or for a walk.

If there isn't a yard, then only one dog at a time should be taken outside. Double leash the dog and bring a plastic bag to pick up feces. Never allow the dog to run or jerk you, if they do then put an anti-jump harness on them for their walks. Never allow a dog to mouth your hand or arm while walking. If they do, then a cage muzzle or leash muzzle is applied before the walk. Never drag or jerk harshly on the collar as this can injure their necks and backs.

If because of weather the dogs cannot be taken outside for their 10-minute walk, allow them to exercise in a run or if available a hallway or room. Anywhere that can be secured with doors that lock or have signs posted that there are animals loose in the area. Throw a ball or play tag with them, whatever is needed to let them thoroughly stretch their legs will help them mentally and physically. Again, if you know two dogs get along and like to play with each other, a supervised play session is also appropriate.

Exercise and socialization is pet dependent. The astute assistant will evaluate and meet the needs of the

individual. A "one size fits all" mentality does not adequately meet patient needs. Let the patient set the tone for the appropriate amount of exercise and socializing. Some may just need you to sit with them on your lap!

Reflection

Think about the types of patients you may see in a veterinary facility – from boarding pets to very sick or injured pets. Describe what you can do personally to ensure their comfort and safety.

Patient Care Based on Reason for Being in the Hospital

Boarding

Pets that are boarded at a clinic may become so lonesome for their owner that they become depressed. This may mean not eating well or at all. Careful records and attention to each pet is vital in order to catch this and take steps to alleviate this behavior. It may involve spending a bit more time with the pet or taking it outside more often or hand feeding. Another comfort would be to ask the owner to bring the pet's bed or an article of the owner's clothing as a comfort item to help them settle in better. Use of the pheromone spray can also help. Some boarding pets may require medications to be given on a regular basis. For example, diabetic dogs will need to be fed at 12-hour intervals and given insulin about 15 minutes later. Keeping them on a strict schedule helps them maintain a good blood sugar level. Careful records of when the insulin was given, where it was given, and how much is very important information to write in the record. Failure to do so may result in a double dose because anyone checking will see that it wasn't done when in fact it was! This can result in dangerously low sugar levels and potential loss of life. Older dogs may require more than a twice daily walk; getting them out for a potty break during the day will reduce anxiety.

Cat housing rules are like those for dogs. They must have room enough to lay down without being inhibited by the presence of litter pan, food, and water dishes. The ideal situation would be a perch that can be placed inside the kennel, allowing them to be up away from the litter

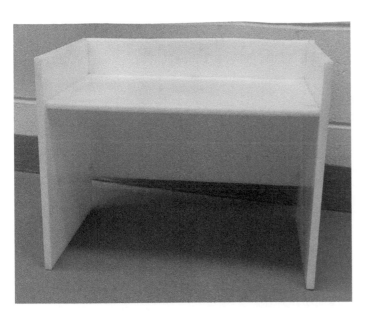

FIGURE 10.1 Cat kennel perch.

box which is tucked under the perch (Figure 10.1). Food and water dishes are placed just inside the door close to the hinge side. This allows the cat room enough to jump off the perch and access the litter box without tipping over the dishes. By placing the dishes to the hinge side you can open the door to remove the cat without working around the dishes.

Cats often become depressed or anxious when boarding. Hiding under towels, crouching in litter boxes, and not eating or drinking can indicate there is a problem. They may also become aggressive and not want you to touch them or clean their kennel. The pheromone spray may help, as well as offering tasty food treats or allowing them to stroll around the ward a bit can help alleviate some of this stress. Offer a paper bag as a toy when out of the kennel. Playing with a toy or feather on a rope is always a welcome relief from the boredom of being kenneled. Make sure there are signs on the doors indicating a loose cat so that it doesn't inadvertently escape.

Reflection

Why would pets that are boarding at a hospital become sick or depressed? What can you do to alleviate these afflictions?

Surgical Patients

Pre-surgical patients should not be fed on the morning of surgery but can have water available. Post-surgical patients are often cold and may need a warming device (Figure 10.2). There are many different types available. Some will not need blankets on top of the pad and some suggest blankets on top. Whatever type is used always make sure the animal can move off the warming pad if they don't need it any more. At that point remove the warming device from the kennel or run. If they cannot move, make sure to shift them every 15–20 minutes. *Never* use a human heating pad to warm a **recumbent** patient. They get too hot and will cause not only devastating burns, but could result in a lawsuit for the clinic. Some surgical patients may need assistance to move from position to position or walking to relieve themselves. Don't attempt this without permission from the veterinarian or technician. With big dogs, always have another person helping to move them or walk them. A sling or long towel is passed under their abdomen, close to the flank, with a person on each side of the dog taking an end and lifting. Lift just to provide support but allow the dog to move under its own power. Care must be taken when moving surgical patients so that they are not jostled excessively. Extra padding for them to lay upon is also a way to offer comfort. Be careful with these patients as pain may make them bite if you inadvertently hurt them. Surgical and ill patients will often have an IV catheter and care must be taken not to dislodge this from the vein. Always handle these patients with care and if they are to be taken outside to relieve themselves you may need another person the help hold the IV bag or to lift and carry them if unable to walk very far. Record the reason for any handling done and at what times. If the handling was for elimination, record what happened, how much, and description as appropriate for feces or urine.

Reflection

Describe some of the ways that caring for a surgical patient is different from caring for a boarding patient.

Recumbent Patient Care

Recumbent patients require extra attention, so they do not develop **decubitus ulcers**, urine scalds, and fecal matting. Decubitus ulcers are caused from the weight of the body putting pressure on the bony parts of the body that are against the floor. To avoid these sores from developing, extra padding under the hips and shoulders will help as well as changing the position of the body every 3–4 hours. Alert the veterinarian if you see any

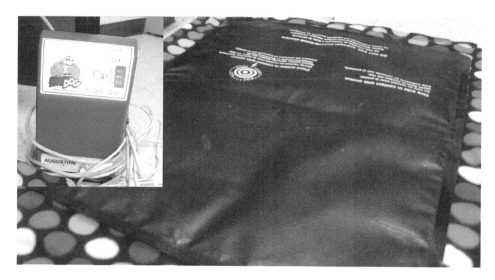

FIGURE 10.2 Patient warmer.

signs of pressure sores or new wounds on a recumbent patient. The sooner these wounds can be treated the better the odds they will not get infected. These are treated much like an open wound from a trauma.

If the patient is incontinent or has diarrhea care must be taken to keep the body dry. There are several techniques for keeping patients dry. Shaving or trimming long hair around the perianal area can help keep the area clean. A thick layer of petroleum jelly or lanolin on the shaved skin on the down side can help prevent urine scald. Place the patient on an elevated grate or rack with padding in all areas except the caudal-most area for female dogs and cats. If the patient is a male dog include an opening in the padding for the prepuce area. This allows urine and feces to fall through the grate, thus avoiding urine scald or the fur from becoming soiled with feces and urine. Utilize disposable diapers, potty pads, or chucks to keep the bedding dry. **Chucks** are great to use with these patients. The wetness is absorbed in an underlayer and a layer of material stays dry between it and the patient. These will still require changing as only liquids are absorbed; fecal material will remain on the surfaces. If a patient gets wet with urine or smeared with feces a wash cloth and warm soapy water to remove the debris is better than a whole body bath. The bath may be too taxing for their weakened condition but being wet and cold will accrbate their condition.

You may also have to feed recumbent patients by hand and give them water with a syringe. The veterinarian or technician will determine whether this should be done, but you can assist with letting them know if the patient isn't eating or drinking. Careful records of eating, drinking, and elimination is just as important with recumbent patients as it is for other patients.

Reflection

What do you look for in a recumbent patient that you wouldn't necessarily think of for a boarding patient?

Constipated Patients – Enemas

Some patients become constipated so if you notice an absence of defecation for more than 1 day alert the veterinarian. He/she may decide an enema is necessary. This is a relatively easy procedure that the assistant can perform. There are two techniques for giving an enema. One is to use a prepared product and the other is to use an enema can and hose (Figure 10.3). The premixed enema is ready to use with a lubricated tip. If you are using the enema can, clamp the hose to prevent the liquid from escaping. Add warm water mixed with a squirt or two of non-degreaser type dish soap (e.g., Dove™ or Ivory™). Depending on the size of the patient, it may be 1–2 pints of water with a squirt or two of the soap. The soap acts as a lubricant so it doesn't have to be a heavy concentration. You will need to apply lubricant to the nozzle tip attached to the end of the hose.

Gather the patient and enema and move to a run. With the patient gently held between your legs and its rear end pointing toward you, lift the tail and gently insert the tip of the enema into the rectum. If using the premixed container, squeeze the bottle until the entire contents have been administered. If using the can enema, insert the tip into the rectum and then release the clamp on the hose then lift the can higher than the

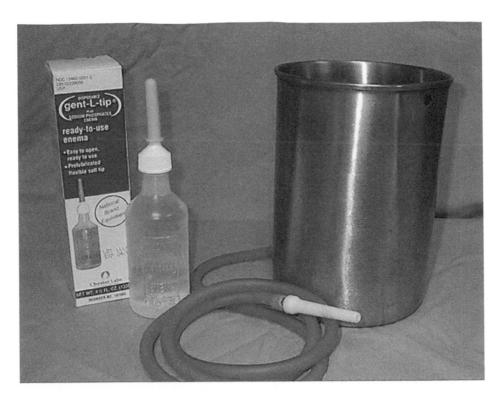

FIGURE 10.3 Premixed enema and enema can.

patient to let liquid flow in with gravity. When it stops flowing the colon is full. Clamp the hose shut and remove the tip from the rectum.

Release the patient, step out, and close the run door. Check back in 10–15 minutes to see if the patient has defecated. If not give it another 15 minutes. If still nothing, alert the veterinarian for further instructions.

Learning Exercise

What personal protection equipment (PPE) would be required for administering an enema?

Contagious Patients

If patients have a contagious disease it is important to care for them last. This prevents the spread of contagious agents through the other wards. It is to be hoped that there is a quarantine ward that is separated from the other wards. Overshoes or booties, a lab coat or apron, gloves, mask, and goggles are all appropriate PPE when caring for these animals. These items are left inside the quarantine room upon exiting; you don't wear the items around the clinic as that can spread contagious agents. Refer to Chapter 4 for a refresher on cleaning isolation or quarantine rooms.

Feral and Quarantine Animal Housing

On occasion, **feral** domestic animals and domestic animals with no prior medical history of vaccinations may be brought to the hospital for quarantine and observation. One such reason for quarantine is a rabies suspect. If a domestic animal has bitten someone, even with vaccinations on records, for legal reasons, they may be quarantined for observation for up to 10 days. Non-aggressive care in handling these patients is important but you should wear gloves and goggles. Feral animals require the use of gauntlets (see Figure 8.54) and capture poles (see Figure 8.44) when having to handle them. This will reduce the possibility of bites and exposure of staff to rabies or other zoonotic diseases. Stringent isolation handling and care as described in Chapter 4 is required to reduce the potential for zoonotic disease transmission and must be in the forefront of everyone one's mind. Skunks, raccoons, and bats are natural carriers of rabies. If they have bitten someone they should never be quarantined. They should be humanely euthanized, and the brains of the animal sent to a diagnostic lab for testing. The person bitten must receive immediate medical attention to start post-exposure vaccinations against rabies. Rabies is almost always fatal and is a horrible way to die.

Remember that zoonotic diseases may be passed through fecal waste, bites, scratches, and fomites. Feral animals often harbor ectoparasites and **endoparasites** that can also be zoonotic. We have already talked about how to check for ectoparasites and how to reduce fomites in Chapter 4; we discuss endoparasites in Chapter 12.

All employees should be aware of the presence of feral or other quarantined patients within the hospital. To protect employees and prevent accidental injury, kennels and cages containing quarantined animals should be prominently labeled. Handling is kept to a minimum with these patients to avoid bites and scratches. Always be on guard against possible "fear biting" with feral animals. Inadvertently backing them into a corner may cause the fight in the flight or fight response.

Reflection

Do feral animals have the same "rights" as a pet? If so, why? If not, why?

Pocket Pets and Birds

Typically, pocket pets are brought to the clinic in a small travel case which is not suitable housing if they need to be hospitalized. If possible, the cage they normally live in should be provided by the owner. Because they are prey animals, being in a dog or cat room may make them very anxious or scared. Finding a quiet countertop or an empty ward is appropriate for these patients. Ask the owner to provide the bedding substrate as some of these pets require specialized bedding. Birds are also brought to the hospital in a travel case which is not suitable for long-term care. Large parrots can be housed in regular kennels with perches provided. Care must be taken to provide a large enough cage to accommodate a long tail and wing span. Smaller birds should be housed in a bird cage.

Food from home and access to water is also very important for these patients. A sick bird or pocket pet will often require warmth. Cover the cage with a towel or hang a towel over the door of the kennel. A heating pad under the entire bird cage, half of the pocket pet cage, or a heat lamp directed into the cage will help.

Treatments and Procedures

Medical Records

Regardless of the reason for an animal to be in the hospital, careful records must be maintained concerning its food and water intake, demeanor, mentation, and elimination. It is important to note this information as it can impact decisions made by the veterinarian on the care the patient may need. These observations may be written in a specific area of the record. If the clinic uses the SOAP format

(**s**ubjective information, **o**bjective of data, **a**ssessment, and **p**lans; see Chapter 3), the appropriate place for that information is in the Plans for daily observations or opinions. If the clinic uses the chronologic format, the date, time, and information is placed on the next available line. Some clinics use the acronym **DUDE normal**, which stands for normal **d**efecation, **u**rination, **d**rinking, and **e**ating. Otherwise, each is marked as good, fair, poor, or none.

Demeanor and mentation is important to note because a depressed animal can become a sick animal. Interaction with each animal in the hospital should include a note about how the animal is reacting to the interaction. The following are some abbreviations that may be used in the medical record to describe the animal's mentation and demeanor:

Bright, Alert, and Responsive (**BAR**)
Quiet, Alert, and Responsive (**QAR**)
Ain't Doing Right (**ADR**) or Not Doing Right (NDR)

If the patient is not doing well or is unresponsive, the veterinarian must be informed immediately.

Learning Exercise

Tigger is boarding at the clinic for a week. Usually he is waiting for you at the front of his kennel. He usually rubs his body along the bars and purrs loudly, but this morning you noticed that he was sitting hunched in the back of the kennel and he hadn't touched his evening meal. When you take the litter pan out to clean it you notice there are no wet areas or feces. What would be your next course of action?

Understanding the Disease Process

Introduction of infection in a patient is a complex cycle of relationships between the infecting organism and the host. Infectious organisms or **pathogens** enter the body through the skin, mucous membranes, **transplacentally**, from vectors and fomites. Likewise, they exit the body through discharges such as blood, vomit, feces, urine, respiratory discharges, wounds, and milk. Transmission is either direct as in animal-to-animal, or indirect as in animal to vector (insects) to animal, or animal to fomite (bedding, dirt, water) to animal.

The first barrier to entry of pathogens are the skin, hair, and secretions of the mucous membranes. The way in which a pathogen enters the patient varies, but once it has invaded the patient, a cascade of responses occurs to try to kill the pathogen. The body's immune defense system kicks in and tries to kill the pathogen. If it fails then the pathogen causes an illness or condition and the patient will show signs of the disease. This is when help with antibiotics, antiparasitics, steroids, chemotherapies, and other pharmaceuticals are used to combat the pathogen or boost the body's immune system to fight it off.

Wellness programs are used to prevent diseases, these usually include vaccinations and deworming programs. These are usually administered to young animals to help them start to build the immunity against these often contagious diseases. However, for rescued patients, where the history is unknown, they may be instituted for these patients as well. There are guidelines for vaccinations for all animals through the various veterinary specialty associations. Every clinic will have their own protocols for when and how often a vaccination program is initiated. Be proactive in learning what your clinic's protocol is for each species of animal it sees.

Reflection

Now that you know the skin is the first barrier to ward off pathogens, what steps will you take to protect your own skin to prevent the possible transmission of diseases?

Treatment Plan Protocols

Treatment plans for all patients begin with the veterinarian diagnosing the disease, condition, or injury. The veterinarian then decides upon the treatments, therapies, medications, and diagnostic tests required. This is placed in the Plans area of the SOAP record format or, if chronologic, written on the next available line. The assistant is a key player in the delivery of the treatment plan and monitoring the patient's response to the treatments. The assistant will use not only her powers of observation, but will also rely on touch, hearing, and smell when monitoring the patient.

Observation of patients occurs throughout the day, however brief, as the assistant works with all hospitalized patients in each ward. If a downward trend is noted, the veterinarian must be promptly notified. Any changes from prior observations are recorded with the time of the observance. Because of the possibility of these changes, the treatment plan should be reviewed several times during the day in the event more tests are ordered or new therapies are introduced. It is also to catch newly admitted patients throughout the day. Many clinics will use a whiteboard, either on the computer or on the wall, to keep tract of each patient's treatment plan. Name, location, and description of the patient is the basic information required. This is followed by what the veterinarian has in mind for diagnostic tests, therapies, treatments, procedures, surgeries, or medications. Completion of each item on the whiteboard is noted with initials and time of completion. Results of tests, notes for completed therapies, procedures, and surgeries are placed in the patient's record either by the person that accomplished them or by you if directed.

Collecting Vital Signs

All hospitalized patients should be "hands on" evaluated at least twice a day. The veterinary assistant may be asked to help the technician do the preliminary evaluations or they may be asked to have these completed before the veterinarian or technicians arrive for the day. Preliminary evaluations are vital signs, weight, body conditioning score, and pain score.

Establish a routine for gathering these evaluations. This reduces time and effort, creating efficiency and preventing oversights. You will need a notebook or the patient's file to mark the readings, you will also need a watch with a second hand, stethoscope, thermometer, and lubricant. Place the baby scale on a level area or cleared area on your cart for your smaller patients. Have your leash ready to move your larger patients to the walk-on scale.

Vital signs are temperature (**T**), pulse (**P**), respiration (**R**), and capillary refill time (**CRT**). It is suggested that these be done while the patient is resting in the kennel or run. Taking them out of their kennel and moving them to a treatment table can elevate the respiration and heart rates. If the patient is naughty or you think they may bite, a cage muzzle for dogs and a cone muzzle for cats are easy to put on to protect yourself. See Chapter 8 for a refresher on muzzles.

Start with the pulse and heart rate, which are not the same thing! Pulse is a palpable measurement created by the combination of **cardiac output** and **systemic vascular resistance**. It is defined as the difference between peak **systolic** and minimal **diastolic** pressures. The heart rate is defined as the number of **beats per minute (BPM)**. It is possible to have a heart beat that does not create a pulse. This is called a **pulse deficit**. For this reason, it is important to compare the two by palpating the pulse while auscultating the heart.

For dogs and cats, offer up some treats and proceed with finding the femoral artery to evaluate the pulse. Place your fingers up high on the medial side of the back leg and press in deep but lightly. Figure 10.4 shows the general location of the femoral artery; the fingers in the photo should be flatter against the thigh. Or use the pedal artery, location indicated by the red oval on Figure 10.4.

The normal characteristic of the pulse is described as a rhythmic thump, against your fingers as the heart contracts. Abnormal characteristics of pulse are faint, thready, bounding, strong, weak, or irregular. Alert the veterinary as soon as possible as this can indicate several serious health conditions. Note the pulse characteristic in the

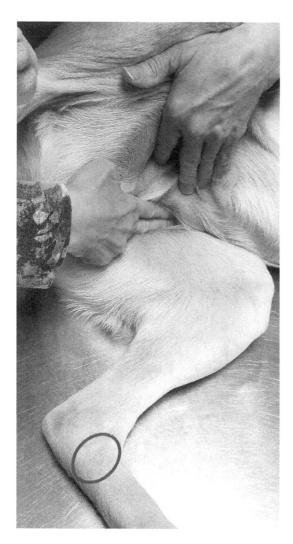

FIGURE 10.4 Femoral and pedal artery positions.

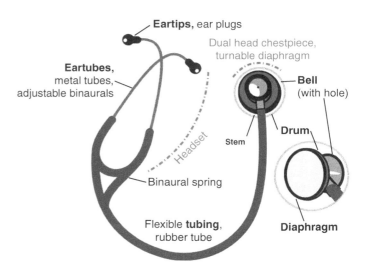

FIGURE 10.5 Stethoscope. Source: Wikimedia Commons. Used under CC-BY-SA 4.0, https://commons.wikimedia.org/wiki/File:Stethoscope.svg.

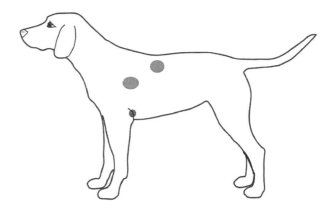

FIGURE 10.6 Auscultation areas for heart (red) and lungs (blue).

patient record. Patient motion, **hypotension**, and patient obesity all play a part in the difficulty of finding the pulse.

Arteries in horses are large and easy to feel but their heart rates are very slow so be patient! The facial artery is the most convenient as it runs along the medial aspect of the mandible. The coccygeal artery runs under the base of the tail or you can try for the dorsal metatarsal artery on the lateral aspect of the hind limb near the hock.

When the artery is found, move to using the stethoscope to **auscultate** the heart. Turn the stethoscope so the ear tips are facing forward in your ear canals. Figure 10.5 indicates the parts of the stethoscope, note how the ear tips are facing backwards. You will want to turn the scope around, so they are facing forward. Check that the large diaphragm is engaged by gently tapping on the diaphragm surface, you should hear a rather loud tap! If not, the bell could be turned to the smaller diaphragm which is used to listen to higher frequencies. Simply turn the entire bell around on the stem and tap again to check. Place the large diaphragm over the left side of the chest just above the sternum, near the

costochondral junction, behind the left elbow (Figure 10.6, red dot). You should hear a solid "lub-dub" as the valves open and close as the heart contracts. On occasion, the heart beat "disappears" and then reappears. Watch the patient as it breaths in the heart beat can't be heard and when it exhales it can! This is called sinus arrythmia and is perfectly normal.

If you hear a whoosh or any sound other than a lub-dub, alert the veterinarian as soon as possible. Heart murmurs and other sounds can indicate a change in the patient's health. If the normal lub-dub is heard, count the heart beats for 15 seconds and multiply by 4, each lub-dub is one beat of the heart. Sometimes you may have to modify the number of seconds you use to count the heart rate. Cats can reach heart rates in the 200s making it very difficult to count. If you use 10 seconds and multiply by 6 or use 6 seconds and multiply by 10 you will get similar results for the BPM. Mark the patient's file with the heart rate and pulse characteristic, as ___ BPM.

TIP BOX 10.2

You should be able to do this math in your head. Practice! If having difficulty with the 15 seconds multiplied by 4, try breaking it down to halves. For example, if the heart rate was counted at 34 beats for 15 seconds add 34 + 34 = 68 and then 68 + 68 = 136.

On occasion you will have a panting dog or a purring cat that obscures the heart sounds. If possible gently close the dog's mouth or offer up a treat and count for 6 seconds to capture the heart rate. Cats can be distracted with treats, running water, or a little isopropyl alcohol on a cotton ball. However, these tricks don't always work so use the pulse points to count the heart rate.

The areas shown in blue on Figure 10.6 are the auscultation positions for the lungs on both sides of the thorax. Listening for a clear whoosh of sound in all four quadrants of the lungs and then move down to listen for gastrointestinal sounds. Dogs and cats should have almost continuous **borborygmi** as you listen for a minute, horses should have 1–3 and should be checked in several spots on the abdomen. Ruminants should have 2–3 contractions of the rumen per minute. This can be heard the best at the left paralumbar fossa. Record the lung sounds and number of gut sounds heard per minute.

The next evaluation is respiration. Respiratory rate is measured by observing the number of breaths, one inhalation and exhalation equaling one respiration. Observe the abdomen just caudal to the rib cage to facilitate visual determination of the respiratory rate or auscultate the patient using a stethoscope over the dorsolateral aspect of the thorax. Count the respirations per minute (**RPM**) for 15 seconds and multiply by 4. A panting or frightened patient can breathe so rapidly that accurate measurement is difficult. In this circumstance, simply note on the medical record that the patient was panting. Note the rhythm, sound, and effort of the respiratory cycle. The rhythm should be regular, there should not be any sound other than the whoosh of air, nor should it seem like the patient is **apneic**. Is it gasping? What color is the tongue and mucous membranes (**MM**)? Normal is pink to light red. If they are brick red, dark red, or blue alert the veterinarian immediately. Is the patient **orthopneic**? The characteristic stance is neck extended, front legs **abducted** from body, and trying to gather in air. Mark the patient file with the respiration rate, as ___ RPM, and any other observations for the respiration.

Temperatures are taken on all animals using a rectal thermometer. This will give you the most accurate core body temperature. However, some animals, especially cats and horses, do not like the thermometer inserted into their rectums. An axial or armpit temperature will work for these animals. There are also ear thermometers that use infrared heat detectors.

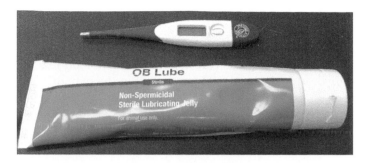

FIGURE 10.7 Digital thermometer and lubricant.

Temperatures taken using an axial location do not give you core body temperature; however, some consider it accurate enough.

Digital thermometers (Figure 10.7) usually give a fast temperature reading in about 10 seconds. Keep your batteries up-to-date as when they run down it will either take longer to get a reading or you will get an inaccurate reading. Mercury thermometers are not used as often because of environmental considerations. The thermometer tip is lubricated with a water-based lube and inserted deep enough to ensure the tip is inside the pelvic canal proper. As you introduce the thermometer, apply a slight twist to ease the pressure and allow for an smoother entry. Push the start button on the thermometer once in place; it will beep to indicate it is ready to be read. Meanwhile, hold the thermometer in place by resting the side of your hand against the patient's rear quarter. You may hold the tail with the other hand. When the thermometer beeps, withdraw it and mark the reading in the patient's file in either degrees Fahrenheit or Celsius depending on the setting. Clean the thermometer with soap and water then spray with a disinfectant and wipe dry with a paper towel.

Digital ear thermometers have a small cone that is protected by a plastic sleeve. The pinna is held straight up and the cone is placed as far into the vertical ear canal as possible. If the ear is showing signs of infection or inflammation, which is indicated by heat, redness, and swelling, do not use the aural thermometer as this ear will be quite painful. Be sure to eject the plastic sleeve into the garbage after each patient.

TIP BOX 10.3

Gathering the TPR normal values of all the animals into a small reference book is a good idea. The *Merck Veterinary Manual* online has a list for almost all domesticated animals.

Capillary Refill Time (CRT)

Capillary refill time in all species of mammals is less than 2 seconds. It is used to check for blood perfusion. It is accomplished by lifting the lip on the side of the mouth and firmly pressing the gum tissue with a finger for a second or two. When you remove your finger count the seconds it takes for the gum tissue to go from white to red. A slow refill time can indicate shock, blood loss, or dehydration. Record CRT in seconds in the patient's file.

Body Conditioning Score and Weight

Body conditioning score (**BCS**) is a subjective evaluation of the patient, whereas weight is an objective evaluation or fact. Weight is useful for calculating calorie requirements and for drug dosage calculations. BCS is used to determine if the weight of the animal fits its frame. Some animals within the same breed can have a very large frame and some are very petite so weight alone when determining if an animal is fit is not enough. There are two scoring scales available, one based on a 1–9 score and the other based on a 1–5 score. Whatever scale is utilized, it is important that everyone in the clinic utilizes the same scale. This moves BCS closer to an objective evaluation.

Figure 10.8 is a sketch of a 5-point scale. The following points are a description of what to look for and what number to select as you evaluate the BCS:

1. *Very thin:* the hourglass shape over the back is very pronounced. The ribs, shoulder, and hip bones are very prominent. When viewed from the side the abdomen is severely tucked up toward the back.
2. *Underweight:* when viewed from above the patient develops an hourglass shape because of the tuck between the thorax and pelvis. No fat is felt over the ribs, shoulder, or hip bones.
3. *Ideal:* the ribs are easily palpated under a thin layer of fat. Ribs, shoulder, and hip bones are visible with only a slight layer of fat over them, muscle is felt in the biceps and biceps femoris areas. A slight hourglass shape or waist is desirable.
4. *Overweight:* the back is slightly broadened when viewed from above. There is a moderate layer of fat over ribs, shoulders, and hip. The ribs are difficult to palpate, and the tail base is thickened. If there is a waist it will be subtle. Cats will have a belly roll.

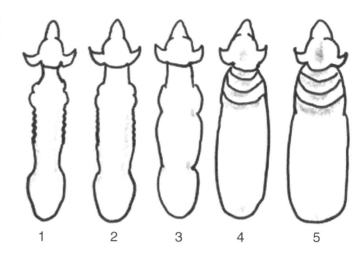

FIGURE 10.8 Body conditioning score drawing.

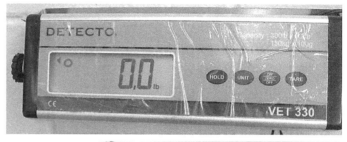

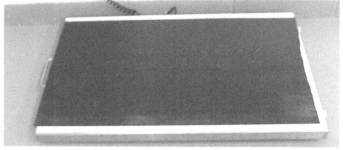

FIGURE 10.9 Walk-on scale. The scale platform sits on the floor and the control head is hung on the wall above it. This has the on–off button, and pound and kilogram units option.

5. *Obese:* the back is broadened and flat when observed from above. It is impossible to palpate ribs because they are covered with a heavy layer of fat; the shoulders and hip are also covered. There will not be a waist. A cat's belly will be **pendulous**.

Weighing Patients

Once the BCS is established it is time to weigh the animal. Animals over 20 lb should be weighed on a walk-on scale (Figure 10.9). It should give you a number in US weight and in metric. Any animal under 20 lb should be weighed on a baby scale (Figure 10.10). If the scales do not have the ability to measure kilograms you will have to convert pounds into kilograms. Refer to the Foundation Skills section in Chapter 1 if you need a refresher. Record both the weight and BCS in the patient's file.

In-hospital Grooming

Grooming by an assistant is limited, focused only on improving the well-being of the hospitalized patient, not necessarily on its appearance. Basic patient care includes keeping a patient clean and mat free. Urine, feces, **vomitus**, blood, and medication may soil the coat. Remove wet debris from fur with warm water on a wash cloth. If it is really messy you may need to place the pet in the wash tub and give a partial or complete bath. Only do so with permission from the veterinarian. If the patient has had surgery the suture line cannot get wet, so a spot clean may be your only option. A very sick patient should not be bathed until well enough to stand. Getting wet and cold will only **acerbate** their symptoms. If that is the case, waiting for the debris to dry and brushing it out is the best option. Blood is often very hard to remove with just soap and water so hydrogen peroxide on a cotton ball can be used to break down the blood cells. Then the area can be cleaned with soap and water on a cloth.

Combing and Brushing

Combing is necessary to remove mats, plant materials, and foreign substances from the coat before bathing. Any patient scheduled for a therapeutic bath or dipping is expected to be combed and de-matted first. Medicinal soaps and dips cannot penetrate a hair coat that is matted.

Combs and brushes come in many sizes, shapes, and materials. A strong comb with widely spaced teeth is used to tease apart mats and coarse tangles. Flea and lice combs have teeth that are very close together and are used to remove flea dirt, lice, and nits. Brushes have either bent wire teeth called a slicker, or stiff metal or plastic bristles which are used to remove loose hair before the bath and after the bath to give the coat a final

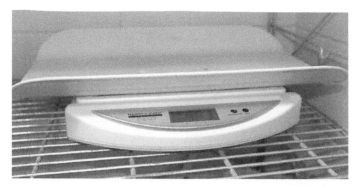

FIGURE 10.10 Baby scale.

fluff. Select the bristle based on length of hair coat; plastic bristle brush for short hair, metal bristle brush for medium to long hair, and wire for double coated dogs. Curry combs with short metal or rubber teeth are also available for dogs and work well on short and medium length hair. Grooming rakes and mat splitters are also available. The rakes are equivalent to a wide-tooth comb with a rake-like handle. Mat splitters have a blade incorporated into a handle and does just what the name implies. Extreme care must be used with this tool.

Starting at the rear of the animal work forward. When brushing out the legs, brush the lateral side of the leg nearest you and then brush the medial aspect of the opposite leg. Small mats are easily teased out with a comb or rake. Grasp the clump close to the skin and starting at the bottom of the mat work up towards the skin. Bracing your fingers against the skin will reduce the amount of pulling on the hair which is painful. Dilute and spray a bit of conditioner on the mat to help the comb go through it easier. Larger mats are more difficult to deal with. If they are loose, use a mat splitter to separate into smaller parts then tease out each part with a comb. If the mat is dense and pad-like it will have to be clipped out with a clipper.

Clipping Hair or Fur

Clipping hair is always done with an electric or battery-operated clipper and *never* with a scissors! Clipping away hair or mats with a scissors is a cut to the skin waiting to happen! Clippers can gouge the skin if held wrongly and although just as painful they usually don't require sutures like a scissor cut. Figure 10.11 shows how the blade end of the clipper is held flat against the skin to prevent gouging the patient.

To clip mats, use the #5 or #10 blade to just remove the matted parts (see Figure 4.13 showing clipper head sizes). Usually the mat is not tight against the body. Lift the mat until you can see the individual hairs, position the clipper blade close to the skin, and move the clipper through the hair. If the clipper binds up as you are going into the mat, try to reposition the clipper to just cut the

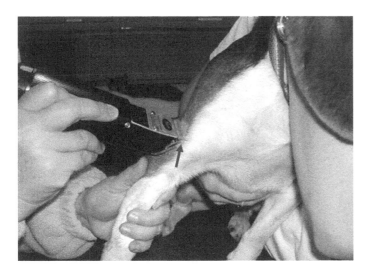

FIGURE 10.11 Clipping hair.

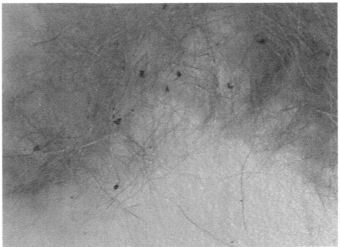

FIGURE 10.12 Flea dirt. Source: Wikimedia Commons. Used under CC-BY-SA 3.0, https://commons.wikimedia.org/wiki/File:Fleadirt.jpg.

individual hairs. Do not fully clip the patient unless directed to by the veterinarian. Be aware that just clipping mats will give the coat a "motheaten" appearance.

Disinfect the grooming tools with hot water and soap, then spray with the disinfectant used on table tops allow to air dry. Clean and disinfect the clipper head as described in Chapter 4. You may have to vacuum or sweep the hair up before starting the bath as wet hair is difficult to capture on a tiled floor.

> ## Reflection
>
> Beside making a pet look nice for a client, what possible benefit could it give to the patient to be clean and mat free?

Identifying Ectoparasites

Note the condition of the skin as you brush, especially under mats. Look for irritated, inflamed areas, any **ectoparasites**, wounds, or tumors. Report observations to the veterinarian. Ectoparasites like fleas, ticks, and lice are not uncommon. Figure 10.12 shows flea dirt, which are the fecal droppings of fleas. It can be found by parting the hair and spritzing with a spray bottle of water then wiping it off with a white paper towel or cotton padding. If the towel shows red streaks it is flea dirt. Fleas are opportunistic parasites and will take a blood meal from humans. Bites around the top of socks and waistbands can indicate there are fleas in the facility! Ticks, if found, should be removed by grasping them as close to the head as possible and pulling in the same direction that they are lying. Check to make sure the head came with the body, as if left in the skin it can become infected. Although ticks prefer the ears and head they can be

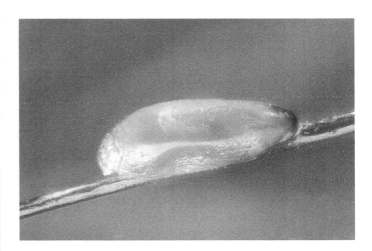

FIGURE 10.13 Lice nit. Source: Wikimedia Commons. Used under CC-BY-SA 2.0., https://commons.wikimedia.org/wiki/File:Human_head_louse_egg.jpg.

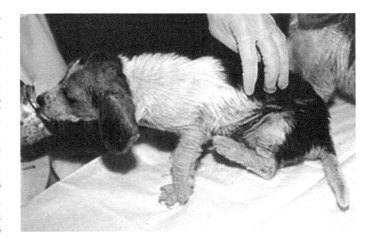

FIGURE 10.14 Sarcoptic mange. Source: Wikimedia Commons. Used under CC-BY-SA 3.0, https://commons.wikimedia.org/wiki/File:Scabies_puppy.jpg.

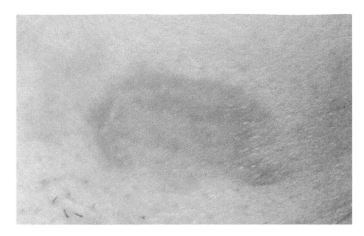

FIGURE 10.15 Ringworm. Source: Wikimedia Common. Used under CC-BY-SA 3.0, https://commons.wikimedia.org/wiki/File:Ringworm.jpg.

attached anywhere on the body. Lice can also be found either as adults crawling on the skin or as **nits**, glued to the hair shaft (Figure 10.13). If any of these parasites are found, alert the veterinarian and follow his/her instructions for treating the patient and in some cases the ward where the patient was house.

Sarcoptic mange is a zoonotic parasite so extreme care is taken to prevent being infected with these mites. Figure 10.14 shows a very advanced condition of **scabies**. Look for any red, raised, sores that includes loss of hair. Alert the veterinarian to any sores found when doing your exam.

Ringworm is another skin disease that is zoonotic. It is a fungal infection that appears with a hairless area that usually has a raised ring of red tissue, thus the name ringworm (Figure 10.15). Older sores will appear scaly as the ring expands and more hair is lost.

Shaving or clipping the hair around these diseased areas are often part of the treatment. If you are asked to clip the hair around a lesion, use a #40 blade to remove all the hair (see Figure 4.13 showing clipper head sizes) Trim the hair about 1–2 inches away from the lesion.

Learning Exercise

Make a small reference book with pictures of the endoparasites and ringworm lesions so that you can compare them to anything you may find while grooming a patient.

Bathing and Dipping

Bathing a patient starts with gathering supplies. You will need two to four towels at least, shampoo formulated for the species you are bathing, cotton balls, artificial tears ointment, wash cloth, and a hairdryer. PPE will include goggles, waterproof gloves, and waterproof apron (Figure 10.16). Place the items near the wash tub and prepare the tub.

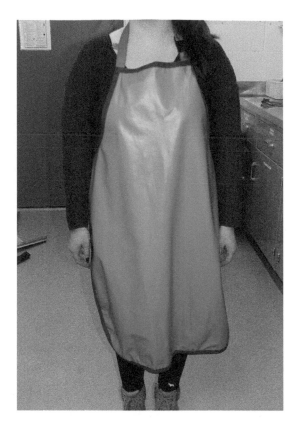

FIGURE 10.16 Waterproof apron.

Often the treatment table doubles as a bathtub. There is usually a grate or solid panel covering the tub. Remove this panel and check for the presence of a non-slip mat on the bottom of the tub. If not present place a towel down on the floor of the tub. Place a drain screen in the drain to capture the hair. Start the water and set it at a comfortable but warm temperature for you, remembering that normal temperature for a dog or cat is 2–3 degrees warmer than a human. Get the patient and ease them into the tub. You might want to distract them with a few treats as they settle in to being near running water. Put a cotton ball into each ear and apply a bead of ointment in each eye. This will protect these areas from shampoo and water.

Use the spray hose to wet the patient down thoroughly, remembering to run the spray a bit before spraying the patient because the water in the hose is often cold. Once the patient is wet put a good amount of shampoo in the palm of your hand and rub it briskly with the other hand. This breaks the shampoo up and will make it easier to spread around the patient's body, and also makes the shampoo cover more surface area of the body. Starting at the neck, rub across the back, down around the abdomen, adding water as needed to disperse the shampoo. You may need another small amount of shampoo to clean the legs and another small dollop of shampoo may be needed for the rear end. Once the shampoo is worked in thoroughly, take the wash cloth, get it wet and add a small drop of shampoo. Work it into the wash cloth. Use the wash cloth to clean the face, being very careful to not get shampoo into the eyes. Rinse the wash cloth thoroughly and then wipe the face again to clear the face of shampoo. You may have to repeat this step to remove all of the shampoo. Once every part of the body is shampooed use the spray hose to rinse thoroughly, again remembering to spray the first bit into the tub as it will be cold. Rinse, rinse, rinse! It is very important to get all the soap out of the coat! Be extra careful not to get water in the ears – the cotton balls will help – or to run water over the head. This is very disturbing for dogs and cats. Dogs will shake their heads and then their bodies spraying water everywhere and cats will try to escape! If a cream rinse is prescribed apply according to directions and then rinse thoroughly once more.

When finished rinsing, squeeze the water out of the coat with your hands, working from the neck along the back and then down all four legs and the tail. Remove the cotton balls from the ears. Towel the patient dry with one towel and, if necessary, use the second towel to get as much water as possible out of the coat. Bring the remaining towels along as you move the patient back to the ward. Put dry towels down on the kennel floor and if available a porous mat or rack to keep them out of the wet is also put down. Some clinics will have cage dryers that hook onto the doors of the cage; if so, set them on low. These work but the patient doesn't dry on the ventral side and you must check frequently for how warm they are, as some can get quite hot and cause the patient great discomfort. They are also very loud, and some patients get very scared. Check on animals every 10 minutes, making sure they have a full water dish as the dryers can cause them to become dehydrated.

The use of a human hairdryer works well to dry the entire patient. You can dry the patient in the drained tub, to avoid electrocution, or set them on the floor and replace the top grate or panel, then place the pet on top of the treatment table to dry them. Again, be very careful not to use the hot setting as this can dry the patient's skin out, a low–medium setting and towel drying as you go is the way to get the patient dry. Use a brush to smooth out the coat when dry, put them in their assigned kennel or run, and mark the patient's file and treatment board that the bath was completed.

Never leave a pet unattended in the bath tub or on the treatment table. They will try to escape and can severely injure themselves in the process.

If medicated shampoo is prescribed it is applied after the first lather and rinse done with a regular pet shampoo. The medicated shampoo may need to be left on for a period of time in order to work. Use a timer or your phone's stopwatch to time the application. Some will instruct you to massage the lather into the coat for the entire length of the application. Rinse thoroughly then dry as already discussed.

Dipping is often a treatment option for the parasites and diseases discussed earlier. Accurate preparation of the medication is very important. Dilution factors and application instructions will be on the container. Read these very carefully and follow the directions accurately. PPE needed includes goggles, waterproof gloves, and apron. Once the dipping agent is mixed up, prepare the area for the animal. Assemble the tub as explained for bathing. Gather at least 2–4 towels, a wash cloth, cotton balls, timer, and artificial tears ointment. Bring your patient to the tub, double checking that you have the right patient, and place the cotton balls in the ears and the eye ointment in the eyes. Apply the dip per the directions, use the wash cloth to apply dip to the face, being careful not to get it in the eyes or ears. Most dip preparations will have you leave the medication on, but you can towel dry the patient and ask about using the cage dryer or hairdryer. Some preparations will want the patient to air dry. After they are dry use a brush to smooth out the coat, and mark the patient's file and treatment board that the bath was completed.

Return to the tub, rinse the hair to the strainer then clean it out with a paper towel. Spray disinfectant spray in the tub, wait the contact time dictated by the disinfectant and then rinse or allow to air dry. Replace the top and if used disinfect that. Sweep and mop around the tub. Disinfect the brushes, put the dryer away, and take the towels to the laundry. Start a load if you can, set a timer on your watch to check on the laundry so you can keep it going.

Reflection

Think of possible ways a patient can get hurt while getting a bath or being dipped. How can you prevent these injuries?

Collection of Fecal and Urine Samples

Remember to check the patient file or the treatment board for required lab specimens. For dogs, if a fecal sample is needed you will simply use the usual plastic bag. After collection use an overhand knot to secure the bag closed and either write on the bag or use a piece of adhesive tape to mark the name of the patient, date, and time sample was collected. Place it in the lab or the lab refrigerator and alert the technician a sample is waiting. Mark the treatment board and patient record with the same information. Remember to use gloves and wash your hands after handling feces.

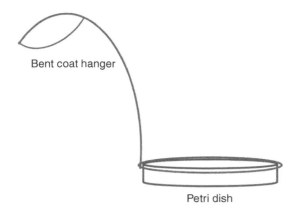

Bent coat hanger

Petri dish

FIGURE 10.17 Urine collection tool.

If a voluntary urine sample is required, a clean water dipper works well to collect the sample without disturbing the patient. A voluntary sample is collected after the first bit of urine is voided. Slip the cup under the stream without bumping the patient. For tiny dogs, you may need to use a modified coat hanger with a Petri dish to catch the sample (Figure 10.17).

After you have collected the urine sample, transfer it to a clean, dry container with a lid. Mark the patient's name, date, and time of collection on the container, treatment board, and patient's record. Put the samples in the lab or refrigerator if the technician cannot get to it right away. Alerting the technician that there are samples available will always be appreciated.

Cat samples are easier to gather because of their use of a litter pan. A fecal sample can be sifted from the litter using the litter scoop or using a gloved hand to gather a piece and place it into a bag. Tie the opening shut with an overhand knot and label it with name, date, and time. Put the sample in the lab or the lab refrigerator and mark the treatment board and record. If a urine sample is required, a little more preparation is involved. Clean, tiny beads are used to replace the litter in a clean litter pan. This is usually left in the kennel only as long as it takes to catch a sample. Once the cat has urinated a strainer is placed over a clean, dry container and the litter box is tilted over the strainer to catch the beads and allow the urine to run into the container. If the strainer is large you may dump all the beads into it; however, you may lose some of the sample as well, so go slow enough to allow the urine to flow into the container. Once you have the sample, tighten a lid on top of the container, label it appropriately, take it to the lab or lab refrigerator, and mark the treatment board and record. The beads and strainer can be washed with a dish detergent, rinsed thoroughly, and allowed to dry before storing them in a container for use with another patient. Put a regular litter box into the kennel. If the cat defecated and urinated in the beads check with the veterinarian or technician to see if the urine sample is acceptable.

Learning Exercise

Describe the different techniques to catch a voluntary urine sample from a dog and a cat. Do you know of other methods? Share those as well.

Pain Evaluation and Monitoring

Pain may or may not be a vital sign depending on the authority cited. Regardless, alleviating pain and suffering is an important and essential job within the veterinary profession. Uncontrolled pain can cause **tachycardia**, **tachypnea**, and **hypertension** which in turn slows healing.

Various pain scales have been deployed to standardize pain evaluation; however, no gold standard has come forth. None are perfect for these reasons:

1. Pain can be chronic or acute. The longer the pain lasts the more difficult it is to assess.
2. How pain is exhibited is influenced by the environment. Prey animals mask pain as a survival mechanism.
3. How pain is demonstrated varies by species, breed, sex, age, and the presence of fear.
4. Pain causes behavioral changes and can increase heart rate, respiratory rate, arterial blood pressure, and cause pupil dilation.

If your workplace uses a specific pain assessment evaluation, then memorize it and apply it to all patients. Usually, veterinarians and technicians are responsible for scoring a patient's pain level, but assistants are vital in recognizing symptoms of pain because of their continued interactions within the wards.

Pain evaluation is a very subjective observation and prone to error. Lack of change in a patient's behavior does not mean pain is absent. A key thought to keep in mind is if what is being done or was done would hurt you it hurts the animal. If you see what you think is an animal in pain consult with the veterinarian or technician. It is always best to error on the side of caution than to let an animal suffer.

In order to alleviate pain, we must first recognize it by monitoring patient's behavior during treatments and while at rest. Changes in behavior can be subtle, so careful observation without letting the patient know you are watching is often recommended. Some signs of pain include diminished eating, drinking, and self-grooming, restlessness, reluctance to move or having difficulty moving, recoiling from touch, shivering, vocalizing, mental depression, constant licking on an area, aggression, panting, and elevated vital signs. Facial expressions such as eyebrows raised and brought together, and a drawing up at the **commissure** of the mouth as if in a grimace.

Remember too that surgery and trauma are not the only things that can cause pain. Infections in ears and eyes, **pancreatitis**, **periodontal disease**, **cystitis**, and **peritonitis** are infections that can be very painful. A slipped disk, cancer, and kidney failure can cause pain. **Arthritis** causes chronic pain. Knowing what your patients are going through will guide you to use extra gentle handling. Record the signs you see in the patient's record and visit with the veterinarian or technician about your observations.

Learn about what pain medications are being used and how long they last. If you notice **break-through pain,** alert the veterinarian immediately.

Learning Exercise

Discuss pain symptoms and treatments with your veterinarian or instructor. Try to get a good picture of what pain may "look like" in dogs and cats. Write a reflection about what you learned and how you will put it to work for you.

Discharging Patients

Before returning a patient to its owner make sure to take a few minutes to brush the medium to long-haired patients out so they look good and to spritz them with a deodorant formulated for pets. Remove the ID collar and pull the cage card, some clinics will have you leave these items inside the kennel or run to indicate that the patient has left the facility and it is OK to clean and reset the kennel or run for the next patient. The patient's file should be marked with the date and time of the pick-up.

Instructions should be explained to owners at the end of the hospital stay, after the veterinarian has completed discussing continuing patient care and before the patient is discharged to the owner. Check with the office manager, the head technician, or the veterinarian regarding the extent of their expectations of the veterinary assistant to review patient care at the time of discharge. Never overstep your boundaries.

It is more effective to provide a written copy of the instructions to the client. Do not just hand it to the client; review it with them. The information to review includes:

- *Medication being sent home.* Discuss why it is being dispensed, how it is to be administered, when it is to be administered, and how important it is to finish all

of the medication unless specified. This is to prevent bacterial resistance to antibiotics.
- *Follow-up care.* Let the owner know if the veterinarian would like a follow-up visit. Offer tips for how to care for the patient at home, for example, only short walks on leash, how to protect a cast, and so on. What to anticipate during recovery and when to call the practice if things are not going well.
- *Environmental care.* Review any dietary changes, food transitions, water volume and frequency measurement if necessary.

Learning Exercise

Select a partner that is willing to act as a client and practice your discharge voice, instructions, and question answering abilities.

Veterinary Hospice Care

As veterinary medicine advances and veterinarians are able to offer more medical options, animals are living much longer lives. Occasionally, a prolonged life leads to an increase in the pet's need for general, sometimes intensive, care.

An owner's denial of the prognosis, personal emotions or fear of losing the pet may play a part in the decision for continued care over euthanasia. For these reasons and many more, hospice care is becoming more and more common in veterinary practice.

The decision for hospice care versus euthanasia can be a heavy burden for an owner. Many people share an indescribable bond with their pets. It can be a difficult decision for an owner to decide when to stop medical treatment. When the decision is made to continue medical treatment, despite the poor prognosis, hospice care begins.

Members of the veterinary team may not always agree with an owner's decision to continue treatment and hospice care. It can be difficult for the team to put aside their personal values and accept the owner's decision during this stressful time. The veterinarian's job is to present and explain the options, the team's job is to provide love and care to the pet and accept the decision as ultimately the owner's.

Owner's may select home care over hospitalization during the hospice period. Opting to take their pet home and performing general nursing, emotional and physical support for the terminally ill is the owner's prerogative. The pet's emotional needs can easily be met, being surrounded by family and familiar surroundings. The veterinary team continues medical care through the owner. For this reason, communication and regular visits with the veterinarian are essential to prevent suffering and unnecessary prolonging of life. Both the owner and the veterinary team must remember the main goal of hospice care is the patient's comfort and quality of life.

Hospice care in the veterinary hospital centers on the emotional well-being of the patient which can and often does affect the physical health of the patient. The veterinary team should consider not only the handling the patient for medical treatment, but also for the tender personal connection a companion pet yearns for. This allows the patient to bond with and trust their caretaker during medical treatments.

"Sunshine therapy" is a positive way to brighten a patient's spirits. Even when a patient is unable to walk or too weak to stand for prolonged periods of time, sunshine therapy is an excellent treatment to provide mental and emotional stimulation. Take the patient outdoors two or three times a day, even if only to lie in your lap and be petted. The patient benefits from the vitamins absorbed by natural sunlight, the physical stimulation of being moved outdoors, and the emotional stimulation from physical contact with the team member.

Visits from the owner can lead to improvement or setbacks in the patient's emotional state. Most often patients are mentally brighter during and following a visit from their owner. Occasionally patients may become anxious about their owner leaving and not taking them. When this occurs, the patient's anxiety may send them into a downward spiral. If the veterinary team finds this occurs after each visit it may be time for the veterinarian to discuss the need to halt the visits or to discuss the option of euthanasia.

Reflection

Can you see yourself as offering hospice care to dying patients? Is so, why? If not, why?

Euthanasia and Post Mortem Protocols

Euthanasia comes from the Greek words *eu* meaning "good or right" and *thanatos* meaning "death." Therefore, euthanasia means a painless or easy death. Certainly anyone who has watched someone die recognizes a natural death is rarely easy or without pain.

When an owner chooses to end a pet's life, it is not always a medical decision but one based on personal or religious values, previous experiences with death, and – the hardest of all – economic reasons. The veterinarian must inform the owner of all the options and then follow the owner's wishes. There are times when a team member may not agree with an owner's decision,

but the pet belongs to the owner and the final decision is theirs. This makes the euthanasia more difficult to perform and is one of the reason for depression and burnout within the veterinary profession.

Once the decision for euthanasia is made an appointment for the procedure is scheduled. The appointment should be scheduled for the end of the day or when the appointment book is at its lightest. It is a good idea to block off the appointment time for the exam room ahead of the euthanasia appointment. This way it can be set up for the procedure, creating an emotionally safe environment for the owner to begin grieving. A box of tissues, cups for water, a nice thick blanket or towel on the exam table and a chair or two for the owners to use will be much appreciated.

If the owner is bringing the pet into the clinic, some clinics will have them check in at the reception desk and then drive around to the back entrance and taken to an exam room from there. Or as they come in the door they are ushered right into the prepared exam room. The veterinarian will meet with the owner, explain how the euthanasia procedure works, and find out if the owner wishes to be present during the procedure. He/she will answer any questions and then give the go ahead for the veterinary assistant and technician to take the pet to the treatment room to prep it for euthanasia. When you enter the exam room make sure to speak to the owner. Convey your sympathies. The receptionist will enter the exam room and go through the paperwork which includes reading and signing the euthanasia consent form, discussion of what is to be done with the remains, and then payment for the procedure and handling of the remains.

Euthanasias are preformed either in the presence of the owner or in the treatment room without the owner. Whichever the case, it is important to remember this is the pet's last moment and it should be treated with every kindness possible. Prepare the treatment table in a similar manner as the exam room table. When handling the patient do so gently, speak calmly and pet gently. Some clinics like to start the procedure by giving the animal a sedative or tranquilizer injection. Know where the injection is going and provide gentle restraint to accomplish the task. If the owner will be in attendance some clinics will put in an IV catheter in which to deliver the euthanasia solution. The IV catheter is usually placed in a back leg to allow the owners to be at the patient's head. Return the pet to the exam room to allow the owner to say their goodbyes privately after the sedative and catheter have been placed. You may ask them to knock on the door when they are ready, at which time you can alert the veterinarian and technician it is time. If you are not needed after this, you may also say a quick goodbye if this is a patient you have had contact with in the past. Otherwise it is best to go gather a cadaver bag and box for the remains.

If you are assisting, your job is to follow the veterinarian's instructions and assist as needed. You will most likely be helping at the rear of the patient while the owners can be petting and talking to the patient. If the owners are not present, you may be asked to talk and pet the patient while the euthanasia solution is being given. The euthanasia solution will be injected into the catheter or into the saphenous or femoral veins in which case you will need to occlude the vessel as described in Chapter 8. The solution works very fast and within minutes the patient will have passed. However, some animals will have what is called **agonal** breathing, muscle twitching, and their mucous membranes will go from **cyanotic** to white. This is a normal reaction and the veterinarian should have explained the possibility of these reactions to the owner if present. The veterinarian will confirm death by listening to the chest for heartbeats.

The owner's reaction to the pronouncement is variable. Some will be stoic, others may be weeping, some may even faint. Be prepared to deal with the owner's reactions whatever they are. Make them feel as comfortable as possible, try to meet their needs which can include taking the collar off and giving it to them, clipping a bit of hair, or just some time alone to say their final farewells. Again, ask them to simply knock on the door when they are ready to leave. If they wish to have the remains, gather the pet up and take it to the treatment area. It is very disturbing to owners if you "bag" their beloved pet up in a "trash bag."

The deceased patient is placed in a cadaver bag or an extra sturdy garbage bag in a curled-up sleeping position. If the owners want to take their pet for burial, place the bag in a cadaver box. This is a box that is coated with a wax to prevent leaks, because the deceased may lose bladder and bowel control. Tape the box closed and take it to the owner's car for them. Many clinics will have the owners park behind the clinic and use the back door to avoid having to go past the reception area full of other clients.

After the Euthanasia

If the patient is to be cremated or buried at a pet cemetery, the box or just the bag is labeled and usually placed in a freezer or cooler to await pick-up. Again, make sure the body is resting in a curled-up position, just in case the owner's change their minds and come back for the remains. If you oversee calling the burial or cremation service do so immediately to arrange pick-up. Many clinics send a sympathy card the next day. If that is your job make sure everyone involved with the patient signs the card and it is put in the mail.

The grief process in clients was discussed in Chapter 1; however, learn to recognize grief and stress in yourself during these times. Seek support from others who are also experiencing these feelings, but always respect the rule of confidentiality. Experienced team members will have more patience with others and themselves during this period. Because of the need to respect patient and owner confidentiality, it is best to limit any discussions about the case with a team member who has also been involved with the patient. A break during the day or activities after work with a team member is helpful in diffusing an emotional day. The depth of feelings will vary depending on how long the team members have known the patient and owner as well as the circumstances bringing the patient to this point. Don't judge if a team member doesn't appear to feel the way you do. People grieve in their own way and some are more demonstrative than others. Some will want to discuss it at length and others won't. Respect everyone's coping mechanism, unless you hear them talk about harming themselves or an increase in destructive behaviors like drinking or taking drugs. These are signs of someone not handling the stress of life and may need an intervention. Realize this: "Several studies have identified a link between suicide and occupation, including the healthcare professions and our own profession. The rate of suicide in the veterinary profession has been pegged as close to twice that of the dental profession, more than twice that of the medical profession, and 4 times the rate in the general population." (Stoewen 2015). If you see something or have a feeling about a team member, speak to them. Don't accuse them of anything, be supportive and let them know you care, as many will be in denial and can become angry. That is OK, don't back down, let them know you will be there if they need you. If you are having these feeling seek help. The **National Suicide Prevention Hotline** is **1-800-273-8255**.

Reflection

Knowing that euthanasia is a service offered to clients what "self-talk" will you use to keep from internalizing the pain of euthanasia, especially with a patient that you may have put a lot of effort into.

Chapter Reflection

The veterinary assistant plays a huge role in providing patient comfort and care, helping with treatments and euthanasias, and helping the patients by being vigilant for comfort and pain control. How do you envision your role in these duties?

Reference

Stoewen DL. 2015. Suicide in veterinary medicine: Let's talk about it. Can Vet J 56: 89–92. Available at: https://www.ncbi.nlm.nih.gov/pmc/articles/PMC4266064/ (accessed July 3, 2019).

Suggested Reading

University of Glasgow. Clinical examination of the cow. [Shows position for heart sounds and checking for gastrointestinal sounds.] https://www.gla.ac.uk/t4/~vet/files/teaching/clinicalexam/examination/left.html (accessed July 3, 2019).

CHAPTER 11

Clinical Techniques

LEARNING OBJECTIVES

- Express anal glands and trim toenails and birds' wings
- Swab ears for parasites and infections, the proper way to clean ears
- Administration of medications: oral, ophthalmic, aural, and parenteral
- Assist with wound care and evaluation
- Apply light bandaging and evaluate for tightness
- Monitor fluid administration and IV catheter sites
- Assist with emergencies and maintain and restock supplies

NAVTA ESSENTIAL SKILLS COVERED IN THIS CHAPTER

IV. Examination Room Procedures
B. Basic procedures
    2. Trim nails (required: cats and dogs)
    3. Express anal sacs using the external method
    6. Perform exam room grooming (i.e., trimming nails, external ear canal cleaning, etc.)
V. Small Animal Nursing (Large Animal Nursing – Optional)
B. Animal care
    3. Monitor/restrain patients for fluid therapy and record observations
III. Pharmacy and Pharmacology
C. Vaccinations
    1. Reconstitute vaccines and be familiar with proper protocols
    2. Describe possible routes and methods of drug and vaccine administration that the veterinarian or veterinary technician may choose and demonstrate appropriate small animal restraint for such protocols

Tasks for the Veterinary Assistant, Fourth Edition. Teresa F. Sonsthagen.
© 2020 John Wiley & Sons, Inc. Published 2020 by John Wiley & Sons, Inc.
Companion website: www.wiley.com/go/sonsthagen/tasks

The National Association of Veterinary Technicians in America (NAVTA) has a specific skill set for veterinary assistants called the essential skills. Many of these essential skills or clinical techniques are the "nursing" skills utilized to care for patients. Whether they are ill or injured, require laboratory tests, a bandage on a wound, surgery or wellness procedures, a veterinary assistant may be asked to perform these skills or to assist the veterinary technician or veterinarian with these tasks. These tasks may be completed in an exam room with a client present or in the treatment room for hospitalized patients.

Toenail Trimming

Toenails are used for traction, defense, and in cats they are used for climbing. Toenails can become overgrown and when they do the toes splay. In companion animals, they can get so long that they grow into the footpad, creating very painful feet and lameness. In livestock and horses, they can start to curl at the tips. Nails of all animals have a similar anatomy; the shape is a little different in livestock and horses. The outer surface is hard and insensitive, the quick or **ungual process** is soft and contains a blood vessel and a nerve (Figure 11.1). As the nail grows in length from the nail bed at the junction of the haired and hairless portions at the end of the toe, the quick extends as well.

If you are lucky the nails will be transparent, and you can see the quick as a pink color as seen in Figure 11.2a of this cat's toenail. Otherwise the nails are black, as shown in Figure 11.2b, and you can't see the quick until you have clipped some of the nail wall away.

Before you begin a toenail trim, gather supplies including treats for distraction, nail trimmer to fit the size of the pet (see Figure 4.14), a cotton ball, and a silver nitrate stick or styptic powder. The silver nitrate sticks (Figure 11.3) are stored in their shipping container and styptic powder is usually in a small jar. If using styptic powder, put a pinch of the powder in a bottle or syringe cap. Never dip the toenail into the jar itself as this can contaminate the jar.

There several tools available to trim nails as described in Chapter 4. Human nail trimmers work well with cats', birds', or lizards' toenails. Cats' nails tend to split easily and so if you realize that either a scissor type trimmer or a human nail trimmer is splitting the nails switch it out for a new one and alert the inventory manager to order new trimmers. A Dremel™ rotary tool with a sandpaper or rough emery board bit can also be used to shorten nails and create a smoother look or surface. Care must be taken when using this tool as it removes a lot of material in a very short period.

If assisting, place the dog or cat in a sitting position or in lateral recumbency. You will either restrain or need assistance to restrain birds and pocket pets as they are restrained on their backs, and rabbits are held in sternal recumbency. If you are trimming a dog's nails by yourself, the dog can be in a sitting or standing position. Cats are held in your lap with their backs to your abdomen and each arm on either side of their body. Some animals are OK with nail trims and others will fight, bite, and struggle. It seems to stem from a bad experience with nail trims; perhaps someone cut one or more too short which is very painful and pets remember! These patients often need a tranquilizer or sedative in order to do a good job on the trim, so it lasts. Always consult with the veterinarian if you have a patient that is struggling. If you over-restrain it until it gives up, this just makes it worse for the next time.

Some poor animals will have very overgrown nails, so overgrown that they are penetrate the foot pad. This will cause lameness and often infection. These patients must be anesthetized to trim the nails short. The quick will be so long that you will cut it as you trim the nail to a normal length, and this is very painful. Also, you will need to clean out the puncture holes as per the veterinarian's orders.

Start trimming a nail by grasping the paw and placing your index finger just above the distal phalanx and your

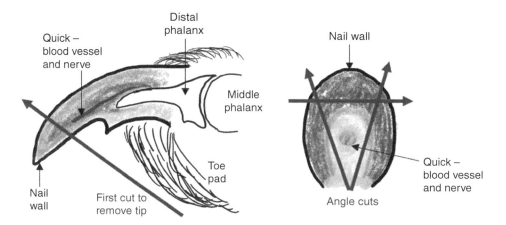

FIGURE 11.1 Anatomy of a toenail and angle of clip.

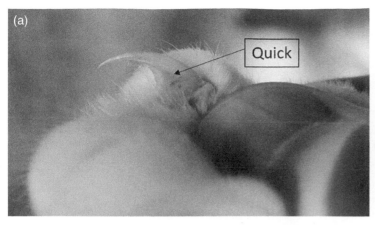

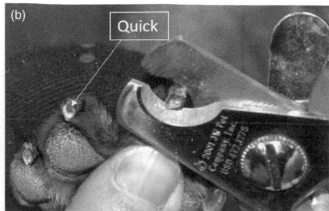

FIGURE 11.2 (a) Cats' and (b) dogs' toenails. Source: (a) Wikimedia Commons. Used under CC BY-SA 3.0, https://commons.wikimedia.org/wiki/File:Cat_claw_closeup.jpg.

FIGURE 11.3 Silver nitrate stick.

thumb under the pad, as demonstrated in Figure 11.2, on either side of the paw. Move in a straight line across the foot so you don't miss any nails. Dewclaws are equivalent to our thumbs and are located a bit further up on the medial side of the foot. Some will have front dewclaws, some will have dewclaws on all four feet. Always look for them as they may or may not be there. Some breeds of dogs will have them removed at 2–3 weeks of age. If they are missed, they can grow into the pad and cause the patient pain. Some cats are **polydactyl** so look carefully for extra toes in between or alongside the usual number of toes.

Figure 11.1 demonstrates the angle of the first clip just deep enough to take the tip off. Then you angle the clipper to either side of the nail and across the top taking more of the wall off around the quick. This allows you to shorten the nail wall and will make the blood vessel and nerve recede giving the owner more time between nail trims. Once you get one nail clipped use that as a guide for the first cut on the next nail. Notice in Figure 11.2b the nail trimmer is positioned almost at the finished level of the two adjacent nails. This will increase your efficiency and reduce the amount of time needed to restrain the pet.

Care must be taken not to clip the quick (Figure 11.2a) which will bleed and cause the patient pain. If you do clip the blood vessel, wipe it off with the cotton ball and apply the silver nitrate stick or styptic powder to the nail. Hold it in place for a count of 10 and then release. If using the silver nitrate stick remember that it stains clothes, skin, and Formica countertops; it also seems to sting. For this reason or because you have clipped the nerve which runs

along the length of the blood vessel, the toe hurts when you touch it. Be ready for the patient to cry out and jerk their foot away, some may even try to bite. If you are restraining for the nail trim, make sure you control the head to prevent biting. Talk soothingly and offer up treats as the procedure progresses. If you have a feeling the pet will bite, apply a muzzle as described in Chapter 8.

Mark the patient's file, indicate if any toes were clipped too short and the patient's behavior during the nail trim. This will help future personnel get ready for this patient if a muzzle or sedative are needed.

Clipping Birds' Wings

Birds are now the fourth most popular pet in the United States. Along with other procedures like nail trims some of the larger pet birds will have their wings clipped. This doesn't keep them from flying, but they won't get far or be very graceful. Some feel this is an unnecessary procedure and psychologically does more harm than good. It takes away the bird's means of locomotion and can make them vulnerable to attacks by household pets. If your clinic does wing clips you may be asked to restrain the bird or to do the actual clipping. The restraint procedure is described in Chapter 8, so we'll concentrate on the clipping procedure.

First spread the wing out (Figure 11.4) to look at the medial side of the wing to check the primary or flight feathers 1–10 for blood feathers. Blood feathers are developing feathers and will have a bright red shaft which is the blood supply to the feather. Blood feathers

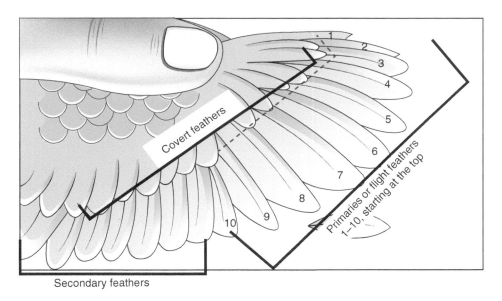

FIGURE 11.4 Birds' wing feathers.

should not be clipped as they will bleed profusely. Feathers are numbered 1–10 starting at the point or top of the wing (Figure 11.4). Take note of which, if any, are blood feathers so that when you are ready to clip the feathers you can count as you go and skip those that shouldn't be clipped. Only the primary feathers are clipped, and the size of the bird will dictate how many are clipped. Smaller birds will have 1–6 clipped and larger birds will have 1–8 clipped. The primaries are clipped shorter (Figure 11.4) than the covert feathers on lateral side of the wing so they blend in and do not look so ragged. Some clinics will not clip primary feathers 1–3 for esthetics, but others say not to do this as it can cause the bird to fly very erratically.

With the bird in sternal recumbency extend the wing out by grasping it at the carpal joint. This is the large joint in the wing where the radius and ulna join the small fused bones of the wing tip. Approach from the dorsal aspect, working proximally slide the scissor blade under the one primary feather at a time. Remember to count so you skip any blood feathers. Clip both wings, if one wing is left with full flight feathers the bird can fly but albeit not very well and injuries can occur.

Expressing Anal Glands

Anal glands are rudimentary scent glands located on each side of the anus (Figure 11.5). To palpate the anal glands, place your index finger and thumb just above the white arrows as shown in Figure 11.5. The location of each glands lies ventrally and slightly caudal at 5 and 7 o'clock to the anus. The black arrows on the Figure 11.5 show the location of the ducts that empty the glands at 3 and 9 o'clock. Ideally, the material secreted by the glands

is forced through the ducts when the animal has a bowel movement. If the material becomes thickened, infected, or the muscles in the area weaken, the glands do not empty properly. The patient will scoot its bottom along the ground and if not expressed glands can become abscessed and rupture. A full anal gland is easily palpated and will feel like a small ripe grape. The material that is expressed from anal glands is malodorous, brown to tan in color, and usually watery to somewhat thicker.

> ### TIP BOX 11.1
>
> Have an extra scrub top at work because if you get anal gland secretions on your scrub top it must be changed because you will be offensive for the rest of the day!

There are two techniques for expressing anal glands: internally or externally. The equipment needed for both techniques include gloves, goggles, cotton batting or paper towels, deodorizing spray, and a lubricant for the internal method. It is thought the internal method empties the gland better than the external method. The external method is used on those patients that are too small to accommodate an index finger.

The internal method involves putting on a glove and applying lubricant to your index finger (Figure 11.6). Place a large cotton ball or a damp paper towel between the index finger and thumb. Gently insert the index finger into the anus and place your thumb on the skin over the gland. Go for the left gland first as that is a natural position for your hand if right handed. Press the thumb towards the index finger, squeezing upwards and together. This forces the material through the duct and hopefully onto the cotton ball or paper towel. Word of caution: the material will sometimes shoot out at high velocity and in a direction unprepared for! Therefore the goggles! Continue to squeeze and move your finger and thumb together until the gland is empty. Rotate your hand so the thumb can reach the right gland and repeat the squeezing (Figure 11.7). The expressed liquid is usually a brownish color and will be quite odorous!

Alert the veterinarian if the material expelled is bloody, grainy, or yellow, pus-like, or if unable to empty the gland. If there is an open sore in the area of the anal gland it could have ruptured; this is also something to tell the veterinarian. He/she will need to flush the impacted anal glands to empty them and treat any ruptured anal glands.

The external method is basically the same technique, except one finger is placed on the skin covering the one gland and the thumb on the skin covering the other gland. Squeezing the fingers together and up, in a "milking" like motion will propel the material up and out of both ducts at the same time.

After expressing the anal glands, wipe any material off the perianal area with a clean cotton ball or wet paper towel. Wrap the items used in one glove as you take it off and then that glove is wrapped inside the second glove (see Figure 2.4 for how to remove gloves safely). Spritz the perianal area with deodorant.

Administration of Medications

Before administering any medication or vaccine to a patient, review the **patients' rights**.

When administering anything to a patient I will check the patients' rights:

Right patient: double check that you have the correct patient
Right medication: double check that you have the right medication
Right strength: read the label to make sure you have the right strength

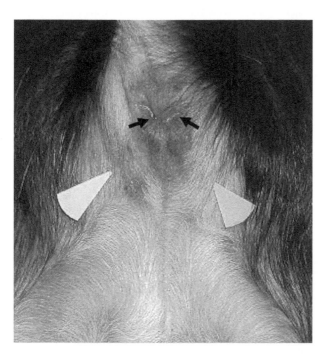

FIGURE 11.5 Position of anal glands and ducts.

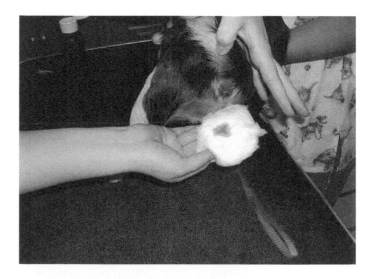

FIGURE 11.7 Expressed anal gland material.

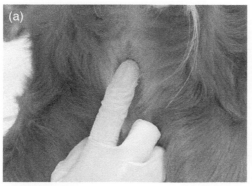

FIGURE 11.6 Internal method of expressing anal glands.

Right dose: calculate quantity or amount to administer, check the dose with a co-worker

Right time/frequency: in which the medications are given on time.

Ear Cleaning and Medicating

Dogs' and cats' ears often require cleaning and sometimes medications for bacterial, yeast, or parasite infections or sores from fly bites, plant awns, or bites from other pets. Patients often vigorously shake their heads, have a head tilt, or are even off balance because of ear infections. These ears can be sore, and the patient may not tolerate the procedure. If necessary, you will need to muzzle these patients or the veterinarian may choose to administer a sedative.

The anatomy of the ear as shown in Figure 11.8 indicates the **pinna**, which on occasion will be dirty or matted. This should be cleaned before starting to clean the internal ear. Brush or comb the hair on the pinna and, if necessary, shave the hair on the inside pinna and over the **tragi** (Figure 11.8). This border of the ear canal is a firm cartilaginous, furred U-shaped projection.

Dogs and cats have an L-shaped ear canal as shown in Figure 11.8. The canal is broken into two parts: the **vertical** and the **horizontal ear canals**. Hair tends to grow inside of the vertical ear canal, and is sometimes plucked if the ears are very infected. However, this should be cleared with the veterinarian first. To pluck the hairs grab them with your fingertips or use forceps to pull the hair out. The **tympanic membrane** is the terminus for the horizontal ear canal (Figure 11.8 inset). The only way to visualize the tympanic membrane is to grasp the pinna and lift up and out, which straightens the canal out enough to see it with an otoscope (Figure 11.9a).

You may be asked to restrain the animal for the technician or veterinarian so use a good sitting restraint with the animal's head pressed into your shoulder and a hand wrapped around the muzzle. If possible, have the owner offer treats or cheese on a stick as the cleaning procedure is started to distract the pet. Try without a muzzle but if the ears are too sore or the patient is wanting to bite, go ahead and muzzle the patient.

Dirty or infected ears smell bad, almost like stale beer or yeast. If they do smell bad, have the veterinarian look at them before cleaning. He/she may ask for an ear swab before the cleaning to determine if the ears are infected with bacteria, yeast, or mites. Supplies needed include four long applicator sticks, two microscope slides, one with a drop of mineral oil on it. One slide will need to be divided in half with a wax pencil line, marking one side with an L for left ear and an R for right ear. Personal protective equipment (PPE) includes gloves.

With the patient in a restraint hold, insert one applicator stick with the cotton end going into the ear, straight down into the vertical ear canal just behind the targi. You should be able to insert the stick at least an inch or more depending on the size of the patient. Gently swirl the stick around and, using a scooping motion, bring it out of the ear. Roll the cotton end of the applicator stick

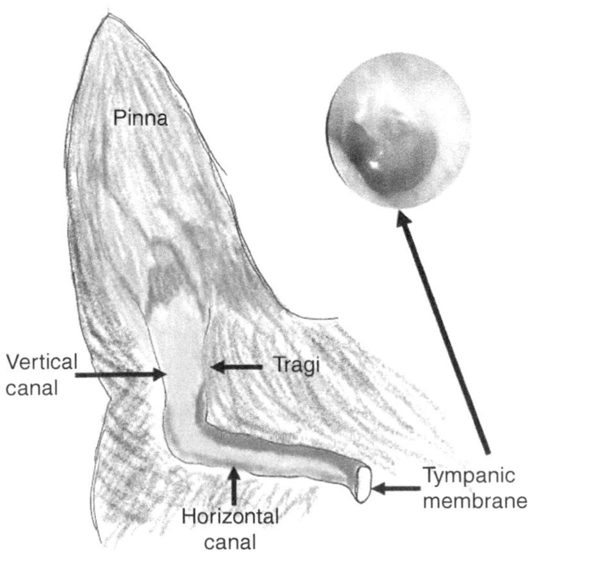

FIGURE 11.8 Anatomy of the ear. Source (inset): Wikimedia Commons. Used under CC BY-SA 4.0, https://en.wikipedia.org/wiki/Eardrum#/media/File:Normal_Left_Tympanic_Membrane.jpg.

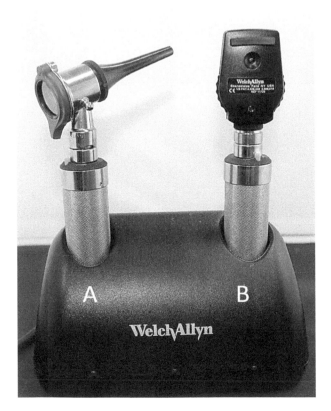

FIGURE 11.9 Otoscope (A) and ophthalmoscope (B).

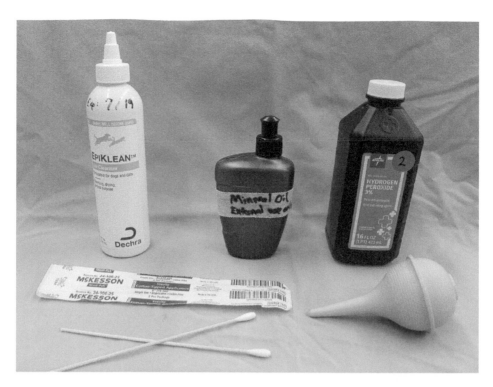

FIGURE 11.10 Ear cleansers and ear swab preparation supplies.

on the appropriate side of the divided slide. Repeat for the other ear and then allow that slide to set for a few minutes. With the other applicator sticks, dip one in the mineral oil on the second slide, go back into the vertical canal, swirl and scoop again. Roll that stick in half the mineral oil on the slide, repeat for the other ear. Give the slides to the veterinary technician to examine. She will use the slide with mineral oil on it to look for ear mites and, after staining the divided slide, look for yeast or bacteria.

The procedure to clean the ear begins with gathering the supplies (Figure 11.10). Ear cleanser or an antiseptic solution, cotton balls, applicator sticks, and an otoscope will be required. Pour a bit of cleanser into a syringe or bottle cap. Dip an applicator stick or cotton ball into the solution and clean the creases of the pinna and exterior ear canal (Figure 11.11).

Use the otoscope with an appropriated sized cannula to see if you can visualize the white translucent membrane of tympanic membrane. Remember to lift the pinna up and out a bit to straighten the canal. If you can't see it because of debris or wax the ear must be cleaned out.

Start with 1–3 mL of cleanser in a syringe (Figures 11.12a-c), gently pull the pinna up and out, and deposit the cleanser into the vertical ear canal by depressing the plunger on the syringe. Place a cotton ball inside the ear canal and then place your thumb just below the targi and fingers on the opposite side of the ear to massage the solution in the ear canal. You should hear squishing sounds as you massage; if not add another

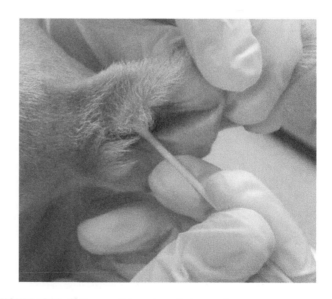

FIGURE 11.11 Cotton swab in external ear canal.

milliliter of cleanser and continue to massage. The cotton ball will soak up some of the solution and grab the debris that comes out of the ear from the massaging. Tilt the head to the side with that ear down to drain more cleanser out. After a minute of massaging use a swiping motion to take the cotton ball out of the ear. Continue adding solution, massaging and wiping until the cotton ball comes out clean. Once it is clean take another cotton ball and pull it about half way apart. Place one piece of the cotton ball over your index finger and try to reach into the vertical ear canal to sop up any

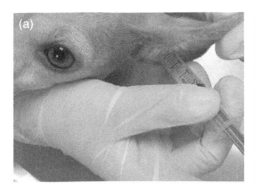
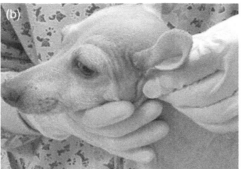
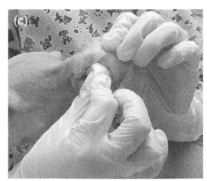

FIGURE 11.12 Cleaning the internal ear canal.

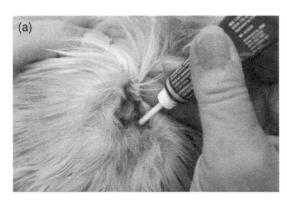
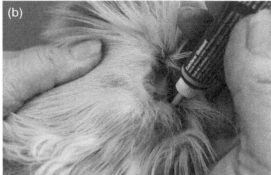

FIGURE 11.13 Medicating an ear.

remaining cleanser or you can twist the cotton ball piece into a cone and put that down into the vertical ear canal. Massage to milk the remaining solution out of the horizontal ear canal. The ear must be dried out thoroughly; moisture in a warm, dark place is an incubator for bacteria and yeast. Check to see if you can see the tympanic membrane using the otoscope. If not repeat the cleaning procedure until you can. Repeat for the other ear.

Once the ear is clean it can then be medicated. **Aural** medications usually have a long tip that can be placed deeply within the ear canal when there is an infection. Remember the "patient s' rights" and read the instructions and medication label before applying. **Oral** and aural are two very different medication routes! They sound similar so double check to make sure you are giving the right medication.

To administer the aural medications, gently grasp the pinna with your non-dominant hand and lift up and out. Slide the tip of the aural medication as far down the vertical ear canal as possible and give the tube a gentle 1–2 second squeeze (Figure 11.13). It is impossible to know exactly how much that is but it should make a satisfying squishing sound as you once again massage the ear. Use a cotton ball to wipe any excess that comes out of ear or into the external ear canal and pinna. If the excess is excessive, reduce the amount of medication applied in the next ear. Repeat on the other ear.

Occasionally, we will see a dog with hanging ears in the clinic with a **hematoma** on the pinna. This occurs from shaking their head so vigorously because of an ear infection and accidentally hitting the pinna on something hard like a coffee table or doorframe. This breaks the blood vessels under the skin and causes the blood to pool under the skin. This is a secondary condition to the primary disease of ear infections so both will have to be treated. The physical sign of a hematoma is a large pocket of fluid under the skin of the pinna which requires a surgical procedure to correct. Hematomas can also be caused by a bite wound.

If you were asked to clean and medicate the ears record what cleanser or solution was used, what medications were used, and if any ear swabs were done. Include a date, time, and your initials.

Topical Medications

Injuries and infections on the surface of the skin may require the application of medications directly to the affect areas. The supplies required will be a hair clipper, cleansing or antiseptic solutions, gauze sponges, and the medication prescribed by the veterinarian. PPE includes goggles and gloves.

Before applying the medication, the diseased skin surface must be cleaned. The first step is usually to shave the hair from around the area with a 1–2-inch border of non-infected skin. This is to ensure that the entire infected area can be treated. If the patient has long hair it needs to be trimmed so it doesn't hang in the wound. Figure 11.14 shows how to hold the clipper to trim the long hair at the edge of the clip.

If the wound is crusty or has dried blood or pus over it, it needs to be soaked to soften before removal. This is accomplished with warm water, warm sterile saline, or an antiseptic solution. Soak a gauze sponge with the desired solution and place it dripping wet on the lesion. This may take several minutes and multiple soakings. Gently rub off the softened material with a clean sponge. If the skin does not have dried-on debris, use the soaked sponges to clean the infected area thoroughly, then dry with paper or cloth towels. Medication is applied to the entire infected area by applying the amount of ointment prescribed by the veterinarian and rubbing it gently

until absorbed into the skin. Application may be twice or three times a day with cleaning of the infected area if seeping or draining. Mark the patient's chart with how the infected area was cleaned, medication applied, and amount used, date, time, and your initials.

> ### TIP BOX 11.2
>
> If the medication prescribed is for "multi-patient" use or in a big jar, use a tongue depressor to remove what you need and lay it on a paper towel until it's needed. This keeps bloody, pus-covered gloved fingers from reaching in and contaminating the jar.

Some skin infections referred to as "hot spots" are bacterial infections that are often found under matted hair or heavily coated dogs that may have gotten wet and then not dried thoroughly. These infections are usually prepared by shaving the area, then treated with an anti-inflammatory and maybe a **poultice**. A poultice for hot spots follows a very specific recipe of household ingredients. It helps to reduce the heat in the area and because it is an **astringent** it will act as a drying agent. Soak a wash cloth with the poultice solution and then hold it on the infected area for 10–20 minutes. This is usually repeated 2–3 times a day until the redness dissipates.

Oral Medications

Oral medications come in a variety of mediums: tablets, capsules, liquids, pastes, and soft chews (Figure 11.15). The way to give the medication is species dependent. Livestock and horse oral medications are often in paste or thick liquid form and are given with a syringe or a stomach tube. With small animals it will depend upon

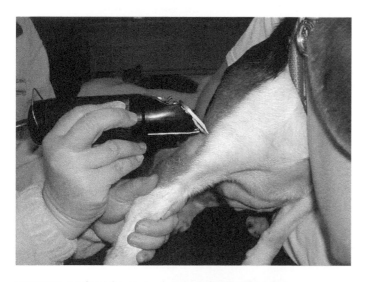

FIGURE 11.14 Straightening edges and clipping long hair.

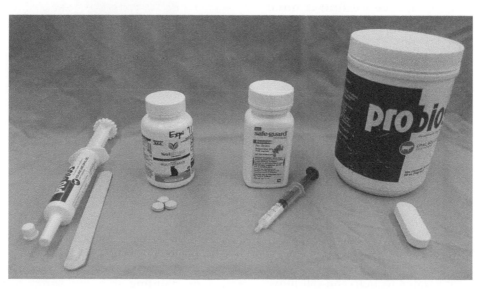

FIGURE 11.15 Oral medications.

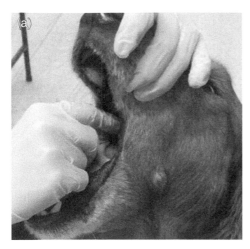
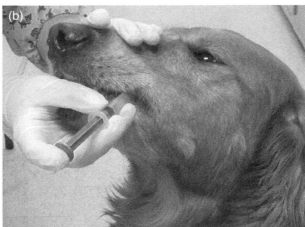

FIGURE 11.16 Administering oral medications.

the medium. Tablets and capsules are usually accepted if hidden in cheese, peanut butter, a piece of meat, or a "pill pocket." These are specially made treats to accommodate pills. However, some medications cannot be given with food and so must be forced down the throat deep enough that the animal can't cough it out.

If you are restraining for oral medications, a sitting or standing restraint works well. If you are giving the medication, there are several methods to use. The following is one method but you may be shown others by experienced personnel.

Hold the pill or capsule in your dominant hand, between the index finger and thumb (Figure 11.16). With the other hand reach over the top of the mouth and curl the lips in over the teeth as you lift the upper jaw. With the pill between your fingers, quickly reach into the mouth at the commissure of the lips and go down the throat as far past the base of the tongue as possible. Release the pill and, if necessary, push it further down with your index finger. Shut and hold the mouth closed, raise the head a bit, and stroke the throat to induce swallowing. If the pill stayed down, a word of encouragement and a treat for the patient is in order.

If the patient wants to bite you may have to resort to a pill gun (Figure 11.17). A pill gun has a split rubber tip that will hold a pill in place on one end; the other end looks like the plunger part of a syringe. The restraint is the same, or you may have to wrap the patient in a towel or place it in a cat bag to control the feet. Tilt the head back as far as possible with your non-dominant hand. Direct the pill gun centrally as far down the throat as possible, depress the plunger, and quickly withdraw the pill gun out of the mouth. Hold the mouth shut and stroke the throat to induce swallowing.

After you have given any pill, either with your fingers or a pill gun, follow it with water to help the pill move down the esophagus; 2–4 mL is adequate depending on

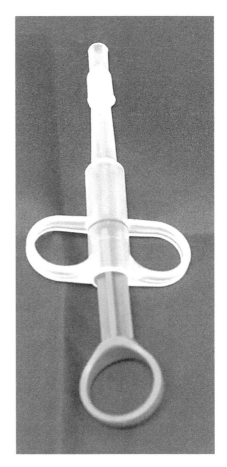

FIGURE 11.17 Pill gun.

the size of your patient. Record the medication given in the patient's file, date, time, and your initials.

Oral liquid medication and water are given with a syringe (Figure 11.16). Locate the patient's file, draw up the prescribed medication, and then retrieve the patient. Sitting or standing restraint works for small animals. Have the restrainer tilt the head up slightly. Gently lift the lip and slip the tip of the syringe between the cheek and teeth back into the cheek pouch. Depress the plunger at a pace to match the patient swallowing. If you give it too fast it may run out of the mouth which creates a dilemma. Did the patient really get its full dose of medicine? How much ran out? This can be very difficult to determine so try not to let it happen. Keeping the head elevated a bit will help and adjusting speed of delivery should also help. If it is bad tasting stuff, try to shoot it down the throat quickly and hold the mouth shut to make the animal swallow.

Oral dosing needles (Figure 11.18) are used on pocket pets and birds. This is a specialized technique that only veterinarians and technicians are trained to do but you may be asked to get the needle and should be able to identify it.

Gastric or nasogastric tubes are used to deliver medication or nutrition directly to the stomach. The veterinarian is usually the person to perform such a procedure. However, the assistant can gather the equipment and medications. Gastric tubes come in French sizes and the larger the number the larger the **lumen** on the tube (Figure 11.19). If in doubt on size, consult with the veterinarian or technician. Set out gloves, lubricant, a syringe with the medication draw up, and a mouth speculum to keep the patient from biting down on the tube. If the tube is nasogastric or directed through the nasal opening into the stomach, then a suture kit and bandaging material to secure the tube end to the neck will be needed.

Hospitalized birds are often medicated or fed using a gastric tube. The trick is to get the beak open and kept open. There are mouth speculums designed for birds but if the clinic doesn't have one you can utilize a paper clip. Small ones for small to medium-sized birds and large ones for the larger birds. The bird is held on its back, the head held between thumb and index finger. Hold the paper clip flat, and approach from the side. Wedge the paper clip between the upper and lower beak, prying it open. Rotate the clip so the top beak is resting on the upper bend of the clip and the lower bend of the clip is forcing the lower beak down. The gastric tube can be inserted through the paper clip and down into the stomach.

Horses are often given pastes that are squirted into the side of the mouth. Start by holding onto the halter with your right hand, slide the tube into the mouth between cheek and side teeth. Depress the plunger a little bit and when the horse starts to move its tongue quickly reposition the tube and squirt the rest of the paste onto the tongue itself. Horses are very adept at working the paste off their tongues so try to spread it out by moving the syringe in and out before pulling it out. If a chunk of paste should land on the floor, scoop it up and smear it on the inside of the cheek with your fingers. Be careful not to get your finger between the molars! They will be squished!

Cattle, sheep, and goats are usually medicated with pastes or liquids given with a multi-dose "gun." They are

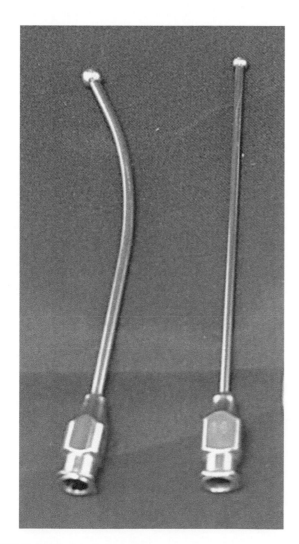

FIGURE 11.18 Oral dosing needles.

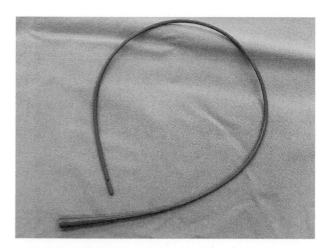

FIGURE 11.19 Gastric tube.

run into chutes or crowded into runs. One hand raises the head under the chin and the other slides the nozzle of the gun into the mouth between cheek and molars. Squeeze the trigger, mark the patient with a wax crayon, and move on to the next. The marking is done so that an animal doesn't get a double dose.

Ophthalmic Medications

Ophthalmic medications are used exclusively in the eye. It is vital that if you are going to put something into an eye you *always read the label!* (Figure 11.20). Medications come in liquid drops or in an ointment form. Both are applied directly to the surface of the cornea. Because of the production of tears these medications are given

more often through the day than other types. It is important to adhere to the prescribed intervals and number of treatments per day. Ophthalmic ointments are prescribed per patient and are not to be used on multiple patients, mostly because of the contagious nature of most eye infections.

To apply ophthalmic medications, gather the ointment or drops, a cotton ball, and the patient. If restraining the patient, put them in a sitting or sternal recumbency, bring your arms around on either side of the animal, placing a hand on each side of the face. Tilt the face up so it is easier to access the eyes and to prevent the drops from rolling off the eye. In the sitting position, reach across the back and snug the patient's side against your front, then reach the other arm around the neck and gently push the patient's head into your shoulder. Because of the proximity of the mouth, care is taken for those patients that may bite.

If you are medicating, the technique is to hold the ointment tube or dropper bottle in your dominant hand with the tip pointing down towards the eye with the side of your little finger placed just below the lower eyelid (Figure 11.21). Gently pull the eyelid down, tuck your fingers holding the medication up close to the palm, and either apply the number of drops prescribed in the center of the eye or squeeze the tube and lay a "bead" of ointment across the length of the eye. Care must be taken to *not* touch the surface of the eye with either the dropper bottle or tube. This can scratch the cornea and contaminate the medication.

Ophthalmic diseases are diagnosed utilizing strips placed onto the cornea. One type of strip is a corneal dye that is used to determine if there are scratches on the surface of the cornea (Figure 11.22). The other is a test strip called a Schirmer tear test that tests for tear production. Another test is for glaucoma, which uses an instrument called a tonometer (Figure 11.23). There are two types of tonometer: manual and digital. Chances are you will only assist with the restraint required for these tests, but gathering the supplies and medications needed will be of great value to the team.

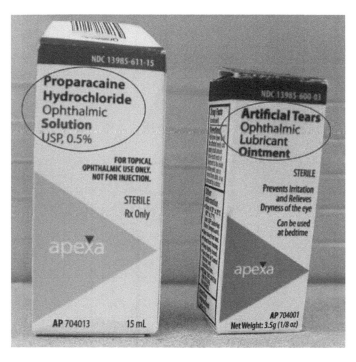

FIGURE 11.20 Ophthalmic medications.

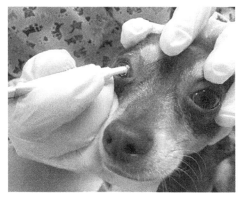
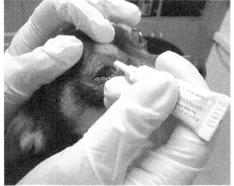

FIGURE 11.21 Administering ophthalmic ointment.

Syringes and Needles

A syringe is a medical instrument used to inject fluids into the body or withdraw fluids from the body. Every syringe has four parts (Figure 11.24). The **barrel** holds the liquid to be drawn and is marked with measurements called *graduations* which are used to fill the syringe to the proper dose. The **plunger** is tipped with a rubber gasket that pulls the solution into the syringe and then pushes the solution into the body by manipulating the plunger with your fingers. The **tip** is where the needle or end of a catheter attaches to the syringe. There are three types of tip available (Figure 11.25):

A. Plain tip or slip tip is centered on the end of the syringe and the needle simply slides on
B. Eccentric tip is off center and is found on 6 mL and larger syringes because the barrels are so large it makes the needles go deeper
C. Luer Lock tip has threads that the hub of the needle or catheter screws onto the tip of syringe, "locking" it in place.

There are two types of syringes used in veterinary practice. The most common are made of plastic and are disposed of after a single use. Plastic syringes come in units for insulin and 1–140 mL sizes (Figure 11.26). Syringes have different-sized graduations depending on the size of the syringe. Insulin syringes come as either 40 or 100 units. This is a smaller measurement than milliliters and is used to deliver minute amounts of insulin

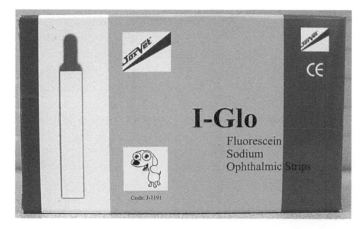

FIGURE 11.22 Fluorescein strips.

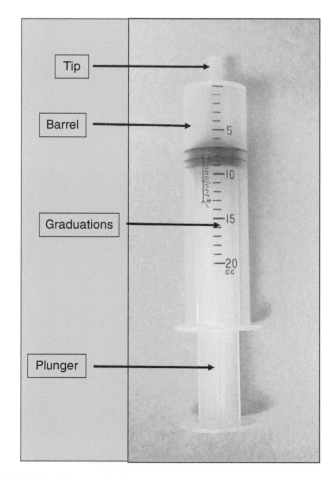

FIGURE 11.24 Parts of a syringe.

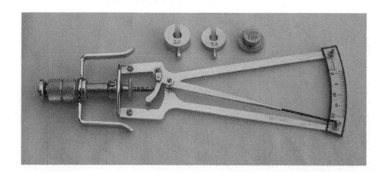

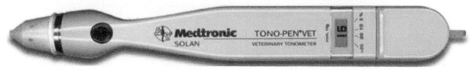

FIGURE 11.23 Tonometers.

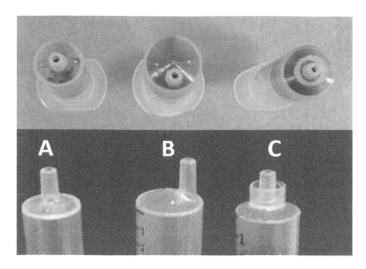

FIGURE 11.25 Syringe tips.

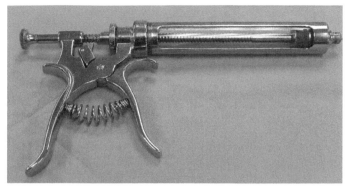

FIGURE 11.27 Automatic dose syringe.

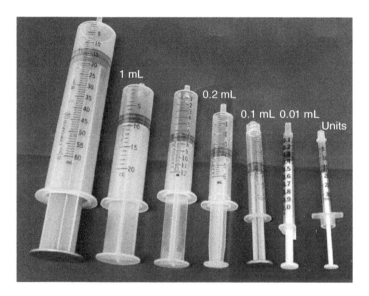

FIGURE 11.26 Disposable syringes with their graduations. The syringes are marked with graduations. Note the smallest unit of measurement each syringe can measure.

accurately. The next biggest syringe is the TB or 1 mL syringe. The total volume is 1 mL and the graduations are marked in 0.1 and 0.01 mL. This syringe is most often used for mixing small amounts of anesthetics and for blood draws on birds, pocket pets, kittens, and puppies. Probably the most commonly used syringe in veterinary medicine is the 3 mL syringe. Its graduations are in 0.1, 0.5, and 1 mL graduations. Six and 12 mL syringes are marked with 0.2 and 1 mL graduations. The 20, 35, and 60 mL syringes are marked in 1 or 5 mL graduations as well as in ounces. The selection of a syringe is based upon the total dose of the medication. You want one that will accommodate the entire amount and accurately measures the medicine. Therefore it is important to be able to determine the smallest unit of measurement for each syringe.

Multiple dose syringes are shaped like a pistol with a trigger handle and glass or plexi-glass barrel housed within a metal chamber (Figure 11.27). They usually have 25–50 mL capacity and a dial that sets the amount dispensed at 1–5 mL per pull of the handle. They are very durable and are used frequently in large animal practices for herd work because they save time by eliminating individual syringe filling time. They are more expensive than plastic syringes and require maintenance. Mineral oil is used to lubricate the rubber stopper on the plunger and O-ring that connects the barrel to the handle as well as careful disinfecting to clean the barrel after each use. This instrument has been known to spread diseases if not disinfected properly between herds.

After a disposable syringe has been used it should be disposed of in a sharps container (see Figure 4.1). Needles should not be recapped as that poses a puncture hazard. Some clinics will have you pull the entire syringe apart and then put it in the sharps container, but that really isn't necessary. The needle cap and the syringe packaging can be disposed of in the general trash. Never leave an uncovered needle lying around. Someone may poke themselves on the needle which can be very dangerous especially if it had been used for a modified live vaccine or vaccines such as brucellosis and leptospirosis.

Hypodermic needles consist of a slender hollow tube called a shaft, a hub on one end designed to attach to a syringe, and a beveled or sloped sharp point on the other end to introduce solutions into a body or to remove fluids from the body (Figure 11.28). The interior of the needle is called a lumen. There are two types of needles available: a disposable type is used once and then disposed of and a stainless steel re-useable needle that can be used multiple times before requiring sharpening. These are most commonly used in large animal veterinary practices where an entire herd may be given an injection with only the use of one needle. The disposable needles tend to get dull going through the rubber stopper on a medication bottle! The only drawback to the re-useable needles is that the points do get thin after multiple sharpenings and

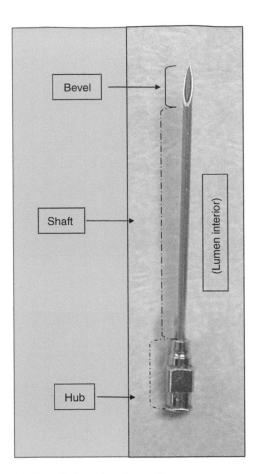

FIGURE 11.28 Part of a hypodermic needle.

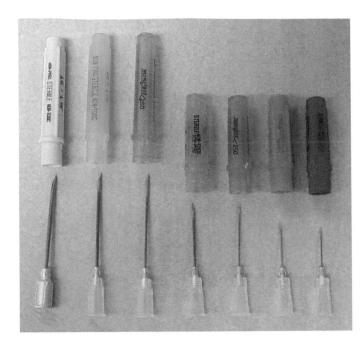

FIGURE 11.29 Monoject™ brand needle sizes.

will bend over creating a burr. They also must be disinfected properly and sterilized between herds.

Needles come in a variety of sizes and lengths. The lumen or circumference of a needle is measured as a gauge and the larger the number the smaller the circumference (Figure 11.29). For example, a 25-gauge needle is smaller than a 14 gauge needle. Selection of size is based upon the size of the animal and the thickness of the solution to be delivered. If the solution to be given is thick like penicillin or euthanasia solution, then a larger lumen is selected. If the solution is watery then select a smaller gauge. Blood cells can be destroyed if pulled through too small a gauge so if drawing blood try to use the largest gauge recommended for the size of patient.

Recommended gauges for each animal group are as follows: 30–25 gauge needles are often used on pocket pets or birds. The lengths are between 5/8 to ½ inch. Small kittens and puppies can handle a 25–22 gauge needle at 5/8 to 1 inch length. Adult dogs and cats can handle 22–20 gauge, 1 inch in length is most commonly used. Livestock and horses can handle a 20–16 gauge needle and usually at 1½ inch in length. The most common lengths used in veterinary medicine are 5/8, ¾, 1, 1½, and 2 inches. Shorter needles are used for more superficial injections. Longer needles are used for deeper injections.

Prepackaged, individually sterilized needles are available in boxes of 100 and each size is color coded. However, the colors are not uniform across manufacturers. Figure 11.29 shows the Monoject™ brand of colors. Learn what brand your clinic utilizes and then memorize the color code so that in an emergency you don't have to stop to read each needle cap for size. Some clinics may purchase syringe and needle combos, this tends to speed up set-up, but it can be a waste if the needle size doesn't match the need.

Guidelines for needle selection; use the smallest gauge needle possible to accommodate the solution. If it is hard to pull a solution into the syringe then try a larger gauge. If you must pass a needle through thick skin use a larger gauge. Use a smaller gauge if you are working on small-sized and young animals. Blood tends to be thick and will become damaged if the gauge selected is too small, usually a 22–20 gauge, 1 inch needle for dogs and cats is appropriate. An 18–20 gauge, 1½ inch needle is appropriate for blood collection on livestock and horses.

Preparing Syringe and Needle for Use

Determine the appropriate syringe for the volume of medication required. Select the appropriate needle based upon the size of the animal and the thickness of the solution being given or drawn out. Check the seals on both the syringe case and needle cover. If they have been broken you cannot be sure they haven't been used, discard those appropriately and select another.

Break the seal on the syringe case and take the top off but leave the syringe in the case until you have broken the seal on the needle, set it down or tuck it between your ring finger and little finger with the top up so the syringe doesn't fall out. Use your index fingers and thumbs to break the seal on the needle by holding the long part of the needle between the fingers of one hand and twisting the short top with the others. Be careful not to touch the hub with your fingers or hand. Pick up the syringe case and turn it so as it drops you can catch the plunger end with your fingers. Be careful not to touch the tip of the syringe with your bare hand or fingers. Hold the needle between your index finger and thumb and carefully slide the tip of the syringe into the needle hub. Leave the cap on the needle at this point.

Solution Bottle Preparation

If using a multiple sample bottle, a bottle that will be used on multiple patients, it is good practice to swab the rubber stopper top of the solution vial or bottle with an alcohol-soaked cotton ball. The only exception would be if it is a single-dose vial that has come right out of the storage container or if the solution in the bottle is a modified or live vaccine. It should say on the bottle or box.

Remove the needle cap and draw an amount of air into the syringe equal to the amount of solution to be withdrawn from the vial. With the bevel of the needle pointing up, you should be able to see the lumen. Pick up the bottle with your non-dominant hand and hold it with the stopper pointing down (Figure 11.30). Insert the needle through the rubber stopper with a slight backward pressure on the beveled side of the needle to prevent coring of the rubber stopper. Always try to center the needle in the top of the stopper. Continue to hold the bottle upside down so the solution falls into the center. Depress the plunger to inject the air into the vial. This prevents pressure from building up in the bottle which in time will make the solution shoot out of the vial through the holes in the rubber stopper. To withdraw the solution, pull down on the plunger drawing the fluid into the syringe. Draw a milliliter or more solution than you need in order to help eliminate air bubbles. Hold the inverted bottle between your index finger and thumb, let the syringe rest against the ball of your palm (Figure 11.31). Then eliminate large air bubbles by tapping or flicking the syringe with your other fingers to make them rise toward the tip of the syringe. Slowly depress the plunger to inject the air bubbles and excess solution back into the bottle until you reach the proper dosage of medication as prescribed by the veterinarian. Withdraw the needle from the vial and recap the needle by sliding the needle into the cap lying on the table. Never pick the cap up to recap the needle, this is to avoid being inadvertently poked by the needle. Label the syringe with a piece of tape if it's not going to be used

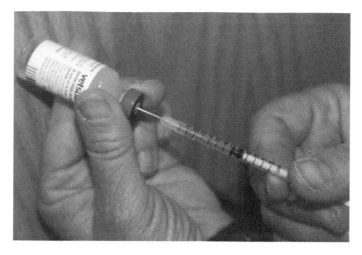

FIGURE 11.30 Inserting a needle into a bottle.

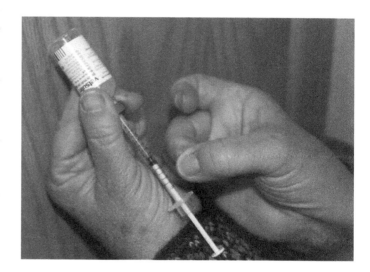

FIGURE 11.31 Ridding the syringe of air bubbles.

immediately on the patient. Patient name, drug, and route should be listed on the tape and put in a spot that doesn't cover the graduations. If you must, tear the tape in half lengthwise to give you a thinner piece. A second technique is to mark the barrel opposite of the graduations with a permanent marker.

Preparing Vaccines

Some vaccines come as a powder and need to be reconstituted with a diluent which can be sterile water or a liquid vaccine that is formulated to be mixed with the powder (Figure 11.32). The most common of these are the feline and canine distemper vaccines. They are packaged in trays with one powder for every one diluent. Always read the packaging to make sure you are getting the appropriate vaccine for each species.

Assemble a needle and syringe, gather one of each vial. Insert the needle into the diluent bottle just inside the stopper in order to aspirate all the fluid, there should

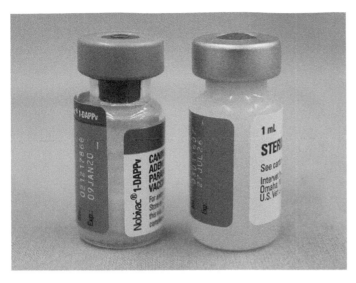

FIGURE 11.32 Vaccine bottles set/powder and dilutant.

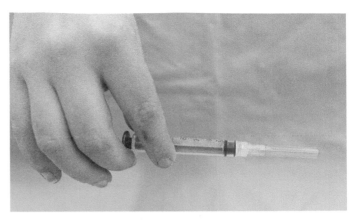

FIGURE 11.33 Proper technique to hold a syringe.

be at least 1 mL of fluid withdrawn. Remove the needle and syringe and insert it into the vial with the powder, and slowly inject all the fluid. Leave the needle in the vial, and gently roll the vial in your palm hanging onto the syringe barrel. When the powder is fully dissolved, invert the vial and withdraw all the fluid. Take the needle out of the vial and slowly push the barrel up to get rid of the air. If there is a "bridge of liquid" in the barrel, tap the barrel with your fingernail to loosen it. If you don't, it will come out of the needle before you get the rest of the air out of the syringe. The vaccine amount should be 1 mL total in the syringe. Label the syringe with the patient's name and vaccine type; they are similarly colored and are easy to get mixed up. It is important to keep them separate because they are given in different locations on the patient's body.

Vaccines are considered biologicals and therefore must be kept refrigerated. If a vaccine is mixed up and then not used it has a "shelf-life" of 1 hour after which time it must be discarded. If there is some question as to whether the patient is well enough for a vaccination, then just set the bottles out with an unassembled needle and syringe. If they are not used, they can easily be placed back into inventory. Never mix different vaccines together, for example a rabies vaccine with a distemper vaccine in the same syringe. They can react, creating a toxin that could harm the patient or inactivate the vaccine, so the patient isn't protected from the diseases.

Some medications will also come in a powder that needs to be reconstituted with sterile water or saline. Read the label carefully to determine which one to use and how much to mix with the powder. Do not mix the medication with the wrong diluent as it can cause a reaction that results in crystals forming and rendering the medication inactive.

Injections

Beware, there is controversy as to whether an assistant should administer injections. If one adheres strictly to many state practice acts, the answer in most states is "yes," the assistant can administer injections under the direct supervision of a veterinarian. If one adheres to the recommendations of the NAVTA, the answer is "no." The administration of an injection is always limited to credentialed veterinary technicians. In truth, the answer is determined by each veterinary practice. If the veterinarian expects the assistant to be able to give an injection and it is not prohibited by the state's veterinary practice act, then the assistant needs to learn how.

The proper way to hold a syringe for all injections and blood draws is between your index finger and thumb at the end of the barrel as close to the "wings" as you can get. Your hand should be "on top" of the barrel (Figure 11.33). This allows you to use your three remaining fingers to aspirate and inject without letting go of the syringe. If you hold it in the middle of the barrel or close to the tip you will always have to let go in order to reposition your fingers for the injection. When you let go of the syringe it can fall out and it wiggles, causing more pain. If you hold the barrel with your fingers underneath the graduations then they are often in the way when trying to get an IV injection or blood draw.

The three most common routes used for injections are **subcutaneous** (SQ or SubQ), **intramuscular** (IM), and **intravenous** (IV). Subcutaneous is used most frequently for vaccinations. An appropriate location for SQ injections on a dog or cat is anywhere there is loose enough skin to lift up so the needle can be inserted underneath. Some veterinarians will prefer the SQ injection to be given anywhere off the midline, which is along the back or back of the neck. This is so if the vaccination causes an **abscess** it can be drained easily. Figure 11.34 shows the sites available for SQ and IM injections.

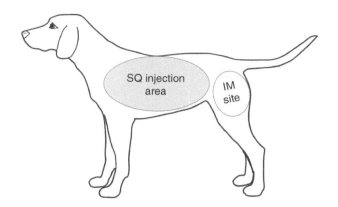

FIGURE 11.34 Subcutaneous (SQ) and intramuscular (IM) injection sites.

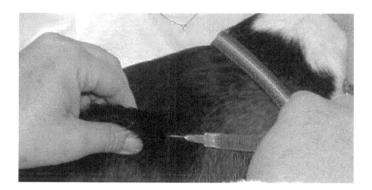

FIGURE 11.35 SQ injection technique.

Subcutaneous Injections

If restraining for a SQ injection, a sitting, standing, or sternal recumbency position works equally well. This tends to be a relatively less painful injection so distraction techniques and a light hold are usually all you will need. This is unless the material being given stings. Then you will want to snug the patient close to your body with an arm around the neck.

TIP BOX 11.3

Practice manipulating the syringe with one hand until you can pull and depress the plunger without excessive movement of the needle within a pillow, orange, or stuffed toy. This will vastly decrease the pain your patient feels when receiving an injection.

If you are giving the injection you will need to gather a syringe and needle, a cotton ball wetted with warm water or alcohol, and the medication or vaccine to be given.

To give a SQ injection properly, assemble and fill the syringe to the prescribed amount of medication or vaccine. Find the area with the loosest skin, gently lift a

pinch of skin up to form a "tent," and wipe the injection site (Figure 11.35), which is the "door of the tent," with the wetted cotton ball. This serves two purposes: it cleans the area and it can be used to part the hair so you can visualize the skin. Put the cotton ball down and properly grasp the syringe in your dominant hand and with the bevel up quickly insert the needle up to the hub through the "door" of the tent. This is usually between your thumb and index finger on your non-dominant hand. Aspirate, which is a quick pull back on the syringe plunger, no more than a tenth of a milliliter, and if no blood or air is seen in the syringe, depress the plunger to deliver the medication. This can be done quickly and with no wiggling! The more you move an inserted needle the more it hurts. Withdraw the needle and give your patient a pat and a treat for being good.

Dispose of the entire syringe and needle in the sharps container. Throw away the needle cap, syringe packaging, and the cotton ball. Put the medications back in the pharmacy if it is a multi-draw bottle. Mark the patient's file with the medication amount given, the location of the injection, the date, time, and your initials.

There is a needle-free, transdermal system of vaccine administration available. It uses a CO_2 cartridge that forcefully propels the vaccine across the skin into the subcutaneous tissues. This provides a more consistent administration of vaccine and is less painful to the patient. Follow the manufacturer's instructions for setup and use of the system.

Subcutaneous Fluid Administration

Subcutaneous fluids are frequently given to patients; the restraint and locations are the same, but the equipment is different. Gather a 20 or 18 gauge needle or butterfly catheter, an IV drip set, the IV bag of fluids or a syringe large enough to accommodate the amount of fluids needed. Mark the bag with the desired amounts divided into the amounts each SQ site can accommodate (Figure 11.36). This will differ depending on the size of the animal. Cats and small dogs can handle 15–25 mL per SQ site. Medium-sized and slender large dogs can handle about 45–50 mL and the giant breeds can handle about 50–75 mL per site. This is a range and the only way to really determine the amount per site is to feel the skin as the fluid runs in. A soft bump will start to rise under the skin, before it becomes tight feeling move to another site, even if not at the amounts provided above.

Once the bag is marked aseptically attach the IV drip set to the IV bag and remove all bubbles from the drip set (see Chapter 12). Attach a needle or butterfly catheter to the end of the drip set and then slip it under the skin in the same way as described for a SQ injection. Instead of pushing the plunger on a syringe, the IV drip

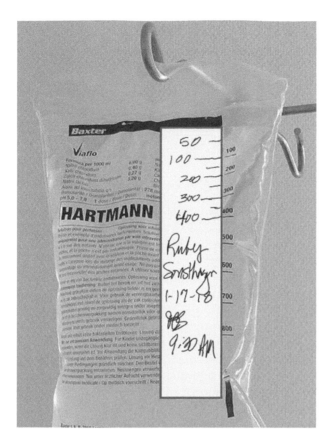

FIGURE 11.36 IV fluid bag marked appropriately. Adapted from Wikimedia Commons.

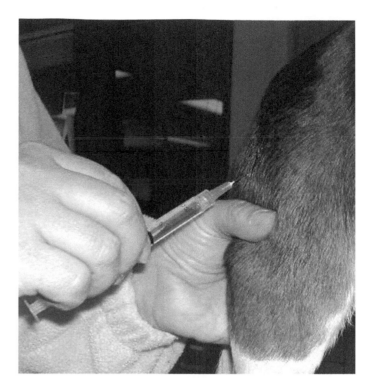

FIGURE 11.37 IM injection.

set is opened by moving the roller clamp down, you should see the fluids running steadily in the drip chamber. Hold the needle or catheter in place and watch the fluid level in the bag, when you've reached the divisions you set up before starting, withdraw the needle *after* you have either closed the roller clamp or bent the IV tubing to prevent the fluid from shooting out! Repeat until all the prescribed fluids are administered. If OK give the patient a treat and a cuddle. Record the number of locations and the amount that was delivered in each location, the name of the fluids given, the date, time, and your initials.

Intramuscular Injections

Intramuscular injections absorb slower than SQ and cannot handle the volumes SQ can. A guideline for IM injections is 1–2 mL for cats and small dogs, up to 5 mL for medium-sized and large dogs. Cattle and horses can handle 10 mL per injection site. If the medication to be given is more than these guidelines, split the dose into two syringes and give on either side of the patient.

Aseptically assemble the appropriate-sized needle and syringe. Check the patient record for the medications as prescribed by the veterinarian and draw up the dose. Wet a cotton ball with water or antiseptic.

The sites for IM injections vary between species (Figure 11.34). Small animal sites are the quadriceps group of muscles, the epaxials, and on occasion the gastrocnemius. For livestock and horses use the neck muscles and the quadriceps group of muscles if necessary.

If you are restraining for the injection, small animals are either kept standing or put in lateral recumbency. Review Chapter 8 for both techniques. If you are giving the injection, double check that you have the right patient and the right medications. Have the restrainer place the patient parallel to your body. Use your non-dominate hand to steady the rear leg and hold the filled syringe with your dominant hand (Figure 11.37). Depending on which way the dog is facing, you will hold the leg right above the knee from the front of the leg or the back of the leg. Give a gentle squeeze, quickly insert the needle approximately half way between the hip and knee running parallel but slightly lower than the femur. Direct the needle toward the opposite hip at a 30-degree angle. This puts the needle deep enough into the muscle without hitting the femur or the sciatic nerve which runs parallel and dorsal to the femur. Aspirate to check for blood and if none go ahead and depress the plunger. If you get blood withdraw the needle, check with the veterinarian to see if you need to get a new dose of medication, if not move to another spot and try again.

IM injections tend to hurt more because the medication can sting and from the pressure of the volume. Be ready for the patient to jump and if you are giving the injection move with them so you don't accidently withdraw the needle as they jump. In which case you would have to poke them again.

Large animals are given IM injections with a 1½-inch needle. It is directed straight into the muscle group chosen, the syringe is aspirated, and if no blood is seen depress the plunger. If blood is seen, again ask the veterinarian for the correct course of action. The neck muscles are usually preferred because those are not expensive cuts of meat! IM injections can cause an abscess in which case that carcass is condemned if found during slaughter and is wasted.

Intranasal Infusion

The third route utilized commonly for vaccinations is the intranasal (IN) infusion. This is where the vaccine is deposited directly into the nostril of the patient (Figure 11.38). It is often no more than 0.5 mL of solution and some clinics will have you divide it and apply half of the dose in each nostril. You must be quick for the second infusion because most patients do not like this and will wiggle to get away from the restrainer! The needle is removed after drawing the vaccine up in the syringe.

Monitoring IV Fluid Administration and IV Catheter Maintenance

IV fluids are administered to rehydrate patients that are **dehydrated**, to maintain fluid balance during surgery to prevent **hypovolemia,** and to treat some illnesses such as kidney failure and shock. IV fluids require a catheter placed into a vein, usually the jugular for long-term treatment or the cephalic or saphenous for short-term treatment. The veterinary assistant will be asked to assist with the placement of IV catheters, the monitoring of the fluid administration, and catheter maintenance.

Fluid administration can be done in two ways. The first method is an IV bag of fluids, hung on an IV pole, which is hooked to an IV drip set that is attached to an IV catheter (Figure 11.39). The IV drip set has a roller clamp that is used to set the rate of fluids going into the vein. When it is rolled open the number of drops in the drip chamber will increase. The rate is determined by the veterinarian or technician based upon weight and percentage dehydration.

The second method is to place the IV drip set into an electronic infusion pump (Figure 11.40). A fluid infusion pump regulates the flow rate of fluids based upon the patient's requirements. Each pump will have instructions for operation and will most likely be set up by the veterinarian or technician. The beauty of the infusion pump is that it has an alarm that will sound if the line is occluded. This allows personnel to move about the room doing other tasks while the patient is lying quietly in its kennel.

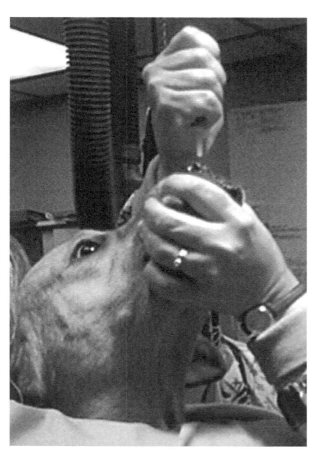

FIGURE 11.38 Intranasal (IN) administration.

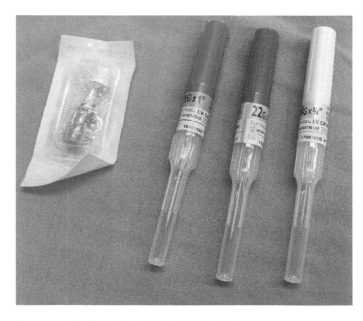

FIGURE 11.39 IV indwelling catheters and end cap.

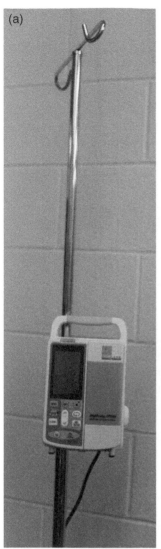

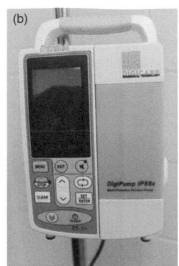

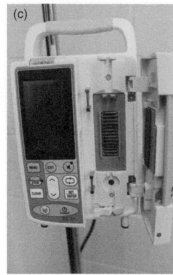

FIGURE 11.40 Infusion pump.

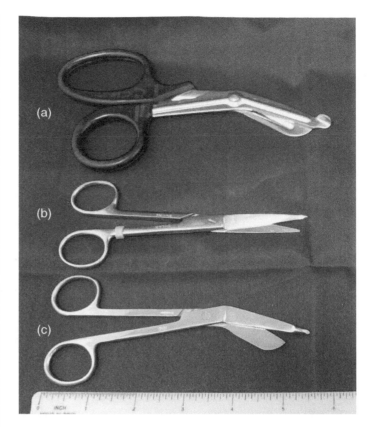

FIGURE 11.41 Utility (a), Knowles (b), and Lister bandage scissors (c).

The assistant's job is to make sure the drips continue at the set rate for the amount of fluids to be given for either method of delivery. This may entail sitting with the patient and holding them still, making sure the tubing and the catheter does not kink. The assistant may also be asked to monitor the IV catheter site or to assist with restraint while the site is evaluated by the veterinarian or technician.

There is usually a bandage placed over the site that will need to be removed in order to check the insertion point and then reapplied after the inspection. Gathering the materials necessary will be of value to the team. The type of bandaging materials will depend on the individual preferences of the veterinarian or technician but will usually be a combination of a roll of self-adhesive bandage material, adhesive tape, antiseptic solution, gauze sponge or cotton balls, and an antibiotic ointment. The bandage is carefully removed to inspect the insertion site. Care must be taken not to cut the IV line or dislodge

the catheter when removing the bandage. Only a bandage scissors can be used to slide under the **tertiary** bandage material (Figure 11.41). Its wedge-shaped tip pushes the skin away from the blades, so it is not cut inadvertently.

Keeping the leg steady while the bandage is removed is very important. The patient should be in sternal recumbency with the leg extended out. This is done by resting the patient's elbow in your palm. This allows you to gently push the leg forward and prevent backward movement if the patient should jerk its leg. If the catheter is in the jugular, sternal or sitting restraint is usually appropriate. When the bandage is off, be very aware that the patient may try to lick the area. This is very strange to them and they will want to investigate. Do not allow them to reach the area. Once the bandage is replaced, an Elizabethan collar or a basket muzzle is usually applied to prevent the patient from chewing on the bandage and pulling out the catheter.

Once the bandage is off, the site should be inspected for **phlebitis**. This is evidenced by a red, swollen, hot, or painful area around the catheter insertion point. Another sign of catheter failure is **pitting edema**, so if there is any kind of swelling, inflammation, or bruising alert the veterinarian immediately. If the catheter is in a leg vein, it is usually changed to another location after 48–72 hours. If in a jugular vein, it can stay in place until it is no longer needed or it shows signs of phlebitis.

Catheters are usually detached from the IV drip set for periods of time throughout the day. In order to accomplish this and keep the catheter patent, an IV cap is placed on the end of the catheter. The drip set is then attached to the catheter with a large gauge needle inserted through the cap. When removing the drip set the catheter must be flushed with a **heparinized saline** solution to remove any backflow blood remaining in the catheter. This reduces blood clot formation and maintains the catheter patency. This is done every time the IV drip set is detached from the catheter and some clinics may clear the catheter every 4 hours if IV fluid are not being given within that time interval. The amount of flush required is just enough to clear the catheter, so paying attention to the length of the catheter before insertion is an important consideration.

When it is time for an IV catheter to be removed, a pressure bandage is usually applied for a few minutes. This usually involves a gauze sponge folded in half twice to make a small square and a roll of self-adhesive bandage material. The square of gauze is placed over the insertion point and held in place with a thumb, the catheter is removed, and the self-adhesive bandage is applied. Three to four wraps of the bandage material and a quick snip with the bandage scissors is all it takes. The bandage should not be very tight, but firm enough to apply a bit of pressure to help the insertion point to clot.

your fingers then turn the clipper so the tip of the blade is pointing at the strands. Bring the clipper down on top of the hair to remove just the long hair strands. If you line the blade up with the edge of the clipped area it will look very neat (Figure 11.14).

After clipping, the wound is flushed clear of the visible debris. This can be accomplished with the spray hose on the sink. However, care must be taken not to drive the debris into the wound if the water pressure is too high. Set the temperature to warm and the water pressure just enough to make the sprayer work. If the water pressure is too high to use the spray hose, a 60 mL syringe with an 18 gauge needle is filled with sterile saline and used to **lavage** the wound. Use a gauze sponge and antiseptic soap to scrub the edges as you go. A more complete flush with antiseptic solutions or saline will be performed by the veterinarian or technician. A surgical scrub begins after the wound is flushed. This is described in Chapter 15.

After the wound has been prepared, the veterinarian will determine if it needs to be **debrided**, lanced, probed, or lavaged some more. Debriding takes place when the wound edges are old and **devitalized**. Lancing is done when there is an abscess. A **Penrose drain** may be placed in a wound to allow it to drain (Figure 11.42). If a drain is in place, careful observation of the skin around the drain exits is important as this area may start to break down because of being wet from the drainage. Drains are

Wound Care and Bandaging

Open wounds are often seen in veterinary practice. They can be small puncture wounds from a bite or large areas where the skin is completely gone or something in between. Wound care starts with clipping the hair from around the edges and cleaning the debris from the wound. Remember that the tissue around and involved in the wound is fragile and further damage can be done while prepping the area. Be as gentle as possible. Appropriate PPE for this procedure are gloves, goggles and a mask would also be added if there is infection present. Materials to gather include clipper with a #40 blade, water-soluble lubricant, gauze sponges, antiseptic scrub or surgical scrub, sterile saline, and hydrogen peroxide. If the wound is to be sutured, a sterilized suture pack and gloves for the veterinarian should also be laid out.

Before clipping the hair the wound must be protected from the falling hair. Place water-soluble lube or saline-soaked gauze sponges inside the wound edges to catch the hair as it is clipped. Clip around the wound edges and clear 2–3 inches of hair around the wound to facilitate suturing and healing. If the patient has long hair that will fall into the wound area it will need to be trimmed. Pull the strands of hair over the wound with

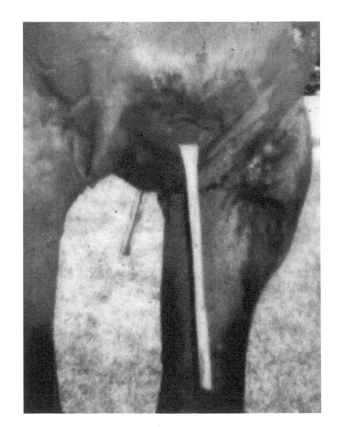

FIGURE 11.42 Penrose drain in place on a wounded horse.

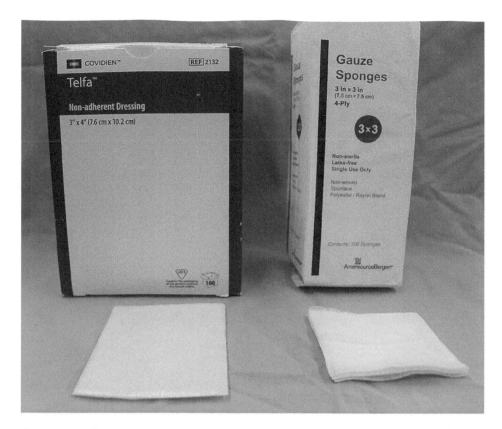

FIGURE 11.43 Non-adherent and adherent primary bandage material.

rotated to keep the exits open; if they should scab over the fluid will accumulate under the skin causing a **seroma**.

After a wound care procedure is completed there is usually a lot of mess to clean up. This is often the duty of the assistant. Clean the clipper! The blades are usually clogged with blood, pus, hair, or all three. Use a blade wash if thick or dried on and spray disinfectant and lube once cleaned. Take all the towels to the laundry and start a load. Clean out the prep sink and disinfect it and the table grate. Put all unused supplies away. If supplies are low be sure to alert the inventory manager.

Apply a Simple Bandage

Bandaging is used to protect a wound from addition injury or contamination. Bandages are also applied to immobilize a minor fracture. There are multitudes of bandage materials and techniques used in veterinary medicine. Always check with the veterinarian or technician as to the bandaging materials needed for the individual patient.

Bandage variations depend on the purpose and the area to which they are applied. Most bandages will have three layers; the primary, secondary, and tertiary. The primary bandage layer is the one closest to the skin and the material used depends on the characteristic of

the wound and the reason for the bandage. A wound dressing is usually non-adherent unless it requires debridement in which case adherent bandage material is utilized (Figure 11.43). The secondary layer is made up of material that absorbs drainage or acts as a cushion layer (Figure 11.44). Its additional purpose is to hold the primary layer in place. It often consists of conforming gauze or padding, with or without a protective layer for the skin (Figure 11.45). It can be thin or quite thick like cotton batting to immobilize a fractured limb. The tertiary layer holds the bandage onto the animal and is either an adhesive tape or a self-adhesive product (e.g., Vetrap™) (Figure 11.46). This product clings to itself and often does not need to be taped to hold it in place. The tertiary layer can be water-resistant, but is not always. It must extend beyond the border of the secondary layer and attach to the patient's skin or fur. A good guideline is that the adhesive tape should be 50% on the patient and 50% on the secondary layer as it is applied.

Bandages are applied taut enough to stay in place, but not so tight that circulation is impaired. A good rule of thumb to check a bandage is to see if you can slide two fingers, held flat against the skin, up to the first knuckle under the bandage before the tertiary layer is placed then it isn't too tight. If you can slide your fingers under the bandage past the first knuckle, then it is too loose.

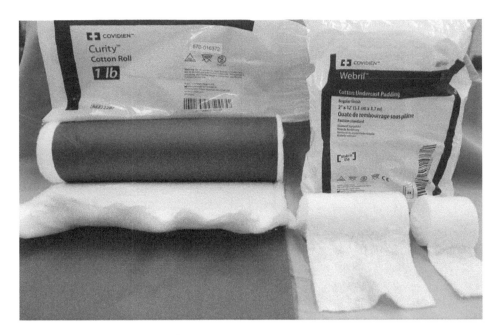

FIGURE 11.44 Secondary absorbent and cushion material.

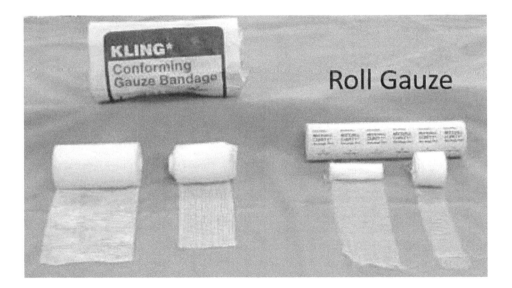

FIGURE 11.45 Kling gauze and roll gauze.

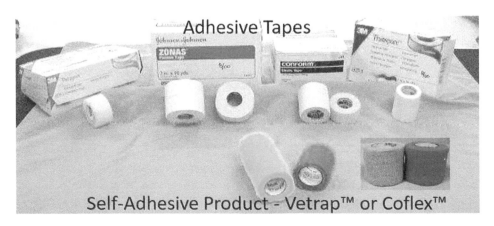

FIGURE 11.46 Adhesive tape and self-adhesive products.

Once the bandage has been checked the tertiary layer is then laid upon the skin and hair without tightness.

The images in Figure 11.47 show the steps to applying a simple paw bandage:

1. Apply "stirrups" to either side of the leg. Place sticky side down, well past the foot, putting the two pieces together once past the toes. One piece should be longer that the other, so a sticky end is available (Figure 11.47a).

2. Apply the primary layer of non-adhesive dressing over the wound, then cover everything with cling gauze or cast padding. Roll off the roll backwards to maintain control of tightness and length of material coming off the roll (Figure 11.47b).

3. Rip the stirrups in half-length wise up to the toes. Take one half of the stirrup and twist it so the sticky side adheres to the fur or secondary layer. Repeat for the other stirrup (Figure 11.47c).

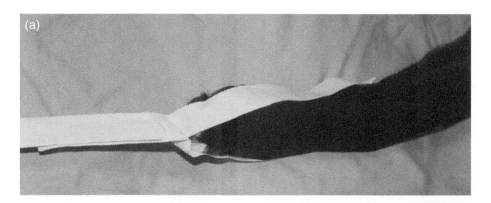

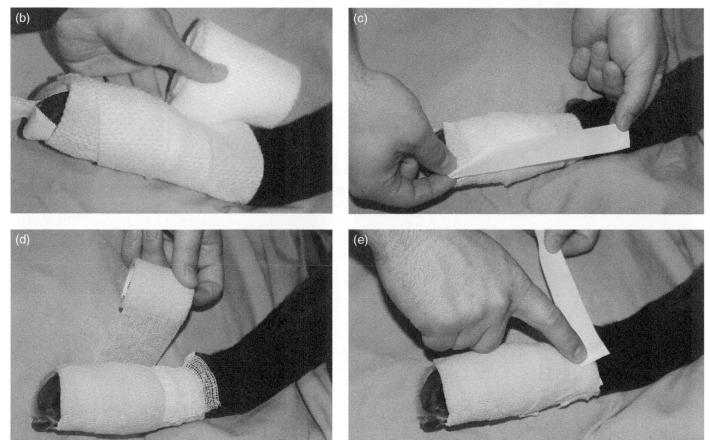

FIGURE 11.47 The steps involved in applying a simple paw bandage.

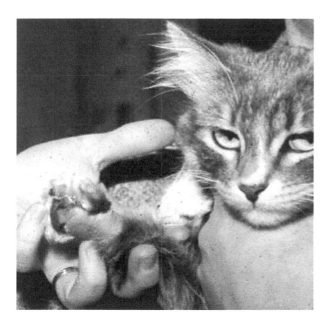

FIGURE 11.48 Damage caused by a bandage applied too tightly.

4. Using a self-adhesive product, apply the tertiary layer over the entire secondary layer and stirrups (Figure 11.47d).
5. Applying adhesive tape half on the bandage and half on the patient's skin/hair to secure the bandage to the leg. Note that you can still see the toes with the bandage which facilitates checking to make sure the bandage isn't too tight (Figure 11.47e).

Indications that a bandage is on too tight include swelling, discoloration, and cooling of the body parts distal to the bandage. Figure 11.48 shows the damage done to a paw from a bandage that was not correctly wrapped or checked for tightness. In this case the secondary layer was not applied properly. The gauze was either twisted or it slipped during application. The veterinarian or technician will most likely apply the bandage, but you can assist by keeping the patient still, helping to hold the bandage material in place, and watching for any signs of bandage failure.

Bandage Failure

Bandage failure is slipping, weeping, or soaked bandage from drainage, a wet bandage from the environment, or a chewed upon bandage. It is important to keep bandages dry as **tissue maceration** occurs and the underlaying tissue becomes fragile. A method of preventing bandages on limbs from getting wet is to place an empty IV bag over the limb. The end with the drip set connector is cut off, then use a scissors to poke holes around the top. Tear off a length of gauze roll that will fit around the leg with some extra to use as a tie. The gauze is threaded in and out of each hole to create a drawstring bag. The

bag is slipped on the limb and the roll gauze is used to tighten the bag around the limb. These are applied only for trips outside and are taken off as soon as possible to avoid impairing circulation. If the bandage is damaged in some way alert the veterinarian or technician.

Multiple bandage changes can irritate the skin as the adhesive tape is removed. To ease removal of the tape an adhesive tape remover product is recommended. Soak a cotton ball or gauze sponge with the remover and apply liberally to the tape surface. Allow it to sit for a minute or two and then slowly peel back the tape from the skin.

A chewed bandage can indicate that it is uncomfortable, but usually it is because animals don't like bandages. An Elizabethan collar or basket muzzle or a spray like bitter apple can be applied to prevent chewing. This is to not only prevent the animal from destroying the bandage, but to prevent possible ingestion of the bandaging materials which can create a whole other set of problems!

Bandage Removal

After the veterinarian has ruled a bandage is ready for removal the veterinary assistant may assist or take the bandage off. A bandage scissor is used by slipping the blade with the blunt wedge adjacent to the skin and under all the layers or each layer individually of the bandage. A slow steady snip and inching forward until the bandage is cut off enough to slip off the end of a limb or to come completely apart.

Emergency Support

Unfortunately, emergencies are a fact of life in every veterinary facility. The arrival of patients with from acute injuries, hemorrhage, respiratory or cardiac distress, shock, or poisoning necessitates life-saving measures. Staff members need to work as a team under the leadership of the veterinarian if these life-saving measures are to be successful.

While the veterinarian and technician are providing the hands-on care, the ancillary staff moves into action. The veterinary assistant is responsible for supplying emergency equipment and drugs to the patient treatment area and providing supplementary support to the team. To be effective, the assistant must:

1. Know where the emergency station is and where the crash cart or kit is stored.
2. Retrieve general supplies as needed if kit supply is used up.
3. Gather gurney, warming blankets, towels, IV stands, monitoring equipment, and other gear as requested by the team.
4. Provide patient restraint, positioning, and moving as needed.

Maintenance of Crash Cart Kit or Emergency Station

One of the primary functions of the assistant to emergency support is to maintain the facility's crash cart or emergency station. It is vital that the crash kit and emergency station be organized and stocked with currently dated materials. All items are to be in their designated places and all equipment batteries charged and ready for use. Establish a weekly routine for checking and changing out the emergency supplies and equipment (Figure 11.49).

If materials and equipment are taken from the cart or station during emergency treatments, they must be immediately restocked or cleaned and returned to the cart or station. When an emergency arises every second counts and there mustn't be time lost trying to locate supplies or dealing with equipment failure. A checklist of required supplies can be drawn up if not already in place. Use this to make sure no item is missed when restocking the crash cart or emergency station.

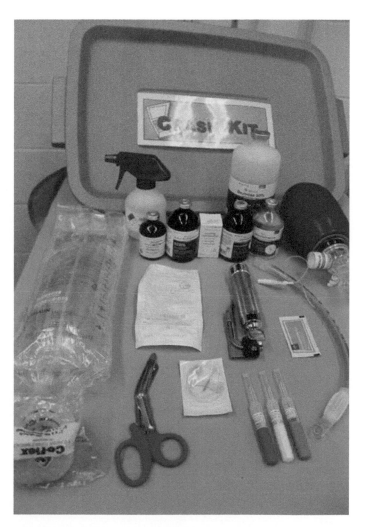

FIGURE 11.49 Contents of a crash kit.

The accessibility of the crash cart or emergency station is important. It should be centrally located within the clinic. In some instances, the ideal area is where anesthesia is induced. Many of the same supplies and equipment are used in this area that are also needed in times of an emergency. Access to oxygen is an absolute necessity for flow-by oxygen, manual ambu bags, or ventilators. Some clinics will have an E tank of oxygen on a small wheeled cart that can be rolled to any location within the clinic. Other items such as clippers, endotracheal tubes, oxygen masks, and assortment of fluids are just the essentials.

Emergency drugs are also needed in the crash cart and because they don't get used as often it is a good idea to check them on a weekly basis for outdates. If outdating soon, see if it can't be moved into the active use inventory and be replaced with a new bottle. Speak to the inventory manager about this concern. There are usually charts with the drugs listed with dosages for the various emergencies. The veterinarians will use these to double check the dosages before administering the medications. If you are asked to draw up a medication, don't let the rush of the moment deter you from checking the label at least twice to make sure you have the correct medication. Even repeating the medication name and dose out loud will confirm that you have the right one. Also show someone else the syringe once it is filled to confirm dose.

Sterile packs that may be required are towel packs, suture pack, and an assortment of suture materials. Other instrumentation may include a defibrillator, monitor for ECG, capnograph, pulse oximeter, and BP monitor.

Emergency phone numbers should be included in the crash kit or emergency station: ASPCA Poison Control, Blood Bank, Disaster and Emergency Response hotlines. Include local numbers that may be helpful during an emergency like local poison control, non-emergency sheriff or police departments, diagnostic laboratories, and so on.

When assisting with an emergency remember these acronyms: **LARK: listen** actively, **anticipate** needs, **respond** quickly, and **know** what you are doing. **A CRASH PLAN** is utilized by the veterinarian and technician when first presented with the patient. These are the things they will assess first to last and include: **a**irway, **c**ardiovascular, **r**espiratory, **a**bdomen, **s**pine, **h**ead, **p**elvis, **l**imbs, **a**rteries/veins, **n**erves.

Suggested Reading

Live Sciences. 2013. What's the most popular pet? https://www.livescience.com/32415-whats-the-most-popular-pet.html (accessed July 4, 2019).

McQuarry AC. 2011.Venipuncture of dogs and cats. https://www.slideshare.net/DrAlana/lec-04-venipuncture-of-dogs-and-cats?next_slideshow=3 (accessed July 4, 2019).

CHAPTER 12

Laboratory Skills

LEARNING OBJECTIVES

- Clean and/or maintain laboratory equipment including binocular microscope, centrifuge, and refractometer
- Recognize common ectoparasites and common internal parasite ova
- Conduct a gross examination of and prepare feces for analysis
- Assist in blood collection, handling, and shipment to a reference laboratory
- Use in-house hematology analyzer to run a complete blood count (CBC)
- Prepare and stain a usable blood smear
- Complete packed cell volume (PCV) and plasma protein tests
- Use in-house analyzers to conduct blood chemistries and electrolyte determinations
- Use assorted serologic test kits
- Assist with urine sample collection techniques
- Prepare urine samples for sediment microscopic examination, urine specific gravity, and urine chemistries
- Assist with sample collection for culture and sensitivity, prepare a Gram stain
- Set up equipment and materials needed to complete a necropsy
- Properly pack samples for shipment to a reference laboratory

NAVTA ESSENTIAL SKILLS COVERED IN THIS CHAPTER

VII. Laboratory Procedures
A. Assistance in the laboratory
   2. Determine physical properties of urine including color and clarity
   3. Assist in the collection of blood samples with restraint and supply preparation

Tasks for the Veterinary Assistant, Fourth Edition. Teresa F. Sonsthagen.
© 2020 John Wiley & Sons, Inc. Published 2020 by John Wiley & Sons, Inc.
Companion website: www.wiley.com/go/sonsthagen/tasks

4. Identify common blood tubes used in veterinary medicine
6. Prepare fecal flotation solutions and set up fecal flotations and direct smears
7. Understand the role of the veterinary assistant in necropsy procedures
8. Explain how to handle rabies suspects and samples safely
10. Identify external parasites: mites, lice, fleas, and ticks
11. Assist in the preparation of various specimen staining techniques
12. Prepare and spin microhematocrit tubes for evaluation by veterinarian or veterinary technician

B. Laboratory record keeping
1. Ensure all laboratory results are accurately recorded
2. Stock laboratory supplies
3. File laboratory reports
4. Maintain laboratory log

In-house laboratories provide test results that aid in the diagnosis, prognosis, and course of therapy for patients. The veterinary technician receives extensive education on running these tests. Entire semesters are devoted to **clinical pathology** which include blood chemistries, urinalysis, serology, cytology, and microbiology testing as well as **hematology** and **parasitology**. The veterinarian depends on the veterinary technician to prepare samples properly for analysis, conduct the tests accurately, and record the results. The veterinary assistant can help with sample collection, set-up, restocking supplies, cleaning and maintaining instruments. It is not the responsibility of either the veterinary technician or assistant to interpret the results of the tests, that is purview of the veterinarian.

These tests measure and monitor changes within the body not otherwise discernible on physical examination. Chemical changes in the body indicate alterations in organ function, which are the hallmarks of disease and its progression. The presence or absence of disease-producing organisms may be determined and drug levels measured. Blood, urine, feces, and other bodily secretions are the source for these analyses. The tasks in this chapter will help the veterinary assistant learn about laboratory work.

Laboratory services are performed either within the veterinary facility, referred to as in-house testing, or sent off-site to a commercial laboratory, referred to as a reference laboratory. The laboratory equipment available in the practice determine which tests are run in-house and which are sent to a reference laboratory. The modern veterinary clinic laboratory is equipped with a suite of instruments. These include hematology, blood chemistry, electrolyte, coagulation, and blood gas analyzers. There are instruments that simply read results like urinalysis strip and serology test readers. You will also find a microscope, centrifuge, and refractometer as common pieces of equipment. The veterinary assistants may use, clean, and maintain these pieces of equipment. The assistant can be of value to the team by maintaining the equipment per the manufacturer's recommendations. Because there are so many companies that produce these pieces of equipment it is beyond the scope of this chapter to describe them all. It is best to read the equipment's user manual if available and if not contacting the manufacturer for a new manual or for an online link.

Watch, read, and learn which piece of equipment performs which test. Learn what kits or disposables are required, as well as what type of sample is required for the test, and have everything ready for the veterinary technician. The following information in this chapter is to educate you on what tests are commonly run in-house, what samples are required, and how to set up some of the basic tests.

Maintenance of Stain Sets

The best veterinary practice cannot obtain reliable results if reliable materials are not used. Stains, reagents, test strips, and miscellaneous equipment need to be available, in-date, and maintained to ensure accurate results. Typical stains are those used for hematology and cytology smears: Gram stain for microbiology stains; new methylene blue for manual reticulocyte counts and cytology specimens like ear swabs. Acid-fast or dip quick stains are used for hematology smears and other cytology preparations.

Stain degradation happens to alcohol fixatives found in the hematology stains. They pick up moisture from the air or evaporate. Stains lose their potency and become contaminated with use. They also tend to precipitate. These make the stains useless and can actually cause misdiagnosis to occur. To take care of them they need to be either refreshed or changed out completely.

Coplin jars are heavy glass jars with tight-fitting lids which are used for most stains. They allow you to see the interior without losing the stain solution to evaporation. Hematology stain sets consist of three solutions that need to be replenished to maintain a depth to completely cover the slide. This is usually based upon the fixative solution. It is first to become low and not cover the entire slide surface. Dump the orange and purple stains out to match the level of the fixative and then add back fresh of each from the source bottles. Usually the stains are refreshed once and then changed out entirely to maintain clear stains. Wash and dry the Coplin jars thoroughly and then add fresh stain from the source containers. Make sure the labels are updated with the dates they were refreshed and when they were changed out. If precipitates develop in a stain they can be removed by allowing the stain to flow through filter paper into a clean container. Wear gloves and work on a non-porous tray. It is a messy process and anything the stain touches will remain that color! To avoid evaporation and keep out moisture, always recap stain bottles after use.

Staining Protocol

The hematology and cytology stains are a three-step process and are often referred to as dip quick stains. The first solution is an alcohol fixative and is usually light blue or clear, the second solution is reddish orange, and the final stain is dark purple, each in its own Coplin jar. It is quick because the slide is dipped into each Coplin jar for 5–10 dips depending on the manufacturer. It is advisable to have two set of stains, one for hematology preparation and one for cytology preparation. The cytology set will have to be changed more regularly because they become contaminated quickly.

Each lab will be stocked with test kits and strips, as well as miscellaneous equipment that are used for a number of tests. Reagents and test strips are used for the variety of tests and for some pieces of equipment. Help out by checking the expiration date, and inventory reorder points on a daily basis. Place the order for more as needed. Help store the reagents properly when new comes in. Keep them tightly capped to avoid moisture in the air from contaminating the chemicals and store them per the manufacturer's recommended temperature. Everyday supplies include microscope slides, coverslips, pipettes, test tubes, and sample containers. These items need to be available at all times. Learn the proper name for each item, how it is used, and where they are stored. Help the team by keeping them in stock by paying attention to the re-order points.

To learn about each instrument in the laboratory you can find and read the user manuals. These manuals contain important information such as directions for use, maintenance, and trouble shooting. The assistant can help the team by maintaining the daily, weekly, monthly, or yearly maintenance on each piece of equipment in the lab. Setting up a maintenance log is a great way to keep track of what has been done to what machine and by whom. It is also a place to log control results and needs to be readily accessible and near the instrument in question.

Learning Exercise

Determine how you will proceed to learn about the stains and test kits available in a veterinary facility. Perhaps starting a lab protocol notebook, or putting instructions and maintenance information on an index card and clipping them together. Whatever your preferred method of learning is, use it to get this information firmly understood.

Laboratory Log Book

Often, auxiliary patient result log books are kept in the laboratory. Some laboratories have one central notebook in which testing information is kept, especially if using paper patient files. This requires laboratory results to be recorded in two places – the patient file and in the laboratory log book – as a way to capture the results if someone forgot to write in one or the other. Test results are entered into the patient file manually for some tests. Other tests can be printed out by the machine and added to the file. If the veterinary practice uses management software, the results from the various analyzers go automatically from the instrument to the patient's electronic file. However, there will still be test results that will have to be typed into the electronic patient file.

When writing in the results learn how they are recorded. Many results have a specific unit of measurement. For example a packed cell volume (PCV) is recorded as a percentage and total protein is recorded as g/dL. The units are always recorded with the numeric value of the test. The lab will most likely have a chart of normal reference ranges, if so they too should be included in the manual entry. Enclose normal reference ranges in parentheses and to the right of the test result. Reference ranges vary by laboratory and instrument. Some test results are not numeric but are positive or negative often indicated by a - or − sign. It is imperative that all test results are recorded in all the places possible. If they are run but not recorded, they weren't run! This costs the clinic time, money, and may endanger an animal's life. Make it your mission to ensure all test results are written down!

Maintenance of the Common Laboratory Equipment in the Veterinary Lab

Binocular Microscope

The binocular microscope (Figure 12.1) is an expensive investment but unfortunately next to the hair clipper is one of the most abused pieces of equipment in the clinic. The veterinary assistant can be of great value to the team if he/she learns how to clean the scope on a daily basis.

The first step is to learn to identify the various parts of the microscope. There are three parts: the head, body, and the base. The head contains oculars and objectives. The **oculars** are what you look in to view what is under the **objective**. Oculars can be adjusted to accommodate looking through both eyes bye sliding them apart or closer together. The objectives are used to magnify the image on the slide There are usually 4–5 objectives; each is designated by a number and an ×. The × stands for a multiplication × 100. So 10× magnifies the image by 1000 times, the 20× by 2000 times, the 40× by 4000 times, and 100× by 10,000 times. The 10× objective is usually used to find the sample, but does not give great detail unless the item being looked at is as large as a flca or tick. The 20× is used for slightly smaller items and the 40× is most often used to positively identify parasite eggs and to focus the scope for the 100× objective. The 100× objective is called the oil objective because it requires a drop of immersion oil on the slide in order to focus. It is used to identify blood cells, and some parasites like cryptosporidia, yeast, and bacteria.

The body of the scope contains the stage; this is what the slide is placed upon for viewing. The stage has a clip

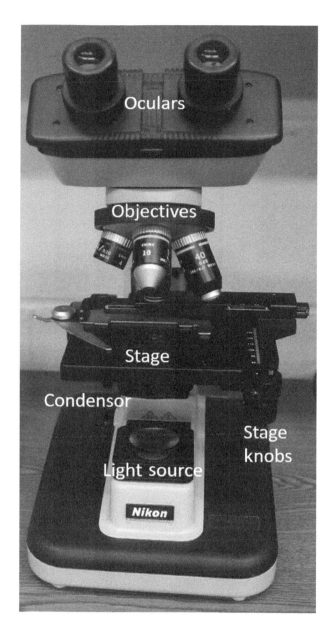

FIGURE 12.1 Parts of a microscope.

that holds the slide in place as the stage is moved. To the right and below the stage are the control knobs to move it left or right or forwards and backwards. On either side and more to the rear of the stage are the focus knobs which moves the stage up and down. This is what will bring the samples into focus. The course focus knob is available on both sides of the scope. This is turned counter-clockwise to lift the stage up in large increments. It is used to find the spot on the slide on which to start. Once the sample is found, the fine focus knob is used. The fine focus knob is centered inside the course adjustment knob and only on the right side of the scope. The fine focus knob brings the image sharply into focus. Directly under the stage is the condenser lens equipped with an iris diaphragm. The condenser can be raised and lowered with a knob usually right under the stage. The condenser controls the amount of light refracted off of the mirrors inside the condenser. The iris directs the light into small or large areas.

The light source control and power switch are on the base. Depending on the manufacturer, these controls are either on the side of the base itself, along the back of the scope, or on the side of the arm of the base. The light source control knob or rheostat is used to make the light brighter or softer. The power switch is of course to turn the scope on and off. The light source located directly below the condenser houses the light bulb. These do burn out after a while and can be changed out by either sliding the entire top of the light source away from the scope or turning it upside down and accessing it from the bottom of the scope. Microscope light bulbs should not be touched with bare fingers. The grease from our hands will make the bulb get too hot and it results in it burning out faster. Use a Kem Wipe or paper towel to remove and replace the bulb. Before replacing the bulb on a scope that won't light up, check the power cord! It has a habit of becoming loosened from the back of the scope. This is especially true if the scope is slid back and forth on the countertop.

The microscope is often abused because no one takes the time to care and maintain it properly. If lucky enough to find a manufacturer's user manual read the instructions for cleaning and maintenance of the microscope. If not available, the following is routine care for the microscope after each use. If taken care of well, this piece of equipment will work forever. If not, it tends to get filthy dirty and will no longer be useable.

The best possible care is to do a quick clean after each use of the microscope. The sample slide is removed and disposed of properly, usually in a sharps container. The oculars are cleaned using a piece of lens paper with a small drop of lens cleaner applied to one end of the paper. Wipe the oculars off with the wet paper; if you have personnel that wears eyebrow pencil and mascara this is very important. The objectives are cleaned using the other end of the same lens paper with another small drop of lens cleaner applied. Let both the oculars and objective air dry. If the 100× objective was used, the oil should be removed after each use again with lens paper. First wipe the 100× objective off and then apply a drop of lens cleaner to the lens paper and clean thoroughly. It never hurts to apply the same care to the 40× objective, as it is long enough to be dragged through the immersion oil by accident.

If either objective has sat in oil for a while it may need a deeper cleaning. This cleaning is accomplished using lens paper and a small amount of alcohol, or xylene substitute as needed. Immersion oil tends to become thick and somewhat crusty if left to dry on an objective lens. The objectives can be turned out of the ring, but care must be taken when threading them back into place. The fittings are copper and bend easily so forcing or threading an objective in wrongly can ruin the entire scope!

"Park" the microscope by turning the light source to its lowest setting, turn the power button off, point the lowest objective toward the stage, lower the stage to its lowest position, and replace the cover over the microscope. This may seem like a huge inconvenience but it is the best procedure for maintaining the microscope. If the microscope is in constant use during the day, the shutdown procedure can be done as one of the last things for the day. A very neglected scope can sometimes be brought back to usefulness by a professional clean. There are companies that travel to clean and fix microscopes. If you happen to have a college or university with a biology department in your area call them to find out who they use and see if you can arrange for them to stop by the practice to clean your scope. It will save the clinic money in the long run as a replacement scope can run up to $2000.

Learning Exercise

Practice working with the microscope. If the school has prepared slides, use one to find, focus, and move the slide. When scanning a slide you look at the entire area under the coverslip. Practice this as well because some people get motion sickness when they first start moving the slide.

Centrifuge

Centrifuges (see Figure 4.24) are used to separate undissolved solids from liquids, resulting in sample material that can be analyzed. Samples centrifuged in the laboratory are clotted blood to obtain serum; unclotted blood to obtain plasma; urine to obtain sediment; and fecal solutions to obtain parasite ova.

There are four rules governing the use of every centrifuge.

1. Always balance the centrifuge before turning it on. An unbalanced centrifuge will "walk" itself off of the counter. It will make a horrible racket and can break or crack the test tubes, which will spin the sample all over the inside of the centrifuge. In short, it makes a terrible mess and can actually damage the centrifuge.

2. Always lock the lid especially on the hematocrit centrifuge. There are two lids: one to hold the hematocrit tubes in place and one to cover the spinning disc. Modern day centrifuges lock automatically when they are started and unlock when the timer goes off. You can stop centrifuges

by pushing the stop button or turning the timer to zero.

3. Never try to stop or slow down a rotating centrifuge with your hand. If you suddenly stop a centrifuge it can remix your sample. Another issue with stopping it by your hand is it's an accident waiting to happen! You can lose a finger or severely burn your fingers by friction. Wait the two minutes it takes for the centrifuge to stop fully.

4. Wipe up any fluids that may have spilled in the centrifuge. Spilled fluids will off balance your centrifuge. If you pull out a test tube that isn't as full as it was when it went in check the tube for fluid. Plastic test tubes are notorious for developing cracks and spilling their contents into the centrifuge tube. Use disinfectant and paper towels twisted enough to reach to the bottom of the tube. Take extra care if the test tubes are glass as they shatter into tiny little pieces that are difficult to remove from a finger!

Practices will often have at least two centrifuges: one for small micro-hematocrit tubes and a standard-sized centrifuge with variable speeds (rpm), a timer, and different-sized centrifuge tubes to accommodate different-sized test tubes. The larger centrifuges can be either fixed slant or swinging bucket heads. Some centrifuges have interchangeable heads, with the heads changed depending on the sample to be run. Whatever the type blood, urine and feces are placed in test tubes and spun in a centrifuge for their various components. By keeping them clean and maintaining them as per the owner's manual you will be of great value to the team.

Learning Exercise

Take a look at the school's or your workplace's centrifuges. Practice balancing and then running them with water in the tubes.

Refractometer

A refractometer (Figure 12.2) is used to determine urine specific gravity, which is an indication of kidney function and to measure total protein in plasma, which can indicate inflammation. Each of these has on its own scale on the refractometer. Refractometry is light passing through a liquid and refracted by dissolved substances in the liquid. Upkeep on the refractometer is easy. Clean it with water from the tap and use a lens paper to wipe the lid and the glass surface dry. The only other maintenance required is to check its calibration once a month. Place a drop of distilled water on the glass surface and gently put the lid over the drop. Hold the refractometer to your eye and under a light source. The ceiling light should be sufficient. The line on the specific gravity scale should

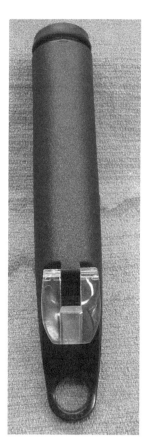

FIGURE 12.2 Refractometer.

read 1.000, which is the specific gravity of water. The smaller scale to the right or left of the large scale is to measure total protein. Don't worry about that number. If the specific gravity scale is off, find the little screw on the refractometer, usually close to the eyepiece and turn it one way to bring the line to 1.000.

If the refractometer is not properly calibrated, invalid results may occur. Record who did the calibration and when it was done in the maintenance log.

Learning Exercise

Put a drop of distilled water on the lens of the refractometer, hold it up to the light and find where the line is to indicate the specific gravity of the water.

Sample Collection

Every sample tested must be prepared according to the directions for testing as per the piece of equipment required to run the test or if it's a manual test. This often includes:

1. Accurate volume or weight measurements. Too little or too much sample will skew results.

2. Time from sample collection until sample is tested. Some samples have to be fresh from the animal in order to obtain accurate results. Giardia, a parasite found in fresh feces, and blood gases measured in blood are examples of time-sensitive samples.

3. Sample handling (refrigerated, room temperature, type of container in which it is to be collected, etc.). If a sample cannot be analyzed immediately, many can be stored in a refrigerator or freezer. In which case they have to be allowed to reach room temperature before running the test. Some samples have to be collected in sterile containers so the normal bacteria found everywhere doesn't give false results.

4. Sample type needed for the test (example: serum versus plasma). There are many types of blood collection tubes available to give accurate blood test results. Failure to utilize the correct tube can result in inaccurate results.

5. Lab procedures are conducted wearing personal protective equipment (PPE) of gloves, goggles, and a lab coat. All tests should be done on a non-porous tray or surface that is easily disinfected. Confining spills and preventing possible staining of the counter. Disinfecting the counter involves letting the disinfectant air dry as discussed in Chapter 4.

6. Follow lab protocols to set up the various tests. Most clinics will have a binder with test "recipes" or protocols used to set the tests up. If they don't, it is a good idea to work with the technicians to set one up. This way everyone runs the tests in the same manner which increases quality results.

Parasitology

Parasitism is the presence of organisms benefiting themselves while harming their hosts, the organisms off whom they live. There are two types of parasites commonly found:

Ectoparasites are external parasites like fleas, ticks, mites, and lice.

Endoparasites are internal parasites like roundworms, hookworms, flukes, tapeworms, and protozoans.

Sampling for and Identification of Ectoparasites

External parasites are commonly reported in animals as they cause and transmit diseases and vary by geographic region. The most common ones found in almost all parts of the world are fleas, ticks, lice, flies, mosquitoes, and mites. All but the mite are visible to the naked eye. Lice and mites are transmitted through **direct contact** and the rest are transmitted by **indirect contact**. The visible ones can be captured and placed into a drop of mineral oil on a microscope slide for identification under 4× or 10×. To determine what kind of mite is present, a skin scraping is required. Treatment and control of ectoparasites begins with identification, then the veterinarian will prescribe appropriate treatment.

The following are descriptions and photos of all but the fly and mosquito.

Fleas

Adult fleas mate and feed on blood from their hosts (Figure 12.3). The average flea is about 5 mm in size, they are a rusty red color, and have large back legs. Fleas spend their entire life on the pet, they mate and lay eggs on the host but many fall off into the animal's environment. They hatch into larvae that resemble fly maggots and will ingest the "flea dirt" (see Figure 10.12) which is fecal material rich in blood. Larvae, after feeding, create a cocoon and develop into a pupae, which later hatches into an adult. that later hatch into adults. Transmission is indirect, occurring when an individual enters a contaminated environment. They have to have a blood meal within two weeks or they die. If a human is the only one available they will take a blood meal from him or her.

Because fleas are fast and great jumpers you may not see them. We discussed how to determine if there are fleas on a host in Chapter 10. If fleas are present, the room needs to be sprayed with an insecticide designed to kill fleas so they don't spread throughout the clinic.

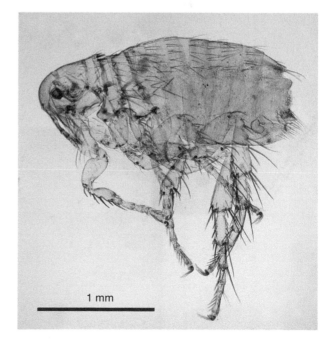

FIGURE 12.3 Flea. Source: Wikimedia Commons. Used under CC BY-SA 2.5 ES, https://commons.m.wikimedia.org/wiki/File:Ctenocephalides-canis.jpg.

Lice

There are two kinds of lice: chewing lice that feed on skin scales and sucking lice that feed on blood (Figure 12.4). The sucking louse has a narrower head than the chewing louse. Lice complete their entire life cycle on their hosts. Lice are about 3 mm in size and are visible when crawling across bare skin. After mating, the female attaches her eggs, called nits (see Figure 10.13), by sticking them on the hair shafts of the host. Nits are white and about 1 mm in size. The nits are also used to identify a louse infestation. A small-toothed comb is used to comb through suspected hair which is then looked at under the microscope. Lice are transmitted by direct contact between an infected host and an uninfected individual. Lice are **species specific**, but there is a species that prefer humans!

Flies

Flies can affect hosts during two phases of their life cycle: adults and larvae. Adult flies vary from the small sand fly, 1–3 mm in size, to the larger horse fly, which can be up to 3.5 cm in length. The different species of adult flies feed on blood, tears, saliva, or mucus. The damage they cause to tissues may indicate their presence. Depending on the fly species, some larvae develop in tissue where they can be seen as white, worm-like creatures called maggots that feed on dead tissue. If not taken care of the maggots will make a small wound quite large. Others will bite and suck blood, making multiple tiny sores often seen on tips of ears or across the nose. Others bite so hard that large welts develop and are quite painful. Flies also spread other parasites.

Ticks

Ticks are bloodsucking, disease-spreading insects that engorge themselves on their host's blood and then fall back into the environment. They lay their eggs in the environment where they hatch and hang out on brush waiting for a mammal to pass by. The unfed nymph may be as small as 3 mm, an engorged adult may be up to three times larger. Their presence is noted when a tick is seen attached to the skin. Favored places are the ears and face. Care is taken when removing ticks that have attached to the host. They are grasped as close to the body as possible and pulled in the direction they are lying. If you lift and pull backwards, the heads break off and cause a sore. Ticks transmit diseases such as Rocky Mountain spotted fever, ehrlichiosis, *Mycoplasma* infections, and Lyme disease. The *Ixodes* sp. or "black legged" tick is the main culprit for Lyme disease (Figure 12.5). This tick as an adult is half the size of other ticks, making it very hard to find. They will attach to any mammal thus making Lyme disease zoonotic.

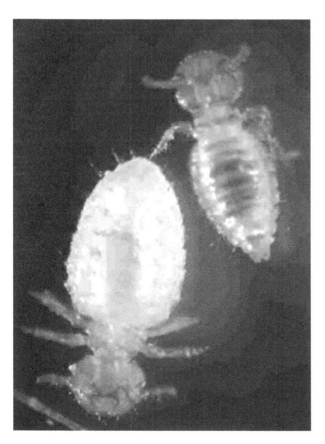

FIGURE 12.4 Chewing louse. Source: Wikimedia Commons. Used under CC BY-SA 3.0, https://commons.m.wikimedia.org/wiki/File:Lice_image01.jpg.

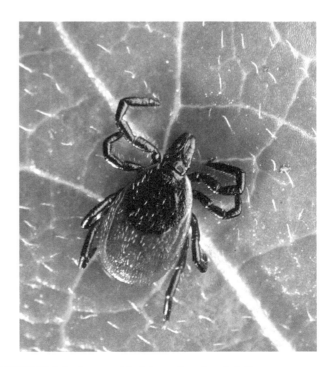

FIGURE 12.5 *Ixodes* sp. or black legged or deer tick. Source: https://commons.wikimedia.org/wiki/File:Adult_deer_tick.jpg. Public Domain.

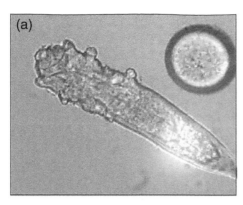 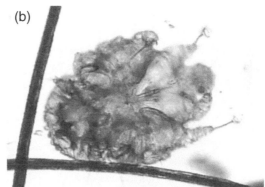

FIGURE 12.6 (a) Demodex and (b) burrowing mite species. Source: (a) Wikimedia Commons. Used under CC BY-SA 3.0, https://commons.m.wikimedia.org/wiki/File:Haarbalgmilbe.jpg (b) Source: Wikimedia Commons. Used under CC BY-SA 2.5, https://commons.m.wikimedia.org/wiki/File:Canine_scabies_mite.JPG.

Mosquitoes

In addition to being irritants and voracious bloodsuckers, mosquitoes are most noted for their transmission of diseases such as *Dirofilaria immitus* (heartworms) and West Nile disease, which is zoonotic. Mosquitoes require water to lay their eggs and different species use different pools of water. They are more active in the evening and early morning hours. Topical and oral medications and vaccines are used as preventatives for the diseases they transmit.

Mites

Mites feed on tissue fluids and skin cells. They can cause severe **dermatitis** accompanied by **pruritus** and **alopecia**. Burrowing mites such as *Demodex*, *Notoedres*, and *Sarcoptes* require a skin scraping to find (Figure 12.6). The supplies needed for this test are a scalpel blade, a microscope slide with a drop of mineral oil upon it, and a microscope. The veterinarian or technician will scrape the area in question with the scalpel blade and deposit the material onto the slide. The *Demodex* are cigar-shaped and the others have eight short legs on rounded bodies. The non-burrowing mites have long legs on rounded bodies (Figure 12.7). Some, such as *Cheyletiella* ("walking dandruff mite") is visible to the naked eye as white flakes of "dandruff" that move! Use a piece of cellophane tape to capture them, then place the tape onto a microscope slide. Diagnosis of *Otodectes* ("ear mites") requires an ear swab as discussed in Chapter 10, although these mites can be seen with an otoscope inside the ear canal.

Sampling for and Identification of Endoparasites

Endoparasites infect internal organ systems and may result in diarrhea, weight loss, or anemia; therefore, the fecal exam is an important and common laboratory test. Collection techniques are discussed in Chapter 10. However, samples need to be fresh out of the patient in

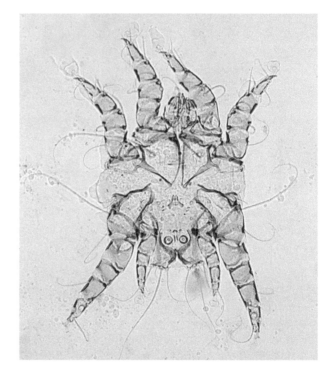

FIGURE 12.7 Non-burrowing mite species. Source: Wikimedia Commons. Used under CC BY-SA 3.0, https://commons.m.wikimedia.org/wiki/File:Otodectes-mite.jpg.

order to find the eggs of the internal parasites. If left outside or at room temperature for even an hour the eggs may hatch and therefore not be found giving a false negative. When collecting a voluntary sample take note of shape; is it formed, semi-formed, soft or watery? Is there any mucus or blood, are there any visible worms? These are things to note on the sample container as the act of collection will distort these physical attributes that may help with a diagnosis.

On occasion the veterinarian may not want to wait for a freely given sample and will utilize a fecal loop (Figure 12.8). This is used to collect a sample internally via the rectum. Items required will be lubricant, fecal

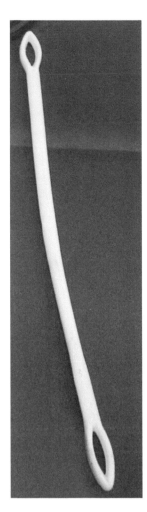

FIGURE 12.8 Fecal loop.

loop, and a microscope slide with a drop of saline or a fecal collection container to take care of the sample after collection. The patient is usually kept standing with one arm around the neck and the other hand to hold the tail up at the base. Once the sample is collected and labeled properly, alert the technician that a sample is waiting. If he/she is not available, place the sample in the lab refrigerator for future examination. Eggs will not hatch as quickly if the sample is refrigerated.

Clients are often asked to bring a fecal sample to the clinic at the time of their appointment or to drop one off for analysis. Instruct the client to watch the animal defecate to be certain it has come from their animal and it is fresh. Have them place the feces into a clean, air-tight, leak-proof container and keep it cool. If the sample is collected the night before the appointment it must be placed in a refrigerator or in an ice chest otherwise the eggs hatch and the larva will die. When delivered to the clinic make sure it has the correct client and patient information on the label. Alert the technician that a sample has been delivered.

To find parasite eggs, the sample is prepared with a concentrated salt or sugar solution. This will float the eggs to the top of a test tube which is captured on a coverslip and then transferred to a microscope slide. There are two standard techniques: a float or a centrifuge preparation.

Fecal Float Technique

Equipment required: 10–12 mL test tube, test tube rack, microscope slide, coverslip, two paper cups, strainer, two applicator sticks, and fecal solution.
  Preparation:

1. Using the applicator sticks, place a "quarter" sized piece of feces into one of the paper cups and add approximately 20–30 mL of fecal solution. You can use the test tube to measure out the fecal solution. Place the test tube into the test tube rack for future use.
2. Mix the feces and fecal solution thoroughly with the sticks. Place the strainer over the second cup and pour the fecal mixture through the strainer. Set the strainer and first cup into the sink.
3. Pour the strained fecal mixture into the test tube until a **meniscus** forms. Don't overfill as this may wash the parasite eggs out of the sample.
4. Carefully place a coverslip on top of the test tube and set a timer for 10–15 minutes. Alert the technician that the time is set.

Centrifuge Technique

The same equipment is required as for the flotation method.
  Procedure:

1. Using the applicator sticks, place a "quarter" sized piece of feces into one of the paper cups and add approximately 20–30 mL of fecal solution. You can use the test tube to measure out the fecal solution. Place the test tube into the test tube rack for future use.
2. Mix the feces and fecal solution thoroughly with the sticks. Place the strainer over the second cup and pour the fecal mixture through the strainer. Set the strainer and first cup into the sink.
3. Pour the fecal solution into the test tube up to the 10 mL mark on the side of the tube. Take the tube to the centrifuge and place it into one of the tubes inside. Then balance the centrifuge by adding a test tube filled with water up to 10 mL opposite the fecal sample. Set the centrifuge at the proper settings and time and push start.
4. Alert the technician that a fecal sample is spinning in the centrifuge.

Each clinic will have their preferred technique for fecal set-up that may differ from the examples given. Find the protocol manual or have the technician show you how to set up a fecal sample. This will be of great help to the team if the technicians are busy with clients.

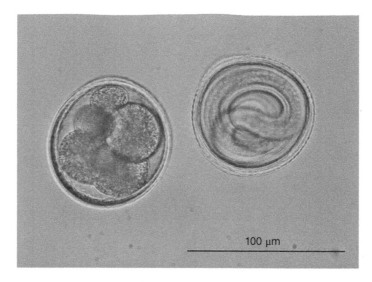

FIGURE 12.9 Roundworm eggs. Source: Wikimedia Commons. Used under CC BY 3.0, https://commons.m.wikimedia.org/wiki/File:Toxocara_embryonated_eggs.jpg.

Endoparasites are encountered worldwide with many more common in certain areas or regions. Some of the most common ones with large geographic territories are roundworms, hookworms, tapeworms, flukes, and protozoans. Most are transferred from one host to another by the oral–fecal route or by consuming an intermediate host that is infected with a stage of the parasite.

Roundworms

Roundworms are very commonly found in young puppies and kittens because the larval stage can cross the transplacental and transmammary barriers. Also, youngsters tend to defecate in their environment and so by walking in the feces and then licking it from their paws infect each other or re-infect themselves. High numbers of adult worms in the young can cause extremely large pot bellies that can be quite painful. The transmission of roundworms to adults is by ingesting the eggs found in the feces of infected animals. The roundworm egg is seen easily under 10× and verified under 40× on the the microscope. It is a round egg, with a thick, wavy cell wall (Figure 12.9). If the microscope has a micrometer it will measure about 70–75 microns. Roundworms are zoonotic so PPE when handling feces are gloves and goggles.

Hookworms

Hookworms can infect both animal and human by skin penetration by larva or ingestion of eggs passed in feces. This sand-loving nematode is why many beaches ban dogs! A heavy infection of hookworms often causes bloody diarrhea or black tarry stools because they attach to the intestines and suck blood. The eggs are seen on 10× and verified on 40× and should measure 75–120

microns. They are oval shaped, have a thin cell wall, and have **morula** inside. There are usually 8–10 morula per egg (Figure 12.10).

Tapeworms

Tapeworms are flat worms that absorb nutrients through their bodies so they get quite large. Their bodies are made up of segments called proglottids that are shed when **gravid**. The proglottids are often found around the anus or in bedding and look like small, white, moving grains of rice (Figure 12.11). The flea is often an intermediate host to the tapeworm and so owners need to take care of those as well as the tapeworm. Take note that some types of tapeworms are zoonotic. The segments are usually found and if an identification is required they are put on a microscope slide with a drop of water. Then, using applicator sticks, are broken apart to spill the eggs. The eggs are usually round, with a thick cell wall that is striated and about half the size of roundworm eggs.

Flukes

Flukes are more common in areas of the country that has lots of wetlands and lakes. They require water to reach their intermediate hosts which are snails, crustations, or fish. If a dog or cat happens to eat an infected intermediate host, the fluke larva migrates to the liver or lungs attaches and starts to suck blood. If the adult population is heavy enough, the patient may show signs of anemia. Otherwise, these parasites take a long time to damage the lungs and liver. Eggs are picked up in the feces and are very large ovals, measuring out at 130–180 microns in length and with an **operculum** on one end (Figure 12.12).

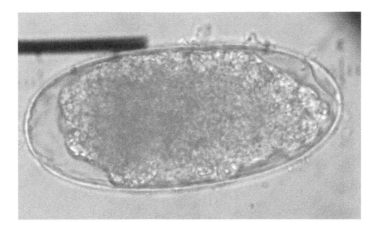

FIGURE 12.10 Hookworm egg.

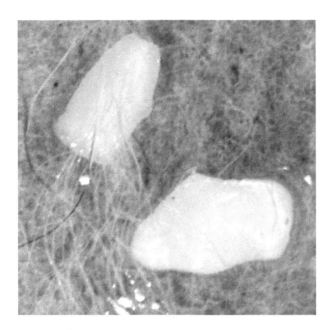

FIGURE 12.11 Tapeworm segments.

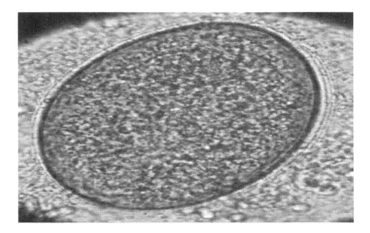

FIGURE 12.12 Fluke egg.

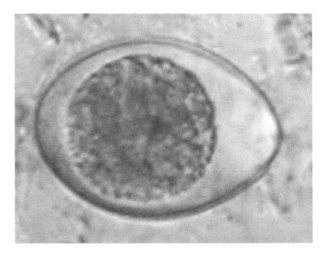

FIGURE 12.13 Coccidia – magnified.

Protozoans

Protozoans are either unicellular or multicellular organisms that for the most part cause profuse diarrhea and sometimes even bloody diarrhea. The most common culprits are coccidia and giardia. Giardia can affect humans usually by ingestion of contaminated water. Coccidia are transmitted by the oral–fecal route. They are found on fecal floats and direct smears. This is where the feces is smeared onto a slide and then looked at under 10×. They are quite small and many technicians will view these **oocysts** using 40× (Figure 12.13). There are also species of protozoans that parasitize blood cells.

Remember to handle feces with care, always use PPE and *wash your hands*! The leftover fecal material is either flushed down the toilet or put in the lab's waste container. The contents of the test tubes used to perform the floats are dumped into the toilet or waste container and the test tubes washed with a disinfectant and then put on a rack to dry. Inspect the tube for cracks and if found throw the entire tube away. Put all supplies away and disinfect the counter. Discard gloves into the waste container when finished.

Learning Exercises

- Make a "recipe" card for the fecal set-up procedure your school or workplace uses. Refer to it until you know how to set-up a fecal sample properly by memory.
- Make flash cards with pictures of ectoparasites and endoparasites. This will help you study for the exam.

Blood Collection and Handling

Blood collection is a two-person process: one to restrain the patient and a **venipuncturist**. Restraint techniques during venipuncture are described in Chapter 8. The venipuncturist will usually be the technician or the veterinarian but knowing the steps involved will be of great help to whomever is drawing the blood sample.

Things to keep in mind:

1. Handle the patient quietly and gently with minimum restraint. Most patients don't know what is going to happen but if you put them into a strong restraint hold it will raise their blood pressure and their stress level. Most fear free clinics will have a policy on how long a hold lasts and how many tries per patient before using other means to collect blood. Stress can actually alter blood results.
2. Some patients do better away from the owner, so ask for permission to take it to the treatment area. Patients are usually more cooperative away from

their owners. Owners are usually less distressed if they do not see the actual blood collection procedure.
3. Blood collection must be done properly to ensure reliable laboratory results.
4. Blood samples are often taken from the jugular vein in order to save the peripheral veins for IV catheterization.

Equipment Set-up

The best blood sample that best reflects the patient's state of health is one that goes directly into a blood collection tube (Figure 12.14). The easiest tubes to use are vacuum sealed and engineered to pull in the right amount of blood for each size of tube. There are different types of tubes that contain different **anticoagulants** within. They are color coded by their caps and are selected based upon the blood chemistry being tested for. There are two tubes commonly used in a veterinary practice. A purple or lavender topped tube and a red topped tube. The "purple tops" contain EDTA which is a good all round anticoagulant and will work for most tests that require whole blood and plasma. Whole blood has all of the components exactly as if flowing through a patient's veins. Plasma is the liquid portion of whole blood and is obtained from a purple top tube by putting it in a centrifuge and spinning it until the solids are packed at the bottom of the tube, usually taking 10 minutes.

"Red topped" tubes also contain a vacuum but no anticoagulant. They allow the blood sample to clot and so are only used if a serum sample is required. Serum is used for most blood chemistry and serology tests. The

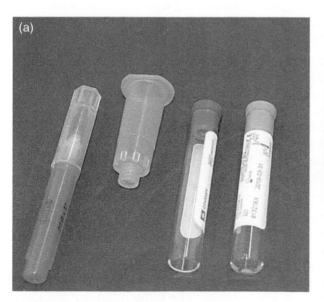
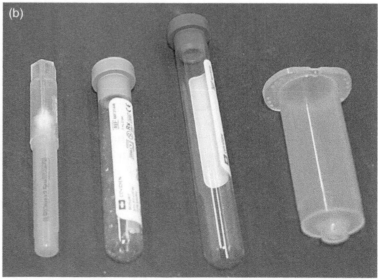

FIGURE 12.14 Blood drawing sets.

sample must sit undisturbed for 10–20 minutes until the blood is fully clotted. The top is removed and an applicator stick is run around the inside circumference of the tube, this breaks the clots away from the glass wall of the tube. Then the tube can be placed in a centrifuge and spun for about 10 minutes.

For plasma and serum samples, the tube is carefully removed from the centrifuge, the cover is removed and using a pipette the liquid is extracted from the cell portion of the sample. Care must be taken to not suck up red blood cells as the liquid is removed. This will contaminate the sample. Serum and plasma should be removed from the tube as soon as possible. The cells within the solid portion of the tube will continue to utilize the components within the liquid, altering the test results. Many tests require either plasma or serum and it will say which in the instructions with the test kits.

To collect the blood using vacuum tubes, a holder and a blood drawing needle is used (Figure 12.14). The needle has two pointed ends. The shortest end, often with a rubber sleeve for multiple tubes, turns into the top of the holder. The other end of the needle has a cap that should remain in place until it is time for the blood draw. The vacuum tube is slid into the holder and impaled upon the needle just until the top of the tube cap reaches a line on the holder. If you push it on too far the tube will lose its vacuum and not work properly. Other supplies to gather are a couple extra tubes just in case, cotton balls, one wetted with water and a dry one, and an ink or sharpie pen to write on the tube.

Once the tube is filled, if it has an anticoagulant it must be gently rocked back and forth 3–5 times to mix the blood with the anticoagulant. Then it can be marked with the patient's name, owner's last name, date, time, and the initials of the venipuncturist. Red topped tubes can be marked right away and then propped at an angle to facilitate clotting. Purple topped tubes can be placed in the refrigerator for 12–24 hours before the blood cells start to deteriorate. Red topped tubes must be processed as soon as the clot forms.

Some clinics use a needle and syringe to draw blood samples and then transfer the blood to a vacuum tube. This requires speed and gentleness! Blood starts to clot the instant it leaves the body, so the blood must be drawn quickly which isn't always easy to do when the patient is tiny! Once sufficient sample is drawn, the needle is removed from the syringe and the cap from the vacuum tube is removed. The blood is gently dispensed into the tube and if there is an anticoagulant, the cap replaced and the tube is rocked gently to mix. The sample must be checked for clots before use. This is done by passing one or two applicator sticks into the sample and swirling them gently to capture any clots. They will look like bumps on the sticks and if present cannot be used as the clots will have changed the makeup of the sample and will not represent the patient's state of health.

Reflection

Envision yourself helping with a blood draw. You are restraining the patient. Write down the procedure as it unfolds, then re-read what you wrote down in comparison to the description in Chapter 8. Did your memory agree with the procedure? If not, re-write the steps to cement the procedure in your mind.

Blood Sample Handling

Improper handling can result in rendering the sample unfit for analysis. Rough handling or use of a needle that is too small can cause hemolysis. Hemolysis is the rupture of red blood cells which imparts a red color to the serum or plasma. Hemolysis may interfere with some test results; consult the instructions that accompany each test.

Tips to prevent hemolysis:

1. Use a needle at least 22 gauge or bigger on either a syringe or in a vacuum tube holder.
2. Handle blood gently. Rock back and forth collection tube to mix with anticoagulant; do not shake blood.
3. Avoid excess pressure when dispensing blood into a vacuum tube from a syringe.

Complete Blood Count

The complete blood count, referred to as the CBC, is run using whole blood collected in a lavender or green topped tube. It is composed of a group of tests that is used in wellness exams, as a screening test before surgery, and as a tool to evaluate disease states.

The individual tests of the CBC are:

1. Total white blood cell count (WBC)
2. Total red blood cell count (RBC)
3. Total platelet count
4. Hemoglobin
5. Hematocrit or packed cell volume, referred to as the PCV
6. RBC indices such as the mean cell volume (MCV)
7. Differential
8. Plasma protein.

Some of the tests that make up a CBC can be run manually but the rest require a hematology analyzer. CBCs run on analyzers are often called hemograms. The tests that can be done manually are the PCV, the differential, and the plasma protein. The PCV reflects the percentage of RBCs in whole blood. The differential is done on a blood smear to determine the percentages of the various types of WBCs; blood cell morphology; WBC and platelet count estimates; and examination for blood-borne pathogens. The plasma proteins are proteins found in the blood and the test is done using the refractometer. This is the only test that an analyzer does not do. Whole blood is sent through the analyzer where the various blood parameters are determined. Blood analyzers take less time to determine the full CBC than doing it manually.

Some clinics will choose to send the blood to a reference laboratory because of costs and small volume of samples run. CBCs sent to a reference laboratory require the following the steps:

1. Complete a requisition form using the patient file to fill in the information.
2. Prepare the blood smear, do not stain it, package in a slide container.
3. Place all the samples from the same patient in a Ziploc bag with the requisition form.
4. Put the bag in the refrigerator.
5. Contact the laboratory to schedule a sample pick-up.
6. Make certain the sample is picked up before the end of the business day.

If the entire CBC is run in-house, the veterinary assistant can start the preliminary set-up of the tests. Ideally, the blood sample is run immediately after being drawn. If not, it should be placed in the refrigerator. If that is the case it needs to be brought to room temperature before running the tests. If the clinic has a rocker it can set on the rocker for 20–30 minutes. If the clinic doesn't have a rocker you can roll the tube between your hands until it feels warmer. This is also done to mix the blood before starting any of the following tests. Once the blood is warm, the blood smear, PCV, and plasma protein can be started for the veterinary technician.

Preparing the Blood Smear

The blood smear is required to perform the differential. The materials required to make a blood smear include: two microscope slides cleaned with a Kem Wipe, a lead pencil used to write on the thick end of the dried smear, blood sample, and a pipette or two applicator sticks. PPE is gloves and goggles.

Check the tube against the patient's file to make sure a CBC has been ordered and to make sure you have the correct sample. Gently rock the sample or roll it between you hands to mix. Then quickly remove the cap and use the pipette to collect a drop or two of blood from the tube. Put a small drop upon one end of both slides. Lay one of the slides flat on the table top and steady it with your fingers on the opposite end of the blood drop. Use one end of one of the slides as a pusher slide to make the smear by laying it flat upon the slide surface at a 45 degree angle (Figure 12.15a), then pull the edge of

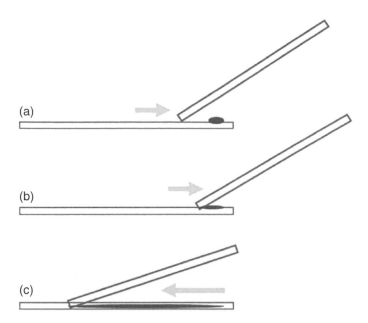

FIGURE 12.15 Making a blood smear steps (a) to (c).

the pusher slide into the blood drop (Figure 12.15b) and allow the blood to wick across the bottom of the pusher slide, then quickly push the slide along the remaining length of the slide (Figure 12.15c) lying on the table, smearing the blood along the length of that slide. Repeat for the pusher slide to make another smear. The end result should be a thin smear of blood that ends in a crescent shape, which when held up to the light has a rainbow appearance (Figure 12.16).

Set the slides aside to dry in order to be stained. The purpose of the blood stain is to facilitate differentiation of white blood cell types and other cellular structures when the smear is examined under the microscope. Hematology stains usually consist of a methyl alcohol fixative a light blue or clear color, an eosin (reddish-orange in color), and methylene blue (purplish-blue color). Most practices use "quick" stains that are modifications of Wright's or Romanowsky stains such as the Dip Stat or Diff-Quick stains, respectively.

The procedure may vary slightly depending on the type of stain used. Always refer to the manufacturer's instructions when staining a blood smear. The immersion of the blood smear in each stain is timed. The steps include fixing the smear using methyl alcohol, then staining first in the eosin stain and then the methylene blue stain.

Open the three jars of Quick Stain and make sure they are in the proper order. Fixative is first, the eosin is second, and the methylene blue is third. Grasp the blood smear by one end and dunk it into the fixative for a full one second count, pull it out and dunk it again, for a total of five times. Then immediately dunk it into the red for a full 5, one-second dunks and then repeat in the purple. Set the water faucet to a thin stream and rinse

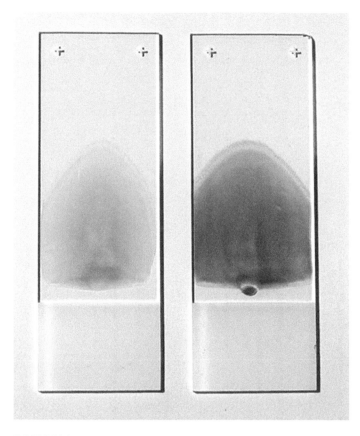

FIGURE 12.16 Unstained and stained blood smear. Source: Wikimedia Commons. Used under CC BY-SA 3.0, https://commons.wikimedia.org/wiki/File:Peripheral_blood_smear_-_stained_and_unstained.jpg.

the stain off of the slide. A good slide should have an overall coloring of purple with pink overtones when examined with the naked eye (Figure 12.16). Set it on a paper towel, leaning against something to hold it upright and allow it to dry fully. When dry, use the lead pencil to write the patient's name, date, and time on the thick part of the smear near the drop.

Some reasons for failing to make good blood smears:

1. Use of slides that are not absolutely clean. Shipping residues on the surface of the slides will not let the blood adhere to the slide so you get big holes in the smear.

2. Blood drops too large or too small. Too large and the smear never tapers down to a monolayer; it is just thick along the entire length of the smear. Too small and the smear isn't big enough to have a representative sample.

3. Not backing the edge of the spreader slide far enough into the drop of blood or backing too far into the drop of blood. The spreader slide is slid into the drop just far enough to have the blood wick across the width of the spreader slide. Then quickly move the spreader slide down the length of the slide on which the smear is being made. Too slow and the

blood doesn't thin out enough and too fast it streaks.

4. Failure to keep the spreader slide at a 45-degree angle. Too steep an angle or too shallow an angle will not give the blood a chance to thin out to the monolayer.

5. Failure to maintain constant pressure on the spreader slide throughout the full length of the slide. This usually results in streaks and or wobbles in the smear.

6. Pulling, instead of pushing the spreader slide. If you put the spreader slide into the blood the wrong way you don't get a good monolayer.

7. Not keeping the stains fresh and free of contaminates. Old stain or stain that has precipitated out will leave small dark marks on the cells. This could be mistaken for blood pathogens and an animal may be treated for something they don't have!

The veterinary technician examines the blood smear under the oil immersion lens of the microscope. This procedure is called the differential cell count. It is done to determine the percentage of each white blood cell type present, the morphology of all cells seen, and the presence of any infectious organisms.

Learning Exercise

Practice making blood smears, then evaluate your smear. Does it have a body, monolayer, and feather edge? Are there streaks or wobbles? Try slowing down, speeding up, or changing the angle of your slide when smearing the blood.

Packed Cell Volume

The packed cell volume (PCV) is a measurement of the percentage of red blood cells in whole, unclotted blood. The red blood cells, called erythrocytes, are the oxygen-carrying component of the blood. The test is simple, rapid, and only requires a small amount of blood. It is referred to as the PCV or "crit," short for hematocrit. These terms are used interchangeably; however, PCV usually refers to the manual method and hematocrit the calculated value from a hematology analyzer.

There are two types of capillary or microhematocrit tubes. A plain tube is used with whole blood containing an anticoagulant. A heparinized capillary tube is used with untreated whole blood. The heparin in the capillary tube keeps the blood from clotting. They can only be used immediately after the blood is drawn otherwise the blood will clot. Often, for a tiny patient just a needle will be introduced into a vein and the heparinized capillary

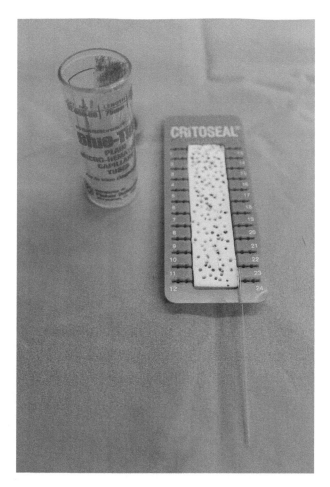

FIGURE 12.17 Hematocrit tubes and tray of clay sealant.

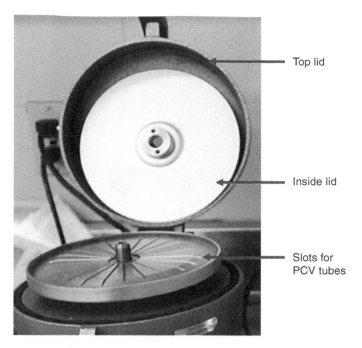

Top lid

Inside lid

Slots for
PCV tubes

FIGURE 12.18 Hematocrit centrifuge lids and slots.

tube will be put into the hub of the needle to draw out just enough blood to fill the tube.

Supplies required for a PCV include two hematocrit tubes, a tray of clay sealant (Figure 12.17), a Kem Wipe, the PCV card reader, the refractometer, and a lens paper. Cap the blood sample and gently mix it once again. Then hold both PCV tubes between your index finger and thumb on your dominant hand. Slide both tubes into the blood and hold them and the sample almost horizontally in order for the blood to flow into the tubes. Once they have filled to about three-quarters full move your index finger over the top of the tubes to prevent the blood from flowing out. Set the blood sample down and wipe the end of the tubes off with the Kem Wipe. Then plunge the ends of the tubes into the clay to seal them. Remove the tubes from the clay and put them into the hematocrit centrifuge. The hematocrit centrifuge will have slots to put the tubes into. To balance the centrifuge, put one tube with the sealed end towards the outside of the circle and then directly across the circle from the first tube lay the second tube into the slot, again with the clay end toward the outside (Figure 12.18), otherwise the blood will be spun out of the tubes. Note the number on the slot in which the tubes are placed. Write

the patient's name on a piece of paper with the tube location. This is especially important if running several samples at the same time. Put the inside cover on the tray (Figure 12.18) and tighten it down with either your fingers or the lid plyers that is usually attached to the centrifuge with a chain. If you forget to put this cover on, the tubes will spin out of the slots and be busted into a fine bloody powder. Close the outside lid (Figure 12.18) and set the centrifuge for 5 minutes.

Once the centrifuge has come to a complete stop, open the first and second lids and remove the tubes. Place them beside the PCV card reader and the refractometer for the technician to read. If there are multiple patients, make sure to keep everyone's sample separate. Some clinics may allow the assistant to read the PCV and perform the plasma protein. If so, the following are the instructions for these two tests.

The tubes will have changed from a homogeneous red color to one with three different colored layers (Figure 12.19). From the bottom up, the clay sealant, a dark red layer composed of red blood cells, just above that and often barely visible a white line is seen. This is called the buffy coat and is composed of white blood cells and platelets. Above that is the clear to golden liquid which is the plasma. If the color is dark yellow, pink or red, or white alert the technician or veterinarian.

To determine the PCV, a microhematocrit reader or PCV card is used. The card can be linear or circular in form. With either type of reader, align the top edge of the sealant on the zero line (Figure 12.19) and the top edge of the plasma on the 100 line. The line running

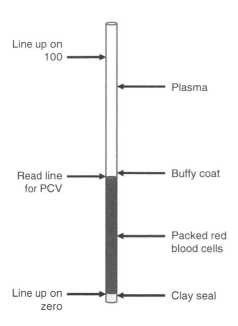

FIGURE 12.19 Hematocrit tube components and reading points.

across the top edge of the red blood cells is the percentage of red blood cells or the PCV. This is recorded as "% RBCs" in the lab log book and in the patient's file.

Plasma Protein

After recording the PCV, retain the hematocrit tube. The plasma from it will be used next to determine plasma protein. Plasma protein is determined using the plasma from the hematocrit tube and the refractometer (Figure 12.2). Remember, refractometers have two scales: one for urine specific gravity and one for serum or plasma protein. Find the scale that shows a number from 0 to 8 or 9 and has the designation of g/dL for units of measurement. It is usually to the lower left or right of the specific gravity scale that starts with a 1.000.

To determine plasma protein, lay the refractometer on the counter and lift the small lid covering the prism. Break the spun capillary tubes just above the buffy coat. Discard the portion with the buffy coat and red blood cells. Take the portion with the plasma and allow it to drip onto the prism or use a small capillary tube bulb to force the plasma out on to the prism. Lower the cover plate, being sure the plasma completely covers the plate. If not, add more from the second capillary tube, as insufficient plasma will not give a proper reading. Also remove any glass chips that may be present from breaking the tube as that will prevent the plasma from flowing over the prism. Use a Kem Wipe to snag the glass pieces without touching the plasma as it will soak it up and you'll lose your sample. Close the lid and hold the refractometer up to your eye, adjust the refractometer up or down to a bright light at a semi-parallel position between the floor and ceiling. Read the plasma protein scale at the interface of the dark and light areas. Record the

results in g/dL (grams per 100 mL) into the lab log book and in the patient's file.

When finished, clean and disinfect the work area, centrifuge, and refractometer, put materials away, and discard blood contaminated materials in a biohazard waste container.

Blood Chemistry and Electrolyte Determinations

In the past, blood chemistries and electrolyte determinations were sent to commercial laboratories, called reference labs. While some veterinary facilities continue to do so, the increasing availability of in-house analyzers has resulted in the expansion of on-site veterinary laboratory capabilities. The advantage is more rapid access to results. With the availability and ease of in-house testing, it is possible to conduct more rapid health screenings of all patients. Pre-anesthetic panels are conducted before routine spays or neuters to detect abnormalities in surgical patients. Geriatric panels can detect developing diseases in older patients before the patient becomes clinically ill. Seemingly healthy patients may have a diagnosable disease identifiable during routine wellness screening.

The in-house chemistry analyzer measures serum samples for glucose, blood urea nitrogen (BUN), creatinine, and others. The electrolyte analyzer measures sodium, potassium, and chloride in serum, plasma, or whole blood. Analyzers for serum chemistries can run single tests or groups of tests referred to as panels. These chemical evaluations provide specific organ function information; for instance, certain values are elevated in liver disease.

Analyzers are increasing in technical capabilities. Expect to see upgrades in the current equipment in veterinary laboratories resulting in expanded capabilities for testing. Tests will be faster, more test types will be available, test errors will be reduced, and ease of use will increase.

There are many manufacturers of instruments in the veterinary field. It is only possible to provide general information about them:

1. Accuracy is essential. Measurements and timing must be exact. Read and follow the directions carefully. The validity of test results is determined by the skill of the person performing the tests.

2. Review the patient record to ascertain which tests or panels are ordered. Then read the test reagent labels to ensure you have the correct test(s).
3. Handle carefully. These are expensive, complex pieces of equipment.
4. Results may be printed out and then secured in the patient record or the instruments may be interfaced with hospital management software and results sent directly to the patient's electronic file.
5. There are reference ranges or normal values for each test for healthy patients of each species. Reference values are dependent on the laboratory or equipment used.
6. Some equipment requires periodic calibration; all require some maintenance and some form of cleaning. Follow the manufacturer's directions for maintenance. Keep a record of who did these procedures and when in the laboratory maintenance log. Carefully follow the manufacturer's directions when doing so.
7. Never use expired reagents as they may not give accurate readings. As with all medical supplies and drugs, reagents must be monitored for expiration dates.

The veterinary assistant may be asked to operate this equipment and may be responsible for its maintenance. Follow the manufacturer's recommendations for use and maintenance requirements or observe an experienced team member using the instrument before attempting it on your own. The first time you run a test, have someone observe your work. Always ask questions if you are in doubt. It is better to ask a question than to make a serious mistake. These instruments will use either liquid reagents or dry test strips of some form, which are usually refrigerated. These reagents are dated and should be checked before use. Keep an adequate inventory of test materials most frequently used on hand.

if the antibody or antigen is present. These are single-use kits although some kits test for the presence of more than one disease. For example, feline leukemia virus antigen, feline immunodeficiency virus antibody, and feline heartworm antigen can all be detected by the same test kit.

These test kits use serum, plasma, and/or whole blood depending on the test and the manufacturer. Use the specified sample type or the one the veterinarian prefers. Most test results are available in 8–10 minutes. Because results are so rapidly available, a test result will be ready by the time the veterinarian has completed the patient examination.

Kits come packaged with all the materials needed for conducting the test. A pamphlet is enclosed that gives step-by-step instructions for setting up the test and interpreting the results. As with other laboratory instructions, a copy of the directions for each kit can be kept in the protocol binder and should be switched out with each new box.

Read all the accompanying information about the test. Read the box when unpacking kits from the wholesaler to ensure proper storage. Some kits need to be refrigerated; others do not. These kits have expiration dates so be sure to check the date before storing the kits and before use.

Be certain to draw the appropriate quantity and type of sample (plasma versus serum or whole blood) needed to run the test. Refrigerate the labeled sample if the test is not run immediately. The veterinary assistant will find these tests easy to run with a minimal margin for error. Because of the differences between test kits, however, the assistant must pay close attention to directions. As with all laboratory work, accuracy and attention to details are the key to success.

Once results have been achieved, mark the patient file and the lab log book. Throw the used test kit into the waste container and disinfect the counter.

Reflection

Read the operation manual for the blood analyzer and blood chemistry machine. What information did you pick up that was perhaps not covered in a lecture?

Learning Exercise

Select a test kit at random. See if you can find what the test is for, what species of animal, what sample does it require, and how long does it take to run the test?

Serologic Test Kits

There are an increasing number of commercial serology test kits available for specific diseases. These tests are quick and easy, ranging from heartworms to Lyme disease. The basis of the test principle is an antigen–antibody reaction followed by a color change on the test pad

Urine Collection

The role of the veterinary assistant may be one of restraint during the process of urine collection. The exception is collection of urine during normal **micturition** (urination) or use of a litter pan. Refer to Chapter 10 for collection of voluntary samples. The following is a brief overview of involuntary urine collection techniques.

The technique chosen for urine collection depends on the reason it is being collected. A sample to check for a urinary tract infection (UTI) can be a voluntary sample, an expressed sample, or a catheterized sample. A sample to be checked for microorganisms and to be cultured is best collected by cystocentesis.

An involuntary collection expresses the bladder manually. The veterinarian or technician applies external pressure to the bladder through the abdominal wall. The assistant may be asked to be ready to collect the midstream sample or help to restrain the patient. As with the voluntary collection, the expressed sample should be midstream unless the bladder contains only a small amount of urine, in which case all the urine is collected.

Catheterization is another technique used for urine collection. This is considered an invasive technique as it introduces a catheter through the vulva or penis and into the bladder. The assistant will most likely restrain the patient while the veterinarian or veterinary technician proceeds with the catheterization. This is an important job as the assistant not only has to control the patient, but has to retract and hold the prepuce back on the male dog while the catheter is placed. If the prepuce is allowed to touch the catheter it contaminates it and another will have to be used. The dog is usually in lateral recumbency with another helper restraining the front legs and head. Using two hands, push the prepuce back with one and with the other keep the top leg out of the way (Figure 12.20).

A urinary catheter is a long, thin tube of rubber or plastic that is inserted into the bladder through the urethral opening. A syringe is attached to the ending of the catheter, and the urine is aspirated. In the female, the catheter is passed through the vulva and enters the external sphincter located on the floor of the vagina.

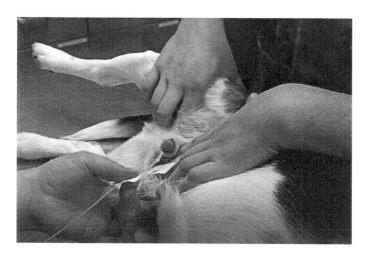

FIGURE 12.20 Restraint for urinary catheterization of male dog.

Usually this is done in the standing position with the assistant holding the base of the tale straight up and out of the way while holding onto the front end to keep the patient from biting anyone!

Cystocentesis is the most invasive procedure but can be necessary as it prevents urine from washing through the urethra and being contaminated by organisms normally residing in that structure. A veterinarian or veterinary technician performs this procedure by inserting a needle through the abdominal wall directly into the urinary bladder. Urine is aspirated into a sterile syringe attached to the needle. The assistant restrains the patient in either lateral or dorsal recumbency. Some clinics will do a surgical scrub at the insertion area while others do not. Ask how the procedure will go and lay out the required equipment.

Cats are usually not as willing to hold still for catheterization and so often have to be sedated. This holds true for those male cats that have plugged urethra. This is usually a sick kitty that doesn't have the patience for being messed with!

Urinalysis

The proper name and spelling for the examination of urine is urinalysis. The urinalysis is divided into four parts: the physical characteristics, specific gravity, chemical assay, and microscopic examinations. The assistant may be responsible for conducting and recording the first three parts of the urinalysis. Ideally, a urinalysis is conducted within 30 minutes of sample collection. If unable to run the sample immediately, place it into the lab refrigerator in a labeled, sealed container. When ready to perform the tests, let it come to room temperature before starting. Indicate on the patient's record and treatment board that the sample has been collected and is in the lab.

Some labs will have a lab form that is filled out as the urinalysis is performed. Others will utilize the management software with a form that is filled out on the computer as the individual parts are completed. If asked to assist with the first three parts of the urinalysis find out which technique is used to record the findings.

The first part of the urinalysis is to record the physical characteristics of the urine: color, clarity, odor, and foam. In the patient's record, create a list: urinalysis: color, clarity, odor, foam. Record your observations after each. Normal urine is yellow and clear. Urine can range from colorless to bright yellow to red and almost brown. Blood, disease states, brightly colored food, and some drugs can alter coloration.

Normal urine is clear but clarity can range from cloudy to flocculent, in which large particles of sediment are suspended in the urine. The odor is usually not diagnostic, but the presence of bacteria imparts an ammonia-like odor and ketones impart a fruity or sweet odor.

Vigorously shake the urine sample (remember to cover the top!). A small amount of white foam is normal. High levels of protein in urine create a larger volume of foam that lasts longer. Bile pigments color the foam greenish-yellow.

The second part of the urinalysis is the urine specific gravity. It is determined using a refractometer and is the comparison of water to other liquids such as urine or plasma. Dissolved substances in the sample determine the specific gravity. Urine specific gravity is used as a measure of hydration state and kidney function. Specific gravity is never less than 1.000 which is the specific gravity of distilled water. The specific gravity is read in decimals on the refractometer, for example 1.023, with no units. The procedure for loading the refractometer is identical to loading plasma for plasma protein, except that the urine specific gravity scale is used to read the result.

Often, the specific gravity is too high to be read on the refractometer scale and the urine must be diluted. Mixing one part urine to one part water results in a dilution factor of two. The specific gravity reading is multiplied by two. (The 1 before the decimal point always remains 1.) For example, if the dilute urine sample reads 1.036, then the correct specific gravity would be 1.072. After the specific gravity has been determined and recorded in the patient's file the third part of the urinalysis is run.

Chemical tests are usually accomplished by using a reagent strip, referred to as a chem strip or dip stick. The number of tests depends on the chemistry strip used – minimally strips with pH, glucose, protein, blood, and bilirubin are used. Each test is no more than a single chemically treated square of paper attached to a plastic strip. There can be from 1 to 10 tests on one strip. The outer label on the container (Figure 12.21) of these strips provides the interpretation of the color changes for each test and a time in seconds when each is read. Each color corresponds to a certain concentration of chemical in the urine. Carefully match the sequence of tests to the sequence on the outer label, at the appropriate times and record the results as you go. Before you dip the stick into the urine sample, record the name of each test on the reagent strip on the patient's record just below the recording of the urine specific gravity. Make a mental note of the time each test square must be read. Dip the strip in urine, saturating each square. Carefully follow the manufacturer's instructions for reading, remembering to align correctly the order of the tests with the order on the label. Record results according to the scale provided. Some tests will have numerical values; others are recorded as negative or 1+, 2+, 3+, and so on. In fully automated veterinary labs, the test strip is placed in an analyzer that reads the strip and prints the results. This provides more consistent results than does just comparing the pictures on the label.

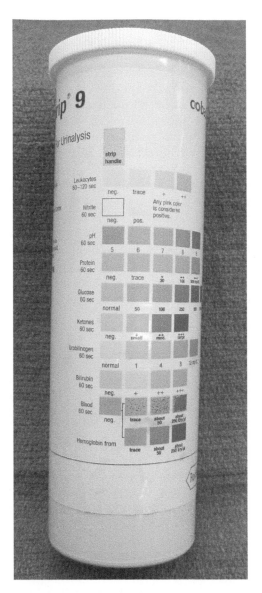

FIGURE 12.21 Chemical test strip container.

Preparation of the sediment is the final test. A test tube with a tapered end is filled with urine and balanced in a standard centrifuge or in a microcentrifuge that uses smaller sample sizes. Run the centrifuge according to the manufacturer's directions as to time and the rotations per minute (rpm) for urine. The recommended rpm is usually 1000–2000 rpm for 3–6 minutes. Once centrifugation is complete, remove the test tube. Decant the urine. This is done by simply turning the test tube upside down, pouring the urine off the sediment at the very bottom of the tube, and turning it back right side up in one motion. Do not tip the test tube on its side or the sediment will pour out! With the tube right side up, gently flick the bottom of the test tube with the end of a finger to mix the sediment with the remaining urine.

At this point, a stain may be added to the urine. This can be a small drop of methylene blue or a commercial stain made specifically for staining urine such as

Sedi-Stain. Some veterinary technicians prefer reading the slide without any stain at all. If a stain is used, mix it well with the urine by flicking the bottom of the tube with a finger.

Using a clean and labeled slide, pour or use a pipette to place a drop of urine on the center of the slide. Place a coverslip over it to minimize the formation of bubbles under it. Place the slide next to the microscope with the patient's medical record. Notify the veterinary technician the slide is ready to read.

Clean the refractometer and put it away. Discard any remaining urine down the drain and flush the drain with lots of cold water. If using reusable test tubes, clean them with hot soapy water and a small bottle brush, rinsing well and drying upside down in a test tube rack. Discard the micro-test tube, if used, and the chemical strip. Put away the chemical assay strips. Clean and then disinfect the counter area. Remove and discard gloves in the hazardous waste container.

Learning Exercise

Take a look at the outside of the Chemstrip container. What does it test for and associate the color changes with each test.

Microbiology – Sample Collection

Accurate diagnosis and the optimal choice of drugs for treatment begin with proper sample collection for microbiology testing. The goal is to collect a sample that contains the causative agent of disease. The identification process and antibiotic sensitivity testing can then proceed to determine the course of treatment.

Most veterinary clinics approach the process in two ways. Preliminary diagnostic work can be done in-house, such as the commonly used Gram stain to determine if the organism is Gram negative or positive and if it is a rod or cocci-type bacteria. The culture and sensitivity can either be sent to a reference laboratory or be conducted in-house. A culture is where the sample is spread upon an agar plate that has a medium that promotes the growth of bacterial organisms. Once the bacteria has grown, further isolation of the different colonies of bacteria can be conducted on different mediums to rule out bacterial strains and move closer to identification of the bacteria. The sensitivity test indicates which antibiotic would be of use against the identified pathogen. The choice depends on the veterinarian's preference, equipment available, and skills of the staff.

The potential for infection to staff handling these samples is high, so use of cautious laboratory techniques and PPE are of the utmost concern. The minimum PPE are gloves, goggles or a face shield to catch splashes or prevent inhalation of infectious materials, and a lab coat to prevent contamination of clothing. Keep the work area clean and uncluttered. Use disinfectant when the work is completed leaving it on the surrounding surfaces to air dry.

Samples must be collected aseptically to prevent contaminants being accidentally introduced into the sample. The veterinarian or veterinary technician will be collecting the sample and inoculating the mediums. The assistant will gather the equipment needed, restraining the patient, prepare the samples for shipping to the reference laboratory if not run in-house and clean up.

When bacterial infections are suspected, the supplies required are two sterile swabs, wax pencil for labeling the microscope slide, and Petri dishes with blood agar which is an all-around bacterial growth medium. Bring all the necessary PPE for the personnel involved.

If the specimen is to be sent to a reference laboratory for work-up, the swabs to use are called culturettes. Culturettes are sterile swabs in sterile plastic tubes. The swab is attached to the inside of the tube top. The top of the tube with swab is removed, the sample is swabbed, and the swab is reintroduced into the tube with the top securely replaced. Pressure is then applied over the end of the tube. Crushing the end releases a liquid nutrient media that soaks the tip of the cotton swab and keeps the bacteria alive while in transit to the reference laboratory. Fill out the appropriate requisition slip. The whole tube is sent to the lab along with the unstained slide. Put the slide in a slide container to keep it from breaking, then put the tube and slide container in a Ziploc bag with the requisition slip. Package the Ziploc in a box with an ice pack and either call for pick-up or ship the box to the lab.

If a fungal infection like ringworm is suspected, the PPE equipment will remain the same. The equipment required is the Wood's light, 10% potassium hydroxide, a clean, labeled slide, coverslip, heat source and DTM or other fungal culturing agar, sterile forceps, and an alcohol-soaked cotton ball.

The veterinarian or the technician will secure the sample. The assistant will restrain the patient and then clean up and put the unused equipment away. Again, allow the disinfectant to air dry on the exam table.

Gram Stain

Gram stain allows the technician or veterinarian to look at the sample under 100×. The stain will help determine if a bacterium is Gram positive (purple uptake of dye) or negative (red uptake of dye) and whether it is a rod or cocci. The stain consists of four solutions and may be performed from the original sample or later from growth on the blood agar plate. The Gram reaction helps determine how to proceed with identification of the bacteria.

Care must be taken when preparing the specimen slide. A common mistake is applying too much inoculum on the slide, resulting in uneven staining. Swabbed samples are rolled onto the slide, one pass per line is all that is needed. If getting the sample from an agar plate, a sterile wire is used to select the desired bacterial colony and a tiny bit of the colony is mixed with a drop of sterile water or saline on the slide.

To stain the slide, start by setting up the stains each in their own dropper bottles or Coplin jars. If in dropper bottles you will need a staining rack. PPE will be gloves and goggles.

1. Fix the sample on the slide by passing it briefly over a hot flame. This is usually accomplished with a Bunsen burner. Fixing adheres the sample to the slide and preserves the morphology (shape) of the bacteria.
2. Place the staining rack over the sink and lay the fixed slide on top of it in a position in which it won't fall off.
3. The first stain applied is the crystal violet. Cover the entire slide with this stain and allow it to remain on the slide for 30 seconds. Gently rinse with tap water.
4. Apply iodine solution in the same manner and let it sit on the slide for 30 seconds. Gently rinse with tap water.
5. Apply the de-colorizer to the slide for approximately 10 seconds or until no more purple coloring washes away. (Do not overdo.) Gently rinse with tap water.
6. Apply Safranin stain and let it sit on the slide for 30 seconds. Gently rinse with tap water.
7. Air dry by propping the slide upright or blot dry using blotting paper. This is different from Kem Wipes and lens paper.

Staining in Coplin jars

1. Use forceps or a spring-type clothes pin to move the slide from jar to jar. Insert the slide and hold it still for the prescribed time.
   Move the slide according to sequence and times listed below. Drain the end of the slide on the edge of each jar before moving to reduce cross-contamination of solutions.
   - Crystal violet stain: 30 seconds
   - Tap water rinse
   - Iodine solution: 30 seconds
   - Tap water rinse
   - 95% ethanol (decolorizer): 10 seconds
   - Tap water rinse
   - Safranin counterstain: 30 seconds
   - Tap water rinse
2. When finished dry in the same manner as described earlier.

When dry, place beside microscope with bottle of immersion oil. If using paper records place the patient record beside slide. Notify veterinarian or technician when slide is ready to read.

Learning Exercise

Write the steps for the Gram stain in your reference book.

Inoculation of Media

Inoculating media is the transferring of a sample or specimen onto media that will support bacterial growth. Culturing (growing) bacteria may take 24–48 hours in an in-house incubator. Blood agar is commonly inoculated initially because many types of pathogens will grow on it. It contains 5% sheep blood. If the specimen is going to be worked up in-house, the first swab taken is used to inoculate the blood agar plate. The quadrant streak method is commonly used to end up with isolated colonies of bacteria growing in the last quarter of the plate. Isolated colonies are necessary so they can be picked out from other colonies as cross-contamination from different bacteria can complicate the identification procedures.

Lift the lid using the free hand (Figure 12.22). Only tip one side of the lid upward enough to slide the culture swab between the upper and lower portions of the plate without touching either part. Removing the lid completely will allow room-air contaminants to settle onto the media. The swab is swept across one-quarter of the plate, with a back and forth motion. Flame a wire loop, rotate the plate a quarter turn, slide the loop into the previous quadrant then sweep it back and forth in the second quadrant. The process is repeated, flaming the loop and streaking material from each quadrant of the plate. In the fourth quadrant, a single squiggled streak is used. Care must be taken to not put too much inoculum (sample) on the plate initially as it may run across the surface as the plate is tilted. Flaming the wire between streaks is essential to thin out the sample enough to get single colonies.

After streaking, the plate is labeled and placed upside down in the incubator to avoid condensation on the agar surface which would cause the bacteria to mix. Enter the date and time that the culture was set up in the patient's file and laboratory log. If there is no growth after 24 hours, the blood agar plate is re-incubated for another 24 hours. If there is still no growth, then the specimen is reported as "no growth." If there is growth, representative colonies from the plate will be selected for Gram staining. Based on the Gram stain

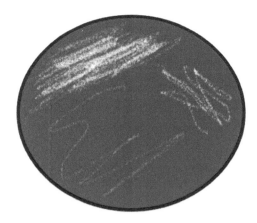

FIGURE 12.22 Quadrant method of steaking a blood agar plate for isolating bacteria colonies.

result, identification procedures using selected media will be started.

Antibiotic Sensitivity Testing

Not all antibiotics work equally well on all organisms. Therefore it is advantageous to test the bacteria isolated from the patient with different antibiotics to determine the best one to use. The efficacy of an antibiotic depends on the sensitivity or susceptibility of the pathogen to it. Isolated colonies of interest from the blood agar plate are selected and tested for antibiotic sensitivity. Identification of the bacteria should proceed at the same time. The key to successful testing is to choose the most likely antibiotics to test because there are so many available. The answer begins with the Gram stain. Some antibiotics are effective against Gram-negative rods, others against Gram-positive cocci, and so on. The veterinarian will determine which antibiotic disks to use for testing after having examined the Gram stain.

First, however, the bacteria need to be grown in a tube of broth media. A few colonies of the bacteria are transferred into a tube of broth media and the tube is incubated until its turbidity matches the turbidity of a standard. (Alternate method: if sufficient colonies are present, prepare the broth by adding enough bacteria to match the turbidity of the standard.) A sterile swab is dipped into the tube and spread evenly over the entire surface of Mueller Hinton agar, this is a special media used for sensitivity testing. Some organisms like streptococci (Gram positive, cocci-shaped bacteria) will not grow well on Mueller–Hinton agar. For these, Mueller–Hinton with 5% blood must be used, and interpretation of results adjusted.

Small paper disks in plastic tubes, each saturated with a single antibiotic, are placed in a disk dispenser. Each hole in the dispenser holds one tube. The dispenser holds multiple tubes. It fits directly over the Petri dish. The lever is pushed releasing one disk of each type onto the surface of the agar. Each disk is coded with the antibiotic it contains. Compare the code on the disk with the code on the tube to determine the name of the antibiotic it contains. The disks are pressed into the agar with a flamed loop or sterile swab. The dish is inverted, labeled, and incubated.

The antibiotic seeps out into the agar surrounding the disk. After incubation, the plate is held to a bright light and zones of inhibition of bacterial growth are noted and measured around each disk. If the bacteria are sensitive to the antibiotic, they will not grow up to the disk. The diameter sizes of the zones are compared with the manufacturer's standardized chart to determine which antibiotic is the best. Some bacteria will be resistant to the antibiotics and will grow right up to the disk.

Record the antibiotic zone sensitivities in the patient's file and alert the technician or veterinarian that the sensitivity results are in. Culture media has to be autoclaved before being discarded. When a Petri dish is no longer needed place it in an autoclavable bag. Seal the bag with autoclave tape and run it through a general autoclave cycle to destroy all of the bacteria. Then it can be disposed of in the regular garbage.

Learning Exercise

If available look at the antibiotic disk dispenser. Write down the types of antibiotics available, then look them up on the internet.

Necropsy: Preparation and Follow-Up

Necropsy is the term used to describe the examination of an animal's body after death. It is conducted in the same manner as a human autopsy. The purposes are to aid the veterinarian in making a more complete diagnosis and to further professional knowledge. Necropsy is performed as soon as possible after death or euthanasia providing the owner has given permission to do so. A delay in the necropsy procedure may result in postmortem **autolysis**, resulting in inconclusive results.

Tissue samples taken during necropsy are sent to a pathologist in a reference laboratory for microscopic examination. The packaging and shipping to the laboratory become the responsibilities of the assistant, as does the preparation for the necropsy. Reference laboratories usually provide containers for submitting tissue samples. If there are to be special requests, contact the laboratory before the procedure to determine how the specimens are to be collected, handled, and shipped.

Lay out all necropsy equipment. This includes:

1. Requisition slip
2. Ziploc bag
3. Formalin-filled vials for tissues
4. Transport media for cultures
5. Bunsen burner and match
6. Flat spatula for searing tissue surfaces
7. Two flat containers for the tissues
8. Slides
9. Suture material – 1 or 1-0 non-absorbable
10. Needle holder and cutting edge needle
11. Large, sharp knife
12. Cleaver
13. Rongeurs for cutting bones
14. Forceps
15. Scissors, operating sharp/blunt
16. Cadaver bag and identification tag.

PPE includes:

1. Heavy rubber gloves and a pair of exam gloves
2. Goggles and mask, or face shield
3. Lab coat and waterproof apron
4. Rubber boots or booties
5. Tape recorder with foot pedal (optional)
6. Patient record and pen.

Completion of the requisition slip must provide a history of the patient and gross description of the tissues. The necropsy is performed in an area away from general clinic activities. It is best conducted on a rack over a sink with access to running water. If that isn't available, layers of newsprint or chucks under the body are alternatives. The canine and feline cadavers are placed in left lateral recumbency with the ventral surface facing the veterinarian.

A thorough necropsy is lengthy and detailed. The veterinarian may wish to have a tape recorder to dictate findings as the necropsy progresses. Ideally, the tape recorder is equipped with a foot pedal. Notes are then transcribed from the tape after the procedure and entered into the patient's record. This reduces the chance for omission of key observations.

In the case of rabies suspects, the whole head is sent to the public health service for evaluation immediately upon the patient's death. While this may seem grotesque, it is necessary for the well-being of all people and animals exposed to the suspect because rabies is a fatal zoonotic disease. The public health service is notified that such a specimen is arriving. Confirm whether the whole head or just the brain is to be sent. Confirm details for labeling, packaging, and shipment.

After necropsy, all remaining tissues and organs are placed within the body cavities. The body cavities are sutured closed. The cadaver is placed in a cadaver bag, sealed tightly, and tagged with the patient's and owner's names and the date of death. Special instructions for burial, cremation with return of the ashes to the owner, and group versus individual burial are entered onto the tag. The body is placed in the freezer designated for storage of cadavers pending pick up by the pet cemetery, animal control authorities, or the owner as is within legal constraints of the county. A log may be kept adjacent to the freezer for entry of each cadaver as it is placed into the freezer. Record date, patient and owner names, and any special instructions for disposition of the body. Contact lab for pick-up of specimens or prepare them for shipment.

After the necropsy put on PPE, exam gloves, waterproof apron, and boots to clean and disinfect the area. Clean instruments using the practice's protocol. Spray disinfectant and allow it to air dry.

Reflection

A necropsy can be a traumatic event, so think about how to prepare yourself for a necropsy mentally. What self-talk can you use to help you through the necropsy?

Preparing Samples for Shipment to Reference Laboratory

Reference laboratories are often utilized by veterinary practices. Samples are sent to reference laboratories for tests that are rarely done in the practice or because it is too expensive to maintain the equipment and reagents. Necropsy samples are sent to veterinary pathologists that are specifically trained to diagnose diseases and conditions from the samples.

It will be the assistant's job to package the samples properly so that they arrive in good shape. This will increase the success of a diagnosis. Fresh tissue samples and body fluids must to be kept cool and packaged in leak-proof containers. Fixed tissue samples are placed in diluted formaldehyde. The reference laboratory will provide leak-proof containers. In addition to the samples, the submission form needs to be completed thoroughly. Regardless of the type of tissue, it all must arrive at the laboratory in the same shape that it was collected.

The shipping container is usually a Styrofoam container with its own lid, inside a cardboard box. Most clinics will save shipping boxes, bubble wrap, or shipping peanuts and ice packs that companies use to ship supplies to the clinic. These are great to use inside the Styrofoam container to keep fresh tissue samples and body fluids cool and to pad them from rough handling. Newspaper or paper towels are often layered on the bottom to soak up any spillage.

To pack the container, secure the completed requisition form in its own Ziploc bag and seal. Line the bottom of the Styrofoam container with several layers of newspaper. Place an ice pack on the bottom of the box if sending fresh tissues or body fluids. Check to makes sure the samples' container lids are on tight and are labeled properly with the patient's identification, the practice name, and date of sampling. Roll bubble wrap or newspaper around each sample container. Place padded samples into the box next to the ice pack.

Add packing peanuts or crumpled newspaper to keep the samples from bouncing around in the box. If it is warm outside add a second ice pack on top of the contents. Place the lid onto the Styrofoam box and put the submission form on top of the lid, then tape the cardboard box shut. Add shipping label on top and place it in the clinic's pick-up location for the shipping company, take it to the shipping office, or if there is a pick-up service call them to schedule a pick-up.

Mark the patient's file and the laboratory log that the samples were sent to the reference laboratory with the date, what tissues/fluids were sent, what method of shipment was used, the tracking number if available, and your initials.

Vaginal Cytology Collection

Dog breeders often like to know where in the reproductive cycle a bitch may be at a certain time. This entails the veterinarian or technician swabbing the inner vault of the vagina. Equipment required for this procedure is vaginal speculum (Figure 12.23), microscope slides, cotton-tipped applicator stick, and lubricant. PPE is gloves. The restraint is standing with an arm around the animal's neck and the other holding the tail out of the way or supporting the abdomen to keep the dog from sitting down. The slides are stained using the Dip Quick set of stains used for blood smears.

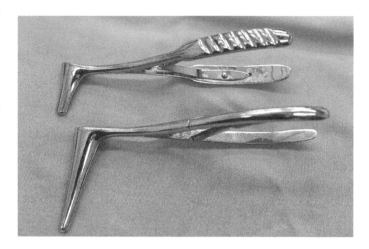

FIGURE 12.23 Vaginal speculum.

Reflection

Explain why it is so important to take care of samples and pack them correctly for shipment to a reference laboratory?

Chapter Reflection

Laboratory work is challenging and very important for determining a disease. How will you maintain the high standards of practice required to turn out quality results for the veterinarian?

CHAPTER 13

Pharmacy Skills

LEARNING OBJECTIVES
- Read primary drug labels correctly
- Interpret a prescription
- Label a dispensing container
- Use a pill counting tray to count pills and capsules
- Calculate correctly the quantity of a drug to dispense
- Demonstrate and explain to a client how to administer patient medication

NAVTA ESSENTIAL SKILLS COVERED IN THIS CHAPTER

III. Pharmacy and Pharmacology
A. Legal issues
1. Recognize legal issues involving all drugs (controlled and non-controlled) in the workplace
2. Recognize general types and groups of drugs and demonstrate proper terminology
3. Differentiate prescription drugs from over-the-counter drugs and describe proper prescription label requirements
B. Filling medications and inventory control
1. Label and package dispensed drugs correctly
2. Store, safely handle, and dispose of biological and therapeutic agents, pesticides, and hazardous waste
3. Perform inventory control procedures including restocking supplies and checking expiration dates

Tasks for the Veterinary Assistant, Fourth Edition. Teresa F. Sonsthagen.
© 2020 John Wiley & Sons, Inc. Published 2020 by John Wiley & Sons, Inc.
Companion website: www.wiley.com/go/sonsthagen/tasks

In general, there are three groups of medications available; one group is referred to as over-the-counter (OTC). These medications can be purchased at pet stores and farm or ranch stores for use by the owner on their animals. Their manufacturing, dosage recommendations, and use is monitored by the Food and Drug Administration (FDA) but not as strictly as the process for prescription drugs. They can be like a prescription drug but at a lower concentration.

The second group is prescribed medications, usually for use on a single animal or by a single heard or flock of animals owned by one person. As we learned in Chapter 2, the veterinarian must establish a client–patient–veterinarian relationship in order to prescribe any medications to any animal. In veterinary practices, only veterinarians can prescribe medications. These medications are supplied to veterinary practices via a distributer or directly from the manufacturer and only veterinarians that are licensed to practice can purchase them for resale to their clients.

Controlled Drugs

The third group is the controlled or scheduled substances that only a veterinarian with a Drug Enforcement Administration (DEA) permit can purchase and utilize for patient care. Permits are issued by the DEA and are renewable every 3 years. A person with such a permit is to post the license in a "visible place" within the facility. These are prescription drugs that have the potential for human addiction. The DEA has specific rules for ordering, storing, and dispensing these medications. All controlled drugs are required to be stored behind two locks. This means they must be stored in a locked box in a safe or other locked, permanently affixed place. Access should be limited to one or two persons within a facility. Careful inventory of controlled drugs within the facility must be recorded as a running total, meaning everything that comes in from the manufacturer and everything that is used on a patient must match. Strict adherence to these rules is absolutely required otherwise the veterinarian could lose not only his/her DEA license but his/her license to practice medicine and possibly have to do jail time.

Careful records of the amounts purchased by the clinic and then dispensed or used for patients are carefully recorded in a drug logbook. Logbooks must be written in ink, with pages numbered and permanently bound so they cannot be tampered with. Drug logbooks are maintained for at least 2 years, but requirements may vary by state. Logbooks are usually set up in a chart format with each controlled substance having its own separate book. The information required for each logbook: name of drug, drug form (liquid, tablet, capsule, ointment, paste), strength, and amount in or size of

primary container. The pages that follow are the running totals of that drug. The inventory headings in the logbook to record the amounts dispensed must include the following:

1. Quantity dispensed – this is the amount used per patient
2. Quantity remaining in the original container – this is a running total with the quantity dispensed subtracted as it is used. For example, ketamine comes in a 20-mL vial, 1.3 mL was used for patient X, 20 – 1.3 = 18.7 mL left in the primary bottle
3. Date and time (optional) dispensed
4. Full name and address of the patient's owner
5. Name and species of animal
6. Signature of the person dispensing – if you use initials there must be a signature with initials page in each book.

The DEA limitations on access to controlled substances lists four categories of individuals who cannot access these items: anyone convicted of a felony related to controlled substances; anyone denied DEA registration; anyone whose license has been revoked by the DEA; and anyone who has surrendered DEA licensure.

Among the processes for new employee orientation is the signing of a statement that the individual is not among the groups denied access to controlled substances. There will be a background check into drug use, so it is best not to lie about this. It is not required by the DEA, but it is permitted. While some may consider this overly cautious, the veterinarian's access to anesthetics and painkillers will be withdrawn by the DEA if strict control of these drugs is not provided and accurate records for use of drugs is not maintained.

Controlled or scheduled drugs are designated with a capital C and a Roman numeral on the primary container. They are "scheduled" from most addictive to least addictive. These medications are recorded in a drug logbook kept on the premises in a central location. The inventory manager will be responsible for entering the quantity of control medications received. It is the responsibility of *everyone* else to enter the amounts used in the drug logbook as it happens.

The following are examples of controlled drugs, their schedule designations, and recording rules:

- *Schedule V:* low addictive potential – CV designation – usually not required in the drug log by law, but the facility may require recording of amounts dispensed (e.g., lomotil, Robitussin AC). *No limits on refills.*
- *Schedule IV:* low addictive potential with limited dependence – usually not required in the drug log by law, but the facility may require recording of amounts dispensed (e.g., diazepam (Valium), phenobarbital). *Limited to five refills in 6 months.*

- *Schedule III:* moderately addictive potential – recording amounts dispensed are required in the drug log by law (e.g., acetaminophen with codeine, ketamine, anabolic steroids). *Limited to five refills in 6 months.*
- *Schedule II:* potential for severe dependence – recording amounts dispensed are required in the drug log by law (e.g., oxymorphone, morphine, pentobarbital injectable, fentanyl). *No refills.*
- *Schedule I:* no medical use. These are not found in a veterinary facility. Their use is limited to research facilities only.

Clients may not receive more than a 30-day supply of a controlled substance. Refills depend on drug classification. Also, beware of clients, particularly those that seem to frequent multiple veterinary clinics, requesting medications for their pets or seeking constant refills. It is not uncommon to find unscrupulous owners who are taking their pet's medication for their own personal use.

Accuracy and safety are vital factors when filling a prescription or administering medications. The patient and client have the right to know that veterinary professionals are following certain standards of practice by ensuring they are getting the correct prescription. Clients can also be reassured that the facility is practicing the best standard of care. When filling a prescription, preparing a label, or giving a medication to a patient *always* double check these against the "Patient's Rights" in Chapter 11. By keeping them in mind we can achieve the goal of best standard of care.

Review

Jot down the "Patient's Rights" discussed in Chapter 11 and reflect on how you can best keep these rights in mind as you assist in the pharmacy.

Reading a Prescription

The veterinarian may ask an assistant to fill a prescription, label the secondary container, and explain to the client how to administer it to their pet. Let's being with the prescription. Filling a prescription presents some major challenges regarding accuracy. The first concern is correctly reading the veterinarian's handwriting. Legibility with handwriting can range from good to indecipherable with anybody, not just veterinary professionals. Learning the scrawl of each veterinarian in a practice takes time. In the beginning, ask an experienced team member to help you. If there is any doubt, it is wiser to ask the veterinarian for clarification than to risk filling a prescription incorrectly. Don't ever assume.

The second challenge arises from the use of abbreviations in a prescription. Remember from Chapter 1 that abbreviations are a combination of Latin and English. There are standard abbreviations recognized within the profession. Some abbreviations have several meanings depending on the context in which they are used. To add further confusion, some veterinarians or practices have *their own* abbreviations. You need to memorize both the standard abbreviations and the ones used within your practice. If you are struggling with the abbreviations it is a good idea to include them in a pocket reference book for a quick review. When you encounter non-standard abbreviations, make a note of these in your book. Never use these abbreviations on labels or when speaking to a client. It is necessary to translate the abbreviations on the prescription to standardized English. For example, most clients don't know what "bid" means.

Review

What do the abbreviations; qd, bid, tid, RX, PO, and q8h mean?

A third challenge encountered when filling a prescription is drug identification. There are brand names for medicines for example, Tylenol® is a brand name of acetaminophen which is the generic name or formulation name. There are many companies that package acetaminophen under their own label and may simply label it as "pain care." This is the same with prescription strength medications. Be aware that one veterinarian in the practice may use the brand name but only the generic formula is in the pharmacy. Usually, this is out of habit. Think of it this way, when you ask for something for a headache do you say, "Does anyone have any acetaminophen?" or do you say, "Does anyone have any Tylenol?"

Medications are made in different concentrations per unit and are packaged similarly, the only difference is the strength. Using our acetaminophen example, they come in 200 or 500 mg tablets. The 500 mg tablets may say something like "extra strength" on the front of the label as your only clue that they may be of a different strength. Reading the label carefully for strength is very important when filling a prescription.

Some manufactures will have a "brand" packaging. For example, all their products have a red and white label. This comes into play when drug names are similar, such as amoxicillin and ampicillin. In this case they are similar antibiotics but work a bit differently and so one may be selected by the veterinarian over another. So, it is very easy to grab the wrong bottle because we went for the color pattern and something that started with an "am." Therefore, it is vital to double check the name of the medication.

Medications can have different brand names but be the same ingredient, for example Heartguard™ and Iverheart™ are both ivermectin soft chews for heartworm preventative – just different manufacturers.

The primary container label will contain information you will need to fill a prescription accurately. Knowing where to look for this information is vital to select and dispense the correct medications as per the prescription. An animal's condition may worsen, or it could die, if these basic rules are not scrupulously followed. Malpractice such as this is detrimental to the patient and the clinic and possibly your job!

On the label you will find:

1. The drug name, this may be a brand, proprietary, or copyrighted ® name such as Heartgard or the generic-compendium name, which in this case would be ivermectin. The generic name may be most familiar. As another example, amoxicillin is the generic name and Amoxi-Tabs® is the proprietary or brand name. Often, in a facility, the generic and proprietary names are used interchangeably.
2. Many drugs have similar spellings. Always compare the spelling on the prescription with that on the drug label. For example, prednisolone and prednisone. They are both steroids but are used for different conditions. Make sure the drug prescribed and the drug on the bottle match and if there is a doubt, ask!
3. The strength of the medication is usually on the front of the label. However, some will have the strength written on the side in the ingredients list. This is especially true if the medication is a combination of drugs.
4. Drugs are marked with an expiration date. *Never* use expired drugs. This is usually printed on the side of the label, on the bottle itself, or on the crimped end of a tube.

On a prescription some veterinarians will write the drug names out completely, while some very frequently used drugs are often written in an abbreviated format. If the name of the drug is abbreviated in the prescription, take the time to identify the drug correctly before filling the prescription. For example, amoxicillin can be abbreviated as amoxi. *Ask* if you do not understand the abbreviation for the drug name. A wise instructor once said, "It's never dumb to ask a question, but it is sure dumb explaining a mistake that could have been prevented by asking one!"

Take multiple opportunities to read the drug label as a double check as you fill a prescription. Here is the sequence as you fill a prescription:

- Read the label the first time you remove the primary container from inventory/pharmacy

- Compare the label with what is written in the patient orders
- Look at the label as you fill the prescription and write/type in the label information for the secondary container
- Read the label as you put the primary container back into the inventory/pharmacy
- Say the name of the medication when the prescription is dispensed or administered to the patient and check it against the patient's file.

Errors in filling a prescription or administering medications compromise patient health or, worse, risk death. Accuracy and hypervigilance are of the upmost importance. This is no time to cut corners, get sloppy or complacent.

Learning Exercise

Use an OTC like acetaminophen or ibuprofen or, if you work in a veterinary hospital, select a primary medicine bottle. Find and then write down the brand/manufacturer's name (if there is one), the generic or formula name, the strength per unit, and the dose.

Labeling a Prescription Container

The purpose of the label is to tell the owner who it is for, what is in the container, and the directions for its use. Most veterinary hospitals have preprinted labels with some of the required information already on them. In that instance, you only need to fill in the blanks whether it be handwritten or on the computer.

Additional cautionary labels should be put on the prescription container with warnings on drug use or storage as necessary. Some examples are labels stating: "Keep refrigerated," "Do not give with dairy products," or "For veterinary use only." These are usually preprinted and come in rolls of peel-off labels. These are important as many medications need to be stored properly or given in a particular way.

When filling a prescription, we often take medications out of the primary bottle and place the pill, liquid, or ointment in a secondary container, or we need to attach a label to an individual use medication like ophthalmic ointment or heartworm preventative tablets. Regardless of the type of container, FDA and/or DEA laws require the following information be included on a prescription label:

1. Name, address, and telephone number of the facility where the prescription is filled

2. Name of the prescribing veterinarian
3. Client name (and address if the drug is a controlled substance [CS])
4. Patient's name and/or identification number
5. Drug name
6. Drug strength
7. Quantity dispensed
8. Expiration date of the drug
9. Number of refills
10. Directions for use in plain English including

    - dose per treatment
    - frequency of treatments
    - duration of treatments

11. *Withholding time.* If the drug is administered to an animal meant for consumption (i.e., food animals such as cattle) or if any of its products are consumed, the withholding time required before processing the animal must be listed. This is the time from the last dose of medication until the time of slaughter or use of products for human consumption. This information is included on the bottle or on the package insert that comes with every medication. If it is missing, veterinarians usually keep a compendium of drugs book that will contain the same information as found on the package insert.

Learning Exercise

The following is an example of a prescription for the antibiotic cephalexin. Break it down and write out a label as you decipher the following prescription.

Rubi, Teresa Sonsthagen, Rx: Cephalexin 250 mg, PO, bid × 10 days, 0 refills

Hospital info: (use your imagination)
Who:
What:
When:
How/where:
Duration:
# of units:
Refills:

Many medications come in more than one strength and so you may need to determine the amount per dose needed because the milligram per tablet in the pharmacy is not equal to the dose prescribed. In our learning exercise above the *what* was 250 mg/tablet cephalexin. If the pharmacy only has 500 mg/tablet cephalexin you can still fill the prescription by doing some simple math.

Dividing the requested strength/unit by the strength/unit available. For example (the requested strength)

250 mg/tablet / (strength available) 500 mg/tablet = 0.5 tablet or ½ tablet per dose. Instead of 1 full tablet twice a day we would send home and mark the label as ½ tablet twice a day. This also works if only 100 mg tablets are available, 250 mg (strength requested) /100 mg (strength available) = 2.5. The patient would need 2½ tablets per dose.

Some medications are dispensed as a dose/body weight. For example, an anesthetic is to be given 0.1 mL/2 pounds and you have a dog that weighs 36 lb. You would take the 36 / 2 = 18 and then multiply by 0.1 = 1.8 mL of anesthetic.

Learning Exercises

- Utilizing the prescription for Rubi above, how many 500 mg tablets would be sent home to fulfill the prescription? How many 100 mg tablets would be sent home to fulfill the prescription?
- Jack needs an antiparasitic and the dose is 4 mL/kg and he weighs 24 lb. How much would you give Jack?

Safe Handling of Dispensed Drugs

Some drugs are hazardous to the people dispensing and administering them. Steroids and chemotherapeutics are examples of the types of drugs that can harm personnel. Pregnant personnel should never handle either of these medications. When handling these drugs, the person *must* wear gloves, goggles, and a mask. Gloves and goggles are the minimum for all the other types of drugs dispensed or administered in the veterinary facility.

Use a pill counting tray to avoid touching any pills or capsules (Figure 13.1). A pill counting tray has a flat surface that pills can be dumped upon, then using a tongue depressor or a flat icing knife the pills can be separated into "twos" – "fives" as they are pushed into the tube section of the tray with the knife. Continue to count the pills until you have reached the required quantity to fill the prescription, then put the cover over the tube. If there are pills remaining on the tray, they can be tipped back into the primary container by tilting the tray toward the small funnel on the corner of the tray opposite to the tube opening. By tipping the tray in the opposite direction you can put the pills into the secondary container utilizing the covered tube with its funnel-like opening.

If you must split pills in half, utilize the pill splitter (Figure 13.1). Count out the number of pills required on the pill counting tray. Place them one at a time into the splitter. If they have score marks or small dents indicating halves and/or quarters, line the dent up with the

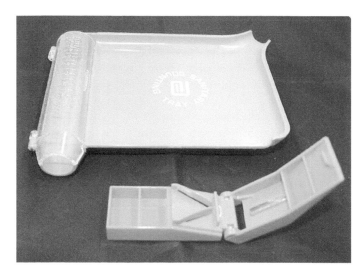

FIGURE 13.1 Pill counting tray and pill splitter.

blade on the lid of the splitter. Close the cover then push down sharply. Some tablets will easily split just using your fingers. For tablets that do not have score marks, set them snuggly into the "V" on the base of the splitter. Carefully close the cover and push down slowly to try to get an even split. You can put your split pills onto the counting tray to make sure you have the right amount before putting them into the secondary container.

If a pill counting tray is unavailable, pour the pills into the palm of your gloved hand. With the other gloved hand, grasp two–five pills at a time and place these in a prescription vial, counting as you go. It is more efficient than counting one pill at a time. Just remember the two, three, four, or fives multiplication table for the number of times you will drop pills into the vial.

Never split capsules! These are designed to melt away once ingested, releasing the medications inside. The medication is a carefully measured dose by the manufacturer.

Prescription Packaging

When dispensing tablets, capsules, or liquids make sure the secondary container is childproof. The only exception is at the request of the owner. Even then, it is best to recommend safety containers to prevent children and pets from opening the container. Persons with disabilities and the elderly may lack the strength and coordination in their hands to open a childproof container and are the most likely candidates for containers that are not childproof. An owner request for a container that is not childproof is documented in the patient's record. Ideally, owners sign a request form documenting their request for dispensing of medication in a non-childproof container. The form is then included in the medical record. If no such form exists in the facility, document the request in the record itself and have the client initial or sign.

Secondary containers are often plastic vials with caps that either twist or snap off and are available in various sizes. Use one that is large enough to hold the entire prescription with a small amount of space left at the top of the vial. It is financially wasteful to fill a prescription in a large vial for 10 tablets. Vials are usually amber or blue colored to protect the medication from deterioration due to exposure to sunlight. Vials are suitable for dry medications such as tablets, capsules, and ointments. Larger ones can be used to dispense smaller items that cannot be fitted with a label such as a tube of eye ointment.

Liquids are dispensed in bottles with twist-off caps or dropper tops. The bottles are often marked on the outside as to the available quantity (in ounce and milliliter, typically) on the inside. This will give you a reasonably accurate amount when filling the bottles. A funnel or a large syringe aids in filling bottles to prevent spillage. Be certain that the funnel or syringe is clean and dry before using.

Some medications begin as a powder and must be **reconstituted** with a specified amount of water to form a liquid; this must be done before sending the medication home with a client. Use a syringe for accurate measurement. Read the label carefully to learn what and how much to use to reconstitute a drug. Mix the medication and replace the mixing cap with one that has a dropper attached to the lid. This is marked in milliliters and is used to give the patient its dose of medication.

Ointments come in tubes either with its own box that may accommodate a prescription label, or if just a tube it should be placed in an amber vial or box that will accommodate the label. If the ointment is in a large multi-use primary container, use a clean tongue depressor to remove the ointment and transfer it to a vial or tin container. Push the ointment in solidly to be certain there are no air pockets within the medication.

Return the primary bottle to the pharmacy or inventory. Take note of the amount left and compare it with the order point card. If it is close or on the order point number alert the inventory manager of the need to reorder. If it is a controlled drug, make sure to mark it properly in the controlled drug log.

Either give the record and medication to the designated recipient (receptionist, veterinarian, and technician) or take it to the designated location (front desk, examination room).

Explaining Prescriptions to the Owner

The veterinarian may have explained to the owner that medication is being dispensed, but it is up to the staff to make certain the client really understands what to do and how to do it. There is always the possibility that the owner's understanding is incomplete or inaccurate, which serves as a basis for failure to comply with the veterinarian's

---

TABLE 13.1	

Categories of Pharmaceuticals Found in a Veterinary Practice with Common Examples of Each

Analgesic/anesthetic (ANST only)	Atipamezole, buprenorphine (narcotic), gabapentin, hydromorphone, medetomidine, morphine, oxymorphone, propofol (ANST), Telazol (ANST), Tramadol
Antibacterial	Amoxicillin, cephalosporin, cefpodoxime, cephalexin, ciprofloxacin, Clavamox, clindamycin, doxycycline, enrofloxacin, ivermectin, marbofloxacin, metronidazole, moxifloxacin, neomycin (oint.), oxytetracycline, ofloxacin, silver sulfadiazine, streptomycin, thiostrepton, trimethoprim, tylosin
Anticoccidial	Ponazuril, roxarsone
Anticonvulsant	Levetiracetam, phenobarbital
Antidepressant	Amitriptyline
Antiemetic	Acepromazine, maropitant, metoclopramide, mirtazapine
Antihistamine	Hydroxyzine
Antifungal	Nystatin
Antimicrobial	Pirlimycin, rifampin
Antiparasitic	Amitraz, clamoxyquine, dichlorophen, fenbendazole, fipronil, levamisole, lufenuron (flea), milbemycin oxime, nitroscanate, nitroxynil, oxibendazole, praziquantel, pyrantel, rafoxanide, selamectin, thiabendazole
Appetite stimulant	Cyproheptadine, mirtazapine
Bronchodilator	Aminophylline, clenbuterol, theophylline (spasm)
Cardiac medication	Atenolol, benazepril (ACE-inhibitor), enalapril, pimobendan, prazosin, theophylline (edema)
Cough suppressant	Butorphanol
Cushing's disease	Trilostane
Diuretic	Furosemide
Emergency drug	Glycopyrrolate
Emetic	Apomorphine
Euthanasia solution	Pentobarbital, phenytoin/pentobarbital
Gastrointestinal medication	Cimetidine, sucralfate
Hepatic medication	Ursodeoxycholic acid
Histamine blocker	Diphenhydramine
Hyperthyroid drug	Methimazole
Hypothyroid drug	Levothyroxine
Insecticide	Nitenpyram
Local anesthetic	Bupivacaine
Muscle relaxer	Butorphanol
NSAID	Carprofen, deracoxib, ketoprofen, mavacoxib, meloxicam, Metacam, nimesulide, phenylbutazone, robenacoxib, tepoxalin, tolfenamic acid
Nutraceutical	Chondroitin and glucosamine
Ophthalmics	Artificial tears (drops and ointments)
Reversal for anesthetic	Atipamezole (dexmedetomidine), yohimbine (xylazine)
Sedative	Acepromazine, dexmedetomidine, diazepam, xylazine
Steroid	Dexamethasone, prednisolone, prednisone, triamcinolone acetonide
Tranquilizer	Alprazolam, ketamine
Urinary and kidney medications	Benazepril, bethanechol, phenylpropanolamine
Weight loss	Mitratapide

ACE, angiotensin-converting enzyme; ANST, anesthetic; NSAID, non-steroidal anti-inflammatory drug.

recommendations for at-home care. The reason these misunderstanding happen are that the veterinarian used terminology with which the client is unfamiliar; the presence of the pet can distract the owner; the owner might be overwhelmed with information; or the procedure can be unfamiliar to the client. Whatever the reason, the result is delay or failure in patient recovery.

If you are asked to explain a prescription to the owner it is done at the very end of the office visit, before the client leaves the examination room with the patient. Have the patient's record, medication, and written instruction form in hand. Greet the client and patient with a smile as you enter the room. Face the owner and start relaying the information at a slow pace, speaking clearly and a bit loudly (especially for older clients). Remember to use layman's terms, not veterinary terminology. Explain to the owner what the medication is and its purpose. Show the drug label and read the instructions to them. Ask if they have any questions. Wait for a reply! Demonstrate how to open and close the container and, if possible, demonstrate how to administer the medication to the patient, or go over how to give the medication if it cannot be given at the appointment. Ask them if they have any questions! For more complicated procedures, you may ask the owner to repeat the procedure after you demonstrate it or explain it.

Review the instruction form with the client and point out the phone numbers to use if they have a question or concern. Ask the owner if there is anything else needed at this time. If not, thank them for trusting their pet's care to the clinic and tell them you will meet them at the reception desk with the prescription and information sheet.

Learning Exercise

Utilize the programs pharmacy and the list provided in Table 13.1. Make a chart and fill in the drug name and what category of medicine it represents.

Classification of Medications

There are many types of medications found within the veterinary practice. They all have specific uses, and some have "off-label" uses meaning it has been found that they may work for unspecified treatment of a condition or illness. It is really beyond the scope of this text and the training of an assistant to learn all of these drugs. However, becoming familiar with the medications may be of some help when starting to work in a facility. Therefore, Table 13.1 provides categories of pharmaceuticals found in a veterinary practice with some examples.

Learning Exercise

Practice explaining a medication with a classmate. Ask for honest feedback and do the same for her/him.

Chapter Reflection

Now that you have learned a bit about pharmacy skills, what are your takeaway points from this chapter?

Suggested Reading

Bill RL. 1997. *Pharmacology for Veterinary Technicians*, 2nd edn. Mosby.

Bill R. 2000. *Medical Mathematics and Dosage Calculations for Veterinary Professionals.* Iowa Press.

Sirois M. 2011. *Principles and Practices of Veterinary Technology*, 3rd edn. Elsevier.

CHAPTER 14

Surgical Room Skills

LEARNING OBJECTIVES
- Preparation of surgical suite in order to provide quality patient care
- Assist with patient prep for surgical procedures
- Set up and maintain anesthesia and surgical equipment
- Assist with inducing anesthesia
- Keep accurate log records of anesthesia, controlled substances, and surgery
- Prepare, sterilize, and set up surgical packs
- Observe and care for recovering surgical patients

NAVTA ESSENTIAL SKILLS COVERED IN THIS CHAPTER

VI. Surgical Preparation and Assisting
A. Assist in performing surgical preparations
   1. Prepare surgical equipment/supplies
   2. Sterilize instruments and sanitize supplies using appropriate methods
   3. Operate and maintain autoclaves
   4. Identify common instruments
   5. Identify common suture materials, types, and sizes
   6. Assist the veterinarian and/or veterinary technician with preparation of patients using aseptic technique
   7. Assist with positioning of surgical patients
   8. Aid the veterinarian/and or veterinary technician with physical monitoring of recovering surgical patients
   9. Maintain the surgical log

B. Surgical suite and equipment cleanliness
   1. Maintain proper operating room conduct and asepsis
   2. Perform post-surgical clean up
   3. Fold surgical gowns and drapes
   4. Maintain operating room sanitation and care

Tasks for the Veterinary Assistant, Fourth Edition. Teresa F. Sonsthagen.
© 2020 John Wiley & Sons, Inc. Published 2020 by John Wiley & Sons, Inc.
Companion website: www.wiley.com/go/sonsthagen/tasks

Cleaning and Maintaining the Surgery Suite

The goal of a surgical procedure is to restore health or function and in veterinary medicine also to stop procreation. All surgeries must be done **aseptically** in order to prevent nosocomial infections. Organisms enter when the skin integrity is altered from the incision made to access the interior of the body. This altered skin integrity increases the risk that pathogens gain access to the body. When the veterinary team adheres to aseptic techniques in preparing instruments, equipment, the surgical suite, the patient, and the personnel, it reduces the risk of infection from a surgical procedure. The veterinary assistant has an important role in making sure the surgical suite is cleaned thoroughly and is ready to be used for surgeries.

Chapter 4 discussed cleaning and disinfecting the wards and treatment areas of the hospital and those concepts are a good starting point. However, the surgical suite must be maintained at a higher level of cleanliness than other parts of the clinic. The surgical suite consists of three areas: the prep room, surgery room, and recovery.

When surgeries are finished for the day, begin your clean with the cleanest to the dirtiest room. The order of cleaning would be the surgery room, prep room, and finally the recovery room. After each daily round of surgeries, the suite must be cleaned from top to bottom.

Start by gathering all of the used surgical packs and towels and take them to the laundry. Take the open surgical packs to the sink where the instruments are placed in cold water to soak until they can be cleaned. When you find the scalpel handle with the blade, carefully remove the blade before putting the handle into the cold water. This is accomplished by using a needle holder or large hemostat to lift a lower corner of the blade up and sliding it forward off the handle. Do not do this with bare fingers as the blade is sharp and contaminated with blood which could lead to a painful and possibly infected cut. Cleaning the instruments will be covered later in the chapter. Sort the cloth wraps and gowns from the towels and start a load as per the instructions in Chapter 4.

Return to the surgical suite with a broom, fresh mop, and bucket filled with diluted disinfectant for later use. Gather the spray disinfectant and paper towels. Start with the surgical lights hanging above the surgery table. Turn them off and using spray disinfectant and paper towels clean the entire light and handles thoroughly. Look for the removeable handles that are autoclaved for each surgery day. Remove them and place them with the other surgical items to be cleaned and sterilized. Move other items to the prep room for cleaning and storing as you clean the surgery room.

Move to the surgical table next. It too must be cleaned thoroughly which may entail lifting the side panels to access the drip tray and the inside edges of the panel.

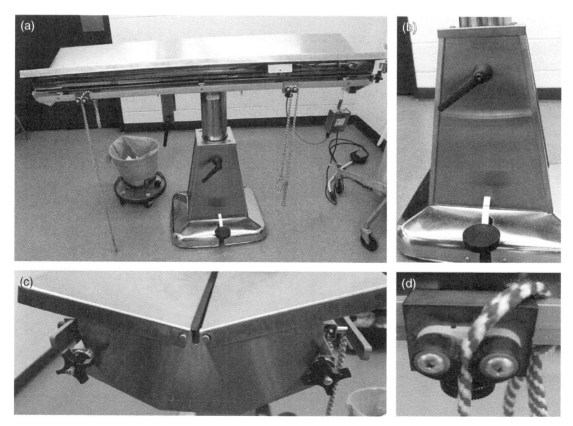

FIGURE 14.1 Surgical table.

Figure 14.1c shows one end of the surgical table. Note the two knobs on each side. These are loosened so that the entire table panel can be removed or, as shown in Figure 14.1a, it can be set at an angle to keep the patient from rolling. This will give you access to the bottom edge. If the table panel is heated, care must be taken not to damage the electrical cords attached at the other end. If that is the case, simply park the table panel in an upright position to clean. Spray disinfectant and paper towels are used over each table panel. While the table panel is up or out, remove the drip tray from the center of the table, centered under the table panels. This catches blood, urine, feces, and other debris during surgery. If there is fluid in the tray, tilt it into the catch bucket under the tray or move the kick bucket under the tray to empty it into that. Otherwise you will dump the liquid all over the place trying to get the tray out. If the tray is full of dried debris, take it to the prep sink to clean with a scrub brush and disinfectant, or spray it with disinfectant and dry with paper towels. Return the clean drip tray making sure it is seated on the pegs that hold it in place. Use spray disinfectant and paper towels to clean the base of the table, as seen in Figure 14.1b. If surgeries are finished for the day, remove the rope restraints seen in Figure 14.1d and run them through the laundry with the towels used for surgeries.

Clean the auxiliary tables and carts in the surgery room in the same manner as the surgical table. Check the suture material, scalpel blades, surgical glue, and other disposables like syringes, needles and tape for adequate supply; restock as needed. The surgical tray (Figure 14.2), surgery tables, and other carts are moved so the floor can be swept and then mopped beneath them. It is amazing how much dust, hair, and debris can collect under them in just one day! Clean the door to the surgical suite on both sides with spray disinfectant and then the light switch panel in the surgical room. Once cleaned it should not be entered without a cap, mask, and shoe covers.

On a weekly basis, the entire room needs to be disinfected. Start with the ceiling using a wash towel and bucket of dilute disinfectant. Pay attention to the pole from which the light hangs from the ceiling, and any oxygen or air lines, which are cleaned with spray disinfectant and paper towels. Use a handheld vacuum to clean the air handling grates, do not spray them with disinfectant, but you can use a paper or cloth towel sprayed with disinfectant to wipe them clean. Remove the room light covers and wipe them off inside and out. Bugs love to congregate in the light fixtures so it is essential to clean them regularly. When finished with the fixtures, wipe off the rest of the ceiling then down the walls with a cloth towel and a bucket of diluted disinfectant. If there are windows in the surgery suite use a window cleaner. Disinfect all of the surgical furniture to remove any dust or debris knocked down from the ceiling and walls. Sweep and mop the floor.

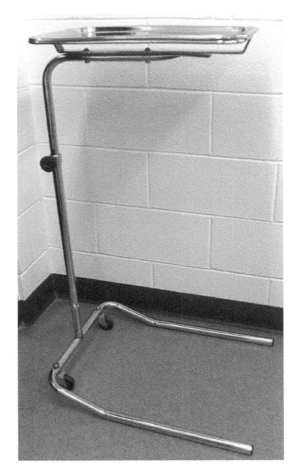

FIGURE 14.2 Surgical tray.

The prep room/recovery room; in some clinics this is the same room or two separate rooms. The prep room is where the patient is prepped for surgery and the recovery room or area is where it recovers from surgery. The prep room is usually equipped with a prep table that has a tub with a rack on top and a spray hose for rinsing (Figure 14.3). This sink is used for baths and cleaning wounds as well as for preparing the patient for surgery. Therefore, it must be cleaned well and disinfected thoroughly after each and every use. The recovery room will have kennels and perhaps a run which are maintained as described in Chapter 4.

As you can see in Figure 14.3, this prep sink has been used and requires cleaning. The clipper is cared for as described in Chapter 4. The warming blanket is sprayed with disinfectant on both sides and dried with paper towels. It is set aside for the next patient or put away if surgeries are done for the day.

The rack is cleaned by scrubbing it with a scrub brush on both surfaces. It is notorious for collecting blood, hair, pus, and other disgusting things on the downside of the bars. Once both sides are scrubbed, rinse it well and then cover it completely with spray disinfectant and allow it to air dry. While it is drying, clean and disinfect the tub portion. Scoop out any large pieces of debris like

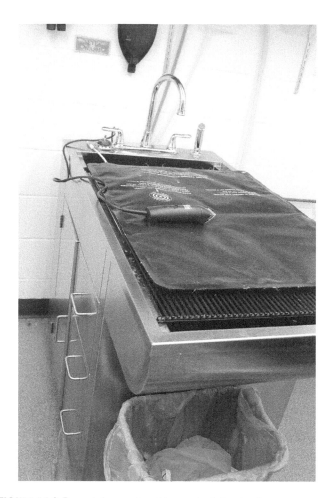

FIGURE 14.3 Prep sink – used and in need of cleaning!

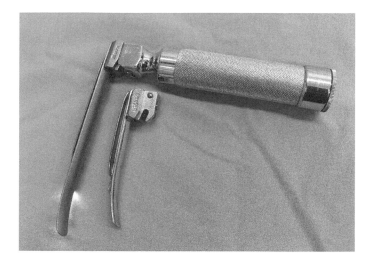

FIGURE 14.4 Laryngoscope and blades.

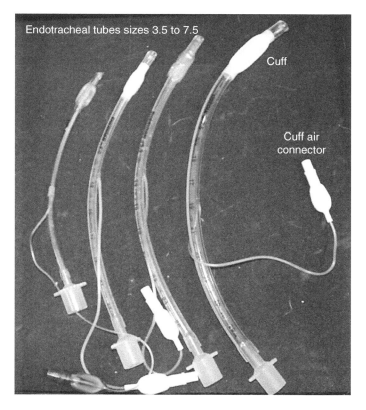

Endotracheal tubes sizes 3.5 to 7.5

Cuff

Cuff air connector

FIGURE 14.5 Endotracheal tubes sizes 3.5 to 7.5.

hair, feces, or toenail clippings with a paper towel then scrub with a scrub brush and soap. Rinse thoroughly and spray with disinfectant and allow it to air dry. Replace the rack on top and then use disinfectant and paper towels to wipe down the outside surfaces of the tub. As seen in Figure 14.3, many prep tables will have drawers or a cupboard in the lower part and these should be checked for hair accumulation and restocked. If there is hair or drips of debris present in the drawers, they should be emptied out, cleaned with a disinfectant, and restocked.

The prep room usually has one or more counters that are utilized for staging anesthetics and other supplies during the day's surgeries. If the surgeries are finished for the day, reusable items need to be cleaned and put away and the disposable supplies restocked. One such item may be the laryngoscope and blades. This is an instrument used to assist with **intubation** (Figure 14.4). It runs on batteries housed in the handle, so it is OK to spray it with disinfectant and wipe it dry with a paper towel and put it in its proper drawer.

Other items include endotracheal tubes (Figure 14.5). The ones that were used for the day's surgeries need to be clean and dry before storing. Check the cuffs to make sure the tube is still useable. They can develop a

spontaneous hole or it can be damaged against a tooth. Use a 6 or 12 mL syringe, pull the full amount of air into the syringe then connect it to the cuff adapter (Figure 14.6), and push the plunger to push the air into the cuff until it is full, but not overfull as that can pop the cuff. Let the tube set for a few minutes to see if the cuff holds air. If it does, then deflate the cuff and proceed to clean it; if it doesn't, throw it away and alert the inventory manager to order a new one.

To clean the endotracheal tube, move to the sink, spray disinfectant into the tube and on the outside of the tube. Use your hand to spread the disinfectant around on the outside of the tube and a small bristle brush to clean the inside. Rinse it thoroughly with warm water and hang to dry, as if put away wet they can develop mold inside of the tube. Do not put fluid down the small air inflation tube as that will wreck the tube and cuff. The endotracheal tubes not used can be put back into storage. They are usually separated by size for easy and quick access so make sure you put them away properly. If there is a doubt as to what tube was used, disinfect them all!

Gas Anesthesia Machine

The gas anesthetic machines are usually assigned to a veterinary technician for maintenance. However, you may be asked to assist with its care. There are parts that can be checked and restocked daily and parts that can be cleaned daily by a veterinary assistant. Figure 14.7 shows the soda lime canister filled with soda lime crystals.

Dr. Donald Sawyer recommends "that at a minimum these must be replaced every two weeks even if not used.

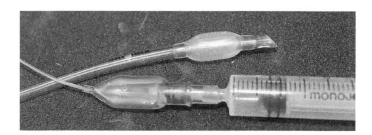

FIGURE 14.6 Syringe connected to endotracheal tube cuff adapter.

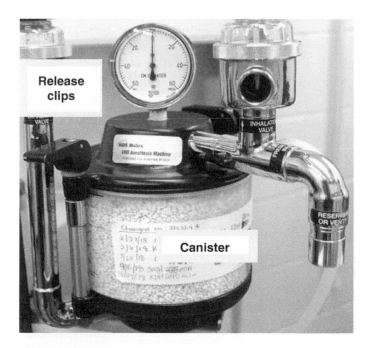

FIGURE 14.7 Soda lime canister.

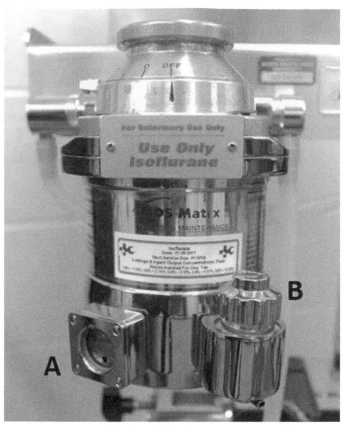

FIGURE 14.8 Isoflurane vaporizer's fill window (A) and fill spout (B).

If the clinic does more than five surgeries a week and/or if you have a large percentage of dog surgeries over 80 lb the crystals should be changed daily" (Sawyer 2016). The canister is removed and the spent crystals are dumped into the trash can. Place a cotton ball in the delivery hole and add crystals up to the fill line on the side of the canister. Put the canister back onto the machine, making sure it is seated into the holder before tightening the knobs or flipping the clamps that make it airtight. Take the trash with the spent crystal out to the dumpster as soon as possible.

Figure 14.8 shows the isoflurane vaporizer's fill window (A) and fill spout (B). Isoflurane is the gas anesthesic used most commonly in veterinary practice. It comes in a liquid form that aerosolizes when exposed to oxygen. Personal protective equipment (PPE) required is a respirator, gloves, and goggles as this is a noxious chemical which can cause headaches if exposed to it for a long period of time. Fill only to the fill line, otherwise it will over run the chamber and dump onto the floor. It will take wax off and it is dangerous to breath the spilled isoflurane. Refer to the chemical waste section in Chapter 4 for cleaning up a hazardous chemical spill.

Another item that the veterinary assistant may be asked to monitor it is the f/air canister (Figure 14.9). This canister traps waste gas if no evacuation disposal system is available. This canister must be changed out

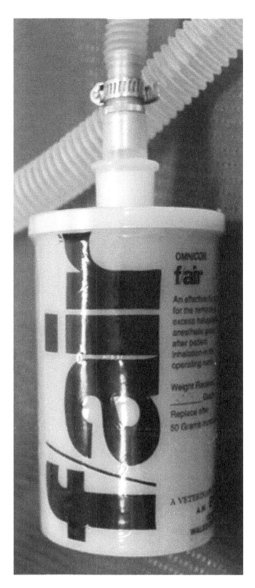

FIGURE 14.9 F/air canister.

after it weighs 50 g. New canisters are weighed and the weight is marked on the side of the canister. After each day's surgeries the canister is weighed and the old weight is subtracted from the new weight and added to a running total that is written on the side of the canister.

The next items to take care of are the air tubes and rebreathing bags (Figure 14.10). Daily maintenance of these include washing them out with warm soapy water, rinsing thoroughly with warm water, and if your spray disinfectant is OK to use on rubber and plastic, spray and let air dry. Hanging them up as shown in Figures 14.10c/d will allow them to drain. If this poses a slipping hazard, a folded towel or plastic boot mat works well to contain the water.

If the medications for surgery are still out, put the non-scheduled drugs into the supply cabinet. Take note of any that have reached the restocking point and if found restock putting the new bottle behind the old, so

it is used up the next day. If the drugs are schedule or controlled drugs, alert the technician or veterinarian who holds the keys so they can be locked up. Check the surgical and control drug logs and update those as required.

Wipe down the countertop with spray disinfectant, check the sharps container and if full replace it with another. Check the disinfectant spray, surgical scrub and alcohol containers and refill so they are available at all times. Restock cotton balls, gauze sponges, tongue depressors, syringes, needles, IV catheters, applicator sticks, adhesive tape, and self-sticking tape rolls. Check the artificial tears ointment tube and if almost gone secure another from central stores and place it under the old tube. Check to see if the bandage scissor got moved and restore it in the proper drawer. Check the IV drip sets and fluid bags and restock as necessary.

Clean the scrub sink where the veterinarians scrub their hands. Make sure you look at the surrounding wall above, below, and to each side. The brush tends to splatter scrub solution everywhere! You can use wet paper towels to clean the area as the surgical scrub is an all-purpose disinfectant. It does suds up so you may have to use several paper towels to get the area and sink clean.

If there are any kennels or runs to clean, take care of those as described in Chapter 4. Then sweep, moving all of the tables and other moveable objects, and mop with the surgical room mop bucket. Remember not to use the general mop bucket or the one for the kennels as this can ruin all of your hard work in cleaning and disinfecting the surgery suite! When finished put the mop head into the laundry and clean the mop bucket, then spray it with disinfectant and allow it to air dry.

Learning Exercise

In your reference book make a step-by-step protocol for cleaning the surgical suite in the manner in which the text dictates or in how your program or facility wishes it to be accomplished.

Cleaning the Surgical Instruments

Veterinary assistants are charged with cleaning the surgical instruments. These are expensive to buy, and their useful lifespan can be extended by proper cleaning techniques. As a rule, they should be cleaned as soon as possible after use. Blood can corrode stainless steel and so it is important to soak them in cold water if they can't be cleaned immediately. To start cleaning, run the sink full of hot water and use a detergent that is formulated for cleaning instruments. The pH must be neutral (5.5–8) so it doesn't corrode or stain the instrument. A brush is

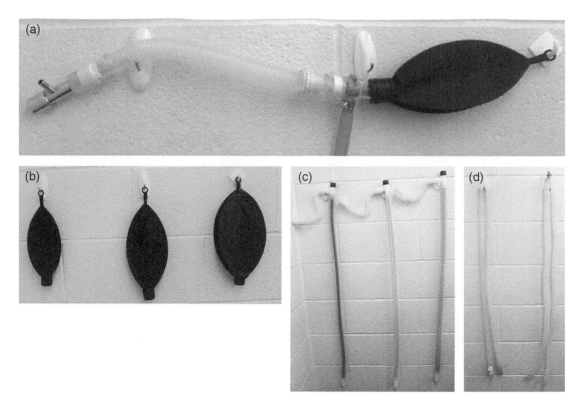

FIGURE 14.10 Non-rebreathing system and rebreathing bags and hoses: (a) non-rebreathing system; (b) 1, 2, and 3L rebreathing bags; (c) "F" rebreathing hoses; (d) "Y" rebreathing hoses.

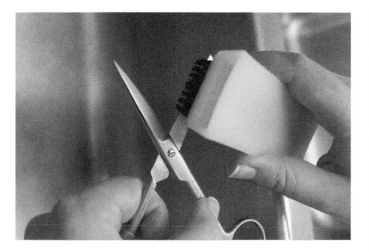

FIGURE 14.11 Brush cleaning a surgical instrument.

used to get all the debris off the instrument (Figure 14.11). It is rinsed thoroughly and if available put into an ultrasonic cleaner (Figure 14.12). This is a machine that produces bubbles that implode on the surface of the instrument knocking the microscopic debris off. This cleaner requires non-suds-producing detergent. The instruments are put into a wire basket with the jaws open, the basket is lowered into the water and detergent. A setting of 5 minutes is set on the dial that also turns the cleaner on. After the cycle, the instruments are rinsed thoroughly once more. The hinges on the instruments should be lubricated and allowed to dry before being repacked or stored. A specially made lubricant for surgical instruments must be used to keep them in good working order. Don't pile the basket too full and don't mix instruments made of different metals because the instruments do not get as clean and the different metals may react with each other causing discoloration or corrosion. Change the water and detergent for each load by unclamping the hose located on the back of the cleaner. Make sure the hose is in the sink before unclamping it!

Learning Exercise

Develop a protocol for taking care of the surgical instruments properly in order to extend their lifespans.

Assembling Surgical Packs

Assembling surgical packs is often delegated to the veterinary assistant. It is important to pay attention to details when assembling these packs as the instruments and materials contained therein are vital to the success of a surgery. In order to select the appropriate instruments, it is important to be able to identify the surgical instruments listed in Table 14.1. Take note of their size and the serrations on the jaws to distinguish one from another.

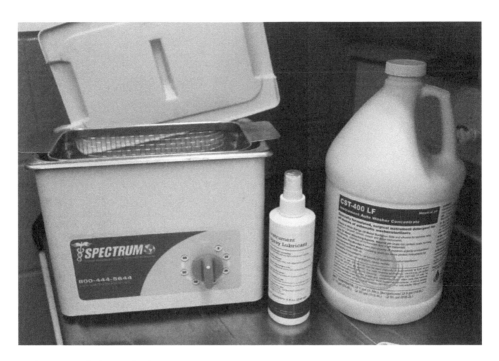

FIGURE 14.12 Instrument cleanser and ultrasonic cleaner.

Instrument Packs

Instrument packs are those that contain the hemostats, needle holders, and other instruments used during a surgical procedure. Every clinic will have their own "recipe" for how many of each is placed in the pack. The following list is just an example of what should be included, which you will have to adjust as per the wishes of the veterinarian (Figure 14.13):

A. 2–3 Rochester–Carmalt forceps
B. 2 Crile or Kelly forceps
C. 4 Halstad Mosquito forceps
D. #3 Scalpel handle
E. Groove director
F. Snook hook
G. Dressing thumb forceps
H. Adson or Adson-Brown or rat-tooth thumb forceps
I. Metzenbaum or Mayo scissors
J. Operating scissors
K. Mayo Hegar or Olsen Hegar needle holder
L. 4 Backhaus towel clamps.

The following are the instructions for packing an instrument pack (Figures 14.14, 14.15, 14.16, 14.17, and 14.18):

Step 1 Gather supplies – all of the instruments required for the pack, two cloth wraps, gauze sponges, sterilization indicator, and autoclave tape (Figure 14.14a).
Step 2 Layout wraps – position the wraps, one on top of the other as shown in Figure 14.14b, with the corners pointing at you.

Step 3 Make sure all the instruments are unlatched. Assemble the instruments as shown in Figure 14.14c, with the sterilization strip positioned as shown. Place the assembled instruments in the center of the wrap.
Step 4 Place the *counted* gauze sponges on top of the assembled instruments (Figure 14.15a). It is important to count the sponges so that none are left inside the patient when they are counted at the end of surgery. Gauze sponges come in a sleeve and if you look closely you will see that every tenth one is hanging out a bit from the stack (Figure 14.16). So you could conceivably just take the gauze in groups of 10. However, you should always count because the sleeve could have been dropped or some taken out for use elsewhere! This would mess up your count and potentially cause the patient to be reopened to look for the missing gauze sponges.
Step 5 First fold – starting with the closest point of the top wrap take it over the instruments then fold it back as shown in Figure 14.15b. The first folded edge must be even with the instruments and the point ends up pointing toward the outside edge or toward you again.
Step 6 Second fold – fold the wrap point on the left so the fold is even with the instruments gathered beneath and point the point toward the outside edge as shown in Figure 14.15c.
Step 7 Third fold – same as step 6 only with the right-hand point – not shown.
Step 8 The fourth corner is brought over the width of the package toward you and the folding point is determined. This would be the edge of the gathered instruments in the wrap (Figure 14.17a). Grasp the wrap at this point and Figure 14.17b shows how the top of the wrap is folded with the point folded under.

TABLE 14.1

Surgical Instrument Names and Uses

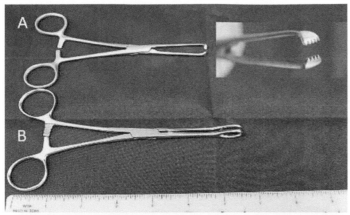

A. Allis tissue forceps	Atraumatic tissue holder
B. Sponge holding forceps	Grasp inanimate objects like sponges and dead tissue

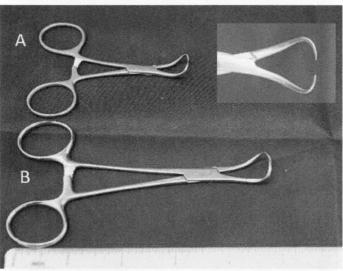

A. Small Backhaus towel clamp	These are both used to keep drapes and towels in place on the patient. The sharp points pierce the material and skin leaving very
B. Large Backhaus towel clamp	small holes

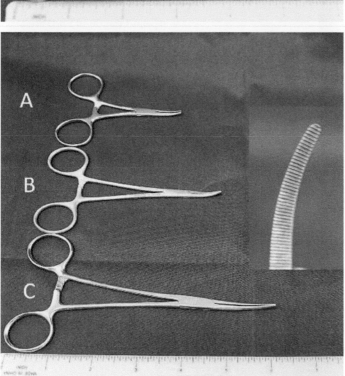

A. Hartman mosquito forceps	All of these forceps are used to clamp off vessels or tissues that will be removed. They crush tissue which cuts off blood supply.
B. Halstad mosquito forceps	The serrations on the jaws are horizontal along the entire length
C. Crile forceps	

(*Continued*)

> **TABLE 14.1**
>
> **(Continued)**

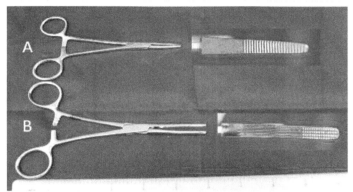

A. Kelly forceps

B. Rochester Carmalt forceps

Both are used to clamp larger tissues for blood control or tissues for removal. The Kelly has horizontal serrations on half the jaw and the Rochester has a combination of vertical on half the jaw and vertical/horizontal serrations at the tips

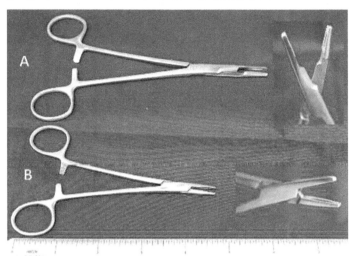

A. Olsen Hegar needle holder scissor combination

B. Mayo Hegar needle holder

Both are used to grasp and manipulate the suture needle while suturing. The Olsen Hegar has a scissor built into the jaws

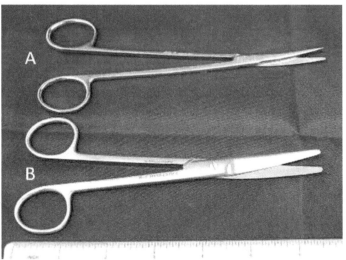

A. Metzenbaum scissors

B. Mayo scissors

These are used to cut tissue and nothing else! They are extremely sharp, and the blunt ends are used for "blunt" dissection

TABLE 14.1

(Continued)

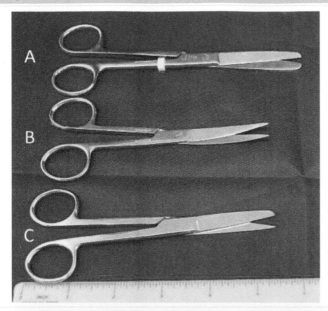

Operating scissors
A. Blunt/blunt

B. Sharp/sharp

C. Sharp/blunt

All three of these scissors are used to cut inanimate objects like sutures

The differences are in the tips as designated. The sharp/blunt scissors are the most common

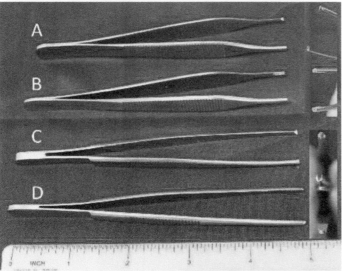

Thumb forceps
A. Adson tissue

B. Adson–Brown tissue

C. Rat-toothed tissue

D. Dressing

The first three thumb forceps are used to manipulate tissue either for inspection or for suturing. D is used for manipulating dressing materials and grasping inanimate objects

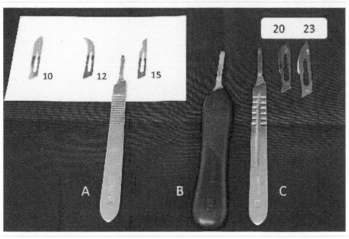

Scalpel blades and handles
A. Small animal with corresponding blades

B. Large animal with corresponding blades

Scalpel handles are packed in with the surgical instruments, but the blades are packaged by the manufacture to open as needed

(*Continued*)

TABLE 14.1

(Continued)

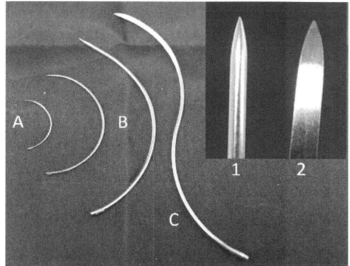

Suture needles
A. Cutting edge – inset 2 close-up

B. Taper – inset 1 close-up

C. Postmortem

Suture needles are either included with the surgical pack or kept in "cold" sterilization trays. The cutting edge needle is used for skin and the taper needle is used for tissues

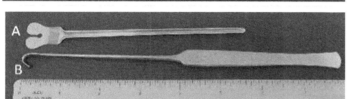

A. Groove director

B. Snook's ovariectomy hook

These are auxiliary instruments and may not be utilized in your clinic. The groove director helps to make a straight incision line and the snook hook is used to find the uterine horn during a spay

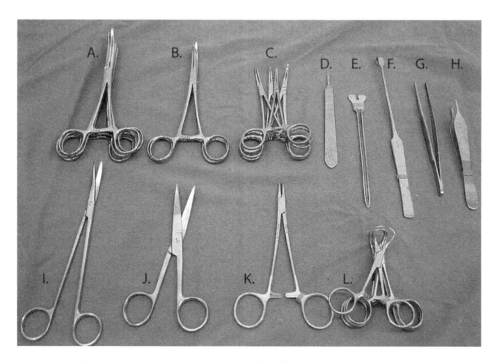

FIGURE 14.13 Instruments to include in an instrument pack. See text for identification.

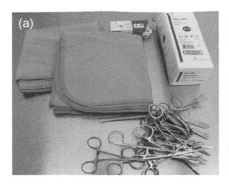
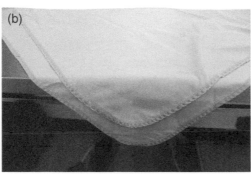
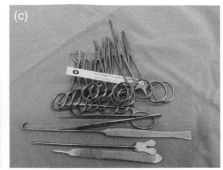

FIGURE 14.14 Steps 1–3 of putting an instrument pack together: (a) Step 1, gather supplies; (b) Step 2, lay out the cloth wraps; (c) Step 3, assemble instruments.

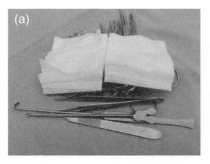
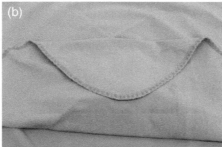
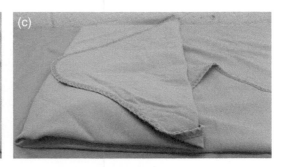

FIGURE 14.15 Steps 4–6 of putting an instrument pack together: (a) Step 4, lay gauze sponges on instruments; (b) Step 5, first fold of wrap; (c) Step 6, second fold with left-hand point.

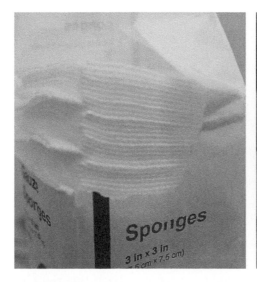
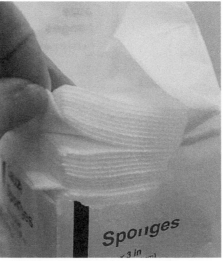

FIGURE 14.16 Sleeve of gauze sponges.

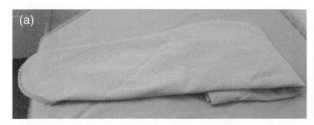
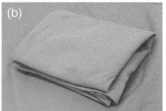

FIGURE 14.17 Step 8 of putting an instrument pack together: (a) finding the folding point; and (b) folding the last point over.

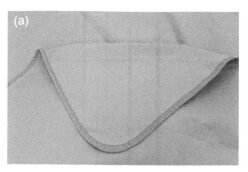
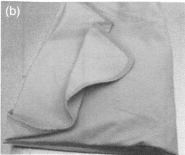
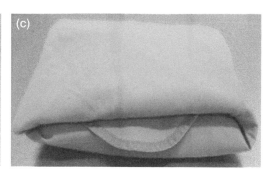

FIGURE 14.18 Step 9 of putting an instrument pack together: (a,b) repeat steps 5–7 to fold the second or bottom wrap; (c) create a tab with the last fold.

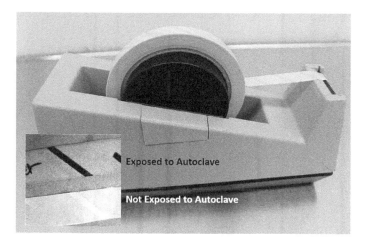

Exposed to Autoclave

Not Exposed to Autoclave

FIGURE 14.19 Autoclave tape. Inset: exposed to autoclave and not exposed to autoclave.

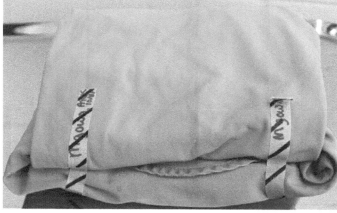

FIGURE 14.20 Autoclaved package showing the autoclave tape turned black.

Step 9 Repeat Steps 5–7 with the second wrap, positioning all of the points so they are pointing to the outside edge (Figure 14.18a,b). This will be important when we open the pack which will be covered later in this chapter. To finish the last point bring it across the entire wrapped package only instead of folding it like in Step 8 the excess material is neatly tucked into folds of this wrap (Figure 14.18c). This holds the pack secure and leaves a tag sticking out which is grasped to start the opening process.

Autoclave tape (Figure 14.19) is then applied to the outer wrap. Autoclave tape is designed to develop black streaks to indicate if a pack has been through the autoclave (Figure 14.19 inset). It is not an indication of sterility. The stripes on the tape turn black when exposed to heat. Tear off 2, 4–5" pieces of tape and bend one end over making a small tab. Then using an ink pen write the date and your initials on one piece and the contents of the pack on the second piece. Apply the tape so the tabs are on top of the last fold. This keeps the fold in place when you are tearing the tape off during the opening process. Figure 14.20 shows an autoclaved pack with the tape in the appropriate

location, note that it has been exposed to the autoclave as the tape has black streaks. It is tempting to use a long piece of tape to make sure the pack stays secure, but if folded as instructed this is unnecessary and wasteful.

Folding a Grown and Wrapping it for Autoclaving

Just like with the instruments, every clinic differs in how they fold their cloth gowns. The following is one way to accomplish this task. To start to fold a gown put it on, making sure you have the right side out. Bring your hands out of the sleeves about 8 inches from the arm pit seam, grasp part of the sleeve, and pull the sleeves inside out (Figure 14.21a). Bring the sleeves together, straighten the arms so they form a circle and straighten the length of the gown, so it is folded in half lengthwise. Make sure the material is smoothed and wrinkle free as going through the autoclave process will make the wrinkles stiff thus making the gown hard to put on.

Step B is folding the gown in half lengthwise one more time (Figure 14.21b). Step C is making the sleeve openings obvious on top of the gown (Figure 14.21c).

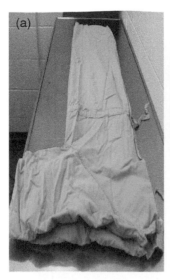
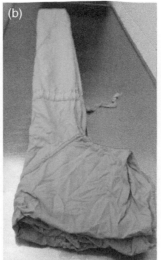
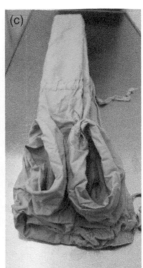

FIGURE 14.21 Steps A–C of folding a gown.

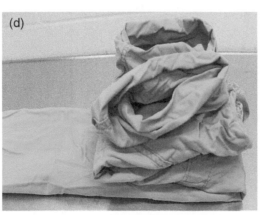
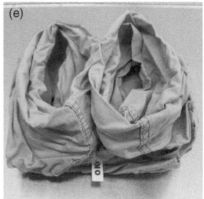

FIGURE 14.22 Steps D and E of folding a gown.

Step D is starting the accordion fold along the length of the gown. Start with the sleeve openings, lift and fold a length of gown under the sleeve layer (Figure 14.22a). Continue until the entire length of the gown is accordion folded under the sleeves as shown in Step E (Figure 14.22b). Insert an autoclave indicator approximately in the middle of the gown material and tuck the ties into the folded gown.

A surgical towel or paper towels are included with the gown. This allows the scrubbed personnel to dry their hands after performing a surgical scrub before putting on the gown. For the steps for folding a surgical towel, see Figure 14.23. Place the towel on top of the sleeves of the folded gown. Gowns are only single wrapped utilizing the technique previously described for the instrument pack (Figure 14.24). Label the tapes with date and initials on one piece and the size of the gown on the other.

Folding a Cloth Drape

Cloth drapes are often used over paper drapes during a surgical procedure. This gives two layers of security and absorption during a surgery. Cloth drapes come with either a rectangle **fenestration** or a circular fenestration. They have to be folded so that the fenestration shows on the bottom of the folded drape. This can be tricky but with a little practice you will achieve this every time. Start by laying the drape out on a table top. The first fold is somewhat of a double fold (Figure 14.25 A.1 and A.2) Grasp the corners with your index fingers and thumbs and pull the cloth over itself so the corners end up pointing out away from the center. A.1 shows the fold completed. A.2 shows the assistant continuing to accordion fold the material until you reach the center of the fenestration. Repeat on the other side of the wrap. Once both sides are folded, start to accordion fold the ends in to meet in the middle of the fenestration (Figure 14.26 B. 1 and B. 2) Note how the folds have almost centered the fenestration on the bottom of the folded drape B.2. As mentioned, paper drapes are often included with the cloth drapes. Most clinics will require four paper drapes folded in accordion style and large enough to cover the chest, sides, and back legs

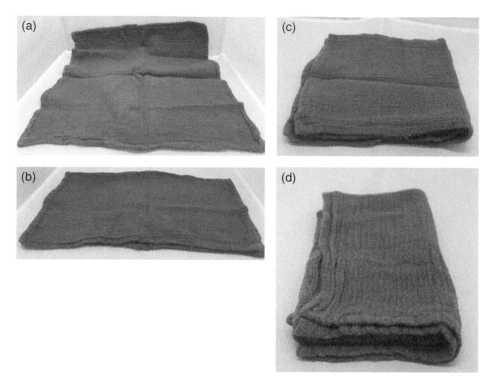

FIGURE 14.23 Folding a surgical towel: (a) Step 1, lay a surgical towel flat; (b) Step 2, fold length-wise; (c,d) Steps 3 and 4, fold in half width-wise.

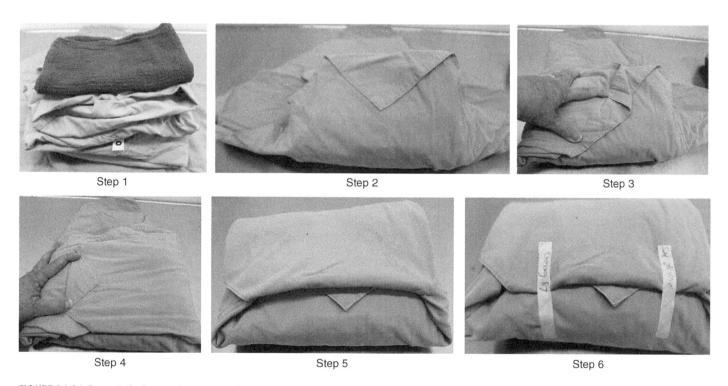

Step 1   Step 2   Step 3

Step 4   Step 5   Step 6

FIGURE 14.24 Steps 1–6 of wrapping a surgical gown.

depending on the size of the cloth drape and the patient (Figure 14.27). Paper drape material usually comes on a large roll so you can match the size of the four paper drapes to the size of the cloth drapes which come in different sizes to accommodate various sized animals. You start by accordion folding the width of the paper drape and then the length until you get an approximate 4 × 4 inch square. Set that one aside and fold the other three the same way. To make a drape pack, set the cloth drape in the middle of a wrap, place a sterilization indicator (Figure 14.28) on top of the cloth drape, and then set the four paper drapes on top. Wrap as demonstrated for

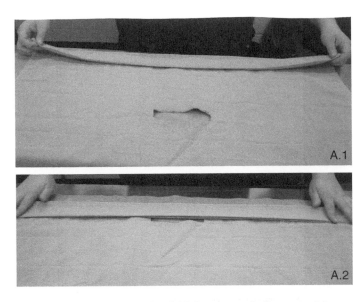

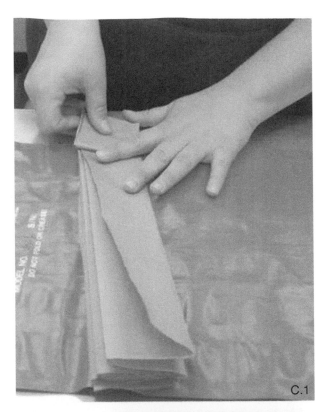

FIGURE 14.25 A.1 and A.2: first folds in a rectangle fenestrated drape.

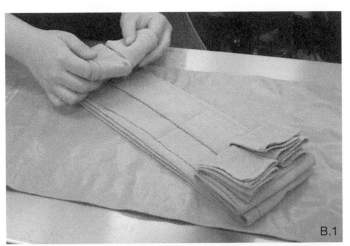

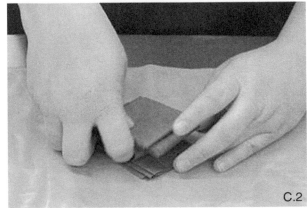

FIGURE 14.27 C.1 and C.2: paper drapes folded accordion style.

the gown. Close with autoclave tape indicating what type and size of drape is inside the pack.

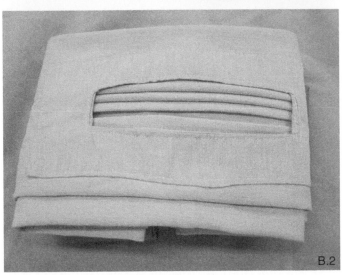

Learning Exercise

Develop a step-by-step protocol for wrapping surgical packs. Complete one for an instrument pack, a gown/towel pack, and a drape pack.

FIGURE 14.26 B.1 and B.2: second folds in a rectangle fenestrated drape.

Ancillary instrument packaging is available in many sizes (Figure 14.29a) They have a see-through side and a solid paper size. They are equipped with their own adhesive tab to secure them closed or you have to bend

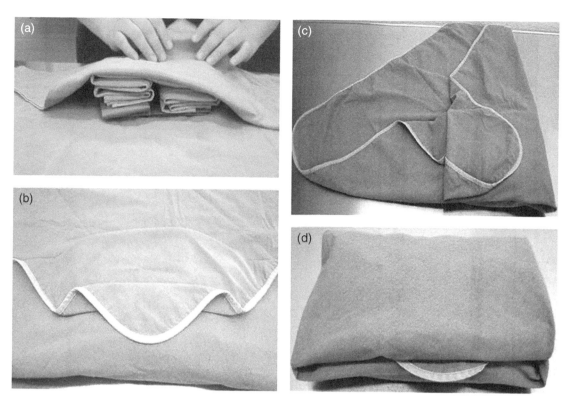

FIGURE 14.28 Wrapping a drape pack.

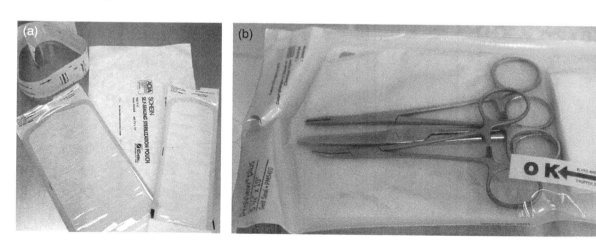

FIGURE 14.29 Ancillary instrument packaging.

the end over and apply a piece of autoclave tape along the entire end. Figure 14.29b shows a small pack of instruments used to neuter cats. Note the autoclave indicator inside the pack; this just as important to include as it is for the cloth wrapped packs. Also note on the left end of Figure 14.29b the tabs located on that end are used to open the pack easily. To open without tearing it randomly first open the two corners a bit. Then, placing both thumbs on each of the tabs, roll your wrists so the paper opens and covers the wrists at the same time. Hold the package steady as the surgeon retrieves the contents.

Once all of the packs are repacked, they need to be run through the autoclave for sterilization. Each autoclave differs in the amount it will hold at a time and the

how long it will take a pack to be sterilized. Consult with an experienced team member for amounts the autoclave will hold and the time requirements. If a new autoclave is purchased, read through the owner's manual for suggested times. Check the times by placing the standardly wrapped packs and running a cycle. Then open the packs and look at the autoclave indicator (Figure 14.30). The indicator at the bottom of Figure 14.30 has been exposed the right amount of time, pressure, and temperature in order for the K and strip to be turned a solid black. The indicator at the top of Figure 14.30 has not been put into the autoclave. Note how dark the O is on this indicator; this is your control. The exposed K and strip should be a solid black like the O after being sent

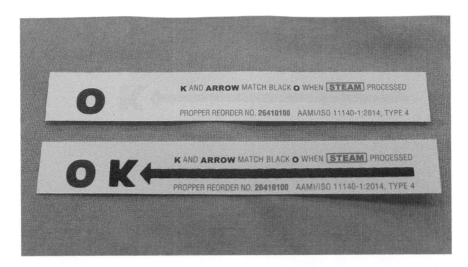

FIGURE 14.30 Autoclave indicator strips.

through the autoclave. The minimum requirement for sterilization is 15 psi of pressure, for 15 minutes at 250°F. Thicker packages will take more time for the pressure and temperature to penetrate to the center of the pack. It will also make a difference if you pack the autoclave tightly. Leaving a bit of space around each pack will ensure that the pressure and temperature get to the center of each item. If your test pack indicators come out lighter in color, you may have to increase the time to achieve sterilization. Remember to place the indicators in the middle of the packs to be sure the entire package has been sterilized.

Reflection

Discuss the differences between autoclave tape and autoclave sterilization indicators, include what they tell you and how they should be used.

Cold Sterilization

Some clinics like to put their sharp instruments, like scissors and needles, into cold sterilization solutions. Some clinics will also use cold sterilization for extra instruments in case one is dropped or contaminated during a surgery. The cold sterilization solutions vary but most are quaternary ammonia compounds and are time sensitive to achieve sterilization, often up to or over 24 hours of exposure. The instruments are cleaned and rinsed in the same manner but are not lubricated. The instruments are then immersed in special containers that have trays that can be lifted out of the solution without touching it with your bare hands (Figure 14.31). This is important as most of these cold sterilization solutions are deactivated by organic material and time. They should be changed out

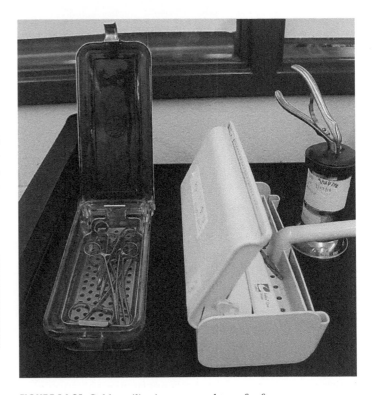

FIGURE 14.31 Cold sterilization trays and transfer forceps.

completely at least once a week and if they are contaminated. In the background of Figure 14.31 you can see a transfer forceps. This allows non-sterile personnel to supply an instrument without touching the solution.

Some clinics may use gas sterilization for items that may be damaged in the autoclave. This method of sterilization utilizes ethylene oxide gas. This is an extremely toxic gas and must be handled with care. Items that are sterilized in this manner need to be "aired" for 12–24 hours before use, so usually they are sterilized well in advance of being required. They too have a type of sterilization indicator and often the individual packaging will have a strip on it that will turn pink when exposed to the gas. There are so many types of gas sterilization chambers that if used in your practice ask for operating instructions from your supervisor.

This concludes your duties for cleaning up after a day's worth of surgeries! It is a lot of work and there are many details to keep straight but with time and experience you will be able to breeze through these important tasks making you a very valuable member of the veterinary health care team!

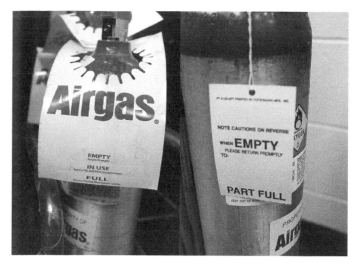

FIGURE 14.32 Oxygen tanks in use and full.

Reflection

Sometimes, cleaning is a "dirty" word. (No pun intended!) As an assistant you are asked to do a lot of cleaning. Why is it so important to clean so carefully in a surgical facility and why should you take pride in doing a good job?

Surgery Skills and Maintaining an Aseptic Environment

Surgical procedures have three phases: pre-surgical, peri-surgical, and post-surgical. Pre-surgical procedures consist of preparing the surgical suite and the patient for surgery. We've talked about the suite in relation to cleaning up after surgeries but now let's discuss the set-up to prepare for surgeries.

Pre-Surgical Phase

The prep room is where the patient is induced with anesthesia, and the surgical site is shaved and scrubbed. Before that occurs, the patient will require a physical exam and blood draw for anesthetic screening tests. Assisting the technician with these tasks could include setting out the required equipment like thermometer, stethoscope, and sample collection equipment. It will also entail restraining the patient for these procedures. Remember, they are going into surgery so *no treats* as a distraction. You'll have to use your voice and gentle pats to calm and distract. Help the technician by verifying that the right patient is being examined for the right surgery!

The order of patients is usually smallest to largest and/or the cleanest to dirtiest procedures; however, emergency surgeries preempt that rotation. So, for example, if you have a cat spay, a medium-sized dog neuter, and an anal gland removal surgery scheduled for the day you would prepare them in that order.

While the tests are being run, the surgical packs can be laid out in the surgery room. The instrument pack

usually goes onto a surgical tray (Figure 14.2) but is not opened yet. A gown and drape pack are usually placed on an ancillary table and opened. Some clinics will want the surgical gloves opened as well, others will wait until after the surgeon is gowned. If OK with the technician, attach the appropriate hoses and bags to the gas anesthesia machine and turn on the oxygen tank if attached to the machine or attach the oxygen hose from the ceiling to the gas machine. This hose is attached to a large oxygen tank that may be kept in another room or part of the hospital. Some clinics never shut them off, but it is a good idea to at least check to make sure there is enough oxygen for the day's surgeries especially in the E sized tanks. E tanks hold only 2000 psi of oxygen (Figure 14.32). These tanks should have an indicator card on them as to which tank is being used. As Figure 14.32 shows, one tag one tank in use and the other is full. When you turn the tank on, look at the oxygen pressure gauge (Figure 14.33, right) to see how much oxygen is left in the "in use" tank. Alert the technician if there is 500 psi or less so he/she can keep an eye on it during surgery. Depending on the size of the patients and the lengths of surgery, that amount may be enough for the day's surgeries. Repeat the process for the gas machine in the prep room.

Once the patients are cleared for surgery the induction phase starts. An anesthesia chart is started with the patient's information and then is placed on a clipboard to record heart rate and respirations as the anesthesia is started (Figure 14.34). The first anesthetic is usually an injection of a sedative/tranquilizer/narcotic "cocktail." Meaning that these drugs are mixed in the same syringe. This may be intramuscular or subcutaneous depending on the mixture and will take 10–20 minutes to take effect. The patient will usually become quite relaxed and may even lie down. It is important to make note of the pulse and respiration before the

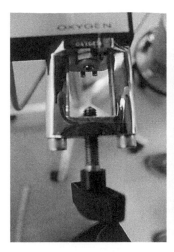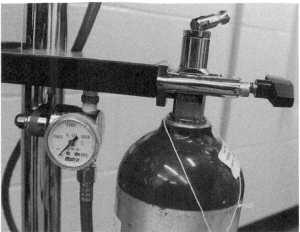

FIGURE 14.33 Left: oxygen tank yoke. Right: oxygen pressure gauge.

injection and then every 5 minutes after the injection on the anesthesia monitoring chart until the patient is moved to the recovery room. Indicate on the chart when the injection was given so the induction agent that follows isn't given too soon. It is during this period that an IV catheter is placed into the cephalic, saphenous, or femoral vein depending upon the species of patient. Be ready to assist the technician by presenting the appropriate leg and occluding the vessel as described in Chapter 8. Once catheterized, the patient will be hooked up to an IV drip set and the fluid rate will either be set manually or via an IV fluid pump as discussed in Chapter 11. The induction agent is given to effect, meaning just enough medication is injected to make the animal slump and offer no resistance to intubation. Depth of anesthesia is checked by utilizing the patient's reflexes. The **palpebral** reflex is evaluated by tapping the fingertip lightly at the **medial canthus** of the eye. If there is a strong blink response, the patient is in a light level of anesthesia and will struggle against intubation. As more induction agent is given, the reflex lessens and finally disappears. The level of anesthesia is sufficient for intubation and prep.

An endotracheal tube is passed through the mouth and into the trachea as demonstrated in Figure 14.35. The assistant's job is to pull the tongue out as far as possible over the incisor teeth and hold the upper jaw up as wide as possible. This makes visualization of the pharynx possible. Once the tube is in place it needs to be secured. There are many methods to do this, Figure 14.36 shows the use of a strip of gauze roll tied onto the tube and then around the upper jaw. Use of a shoe lace tie is appropriate in case the tube has to be untied quickly. Figure 14.36 also shows the cuff being inflated with a syringe. The cuff is inflated until you can hear the patient breath through the tube and not around it. Care must be taken not to over inflate the cuff as it can damage the trachea. The oxygen and

vaporizer settings on the gas anesthetic machine are adjusted for that patient and it is attached to the endotracheal tube via the rebreathing or non-rebreathing hoses (Figure 14.10a-c).

If available, the multifunctional monitor is attached to the patient (Figure 14.37). The respiratory/capnography adapter is attached between the air hose and endotracheal tube. This measures the respirations via a sensor and the capnograph measures the carbon dioxide. The pulse oximeter is attached to the patient to measure the amount of oxygen in the blood and read the heart rate. The clip is attached to the tongue or any place without a lot of hair. The clip has a light that picks up the arterial blood flow and the color of the blood. The flow is recorded as the heart rate reading, the color is the amount of oxygen in the blood. We like to see the oxygen saturation stay about 95% and if it drops the veterinarian should be alerted immediately. Drops in heart rate are important to alert the veterinarian about as well. A guideline to use is to take the resting heart rate and multiply it by 35%. Take that number and subtract it from the resting heart rate for the lowest tolerable limit. For example, a patient's resting heart rate is 75 bpm × .35 = 26. 75 − 26 = 49. The lowest tolerable limit for this patient is 49 bpm.

A blood pressure cuff, applied to any leg that doesn't have a catheter in it, measures blood pressure. The blood pressure cuffs come in a variety of sizes to accommodate small to large companion animals (Figure 14.38). To make sure the fit is right either use the tape measure provided or place the cuff around the leg and see if it can be secured within the arrows indicated on the cuff.

The monitor may also have a thermometer attachment in which case it is inserted into the rectum and using self-adhesive tape secured to the tail. Otherwise, checking the temperature will have to be done with a regular rectal thermometer. Expect the temperature to drop to 99°F in most cases; lower than that and the

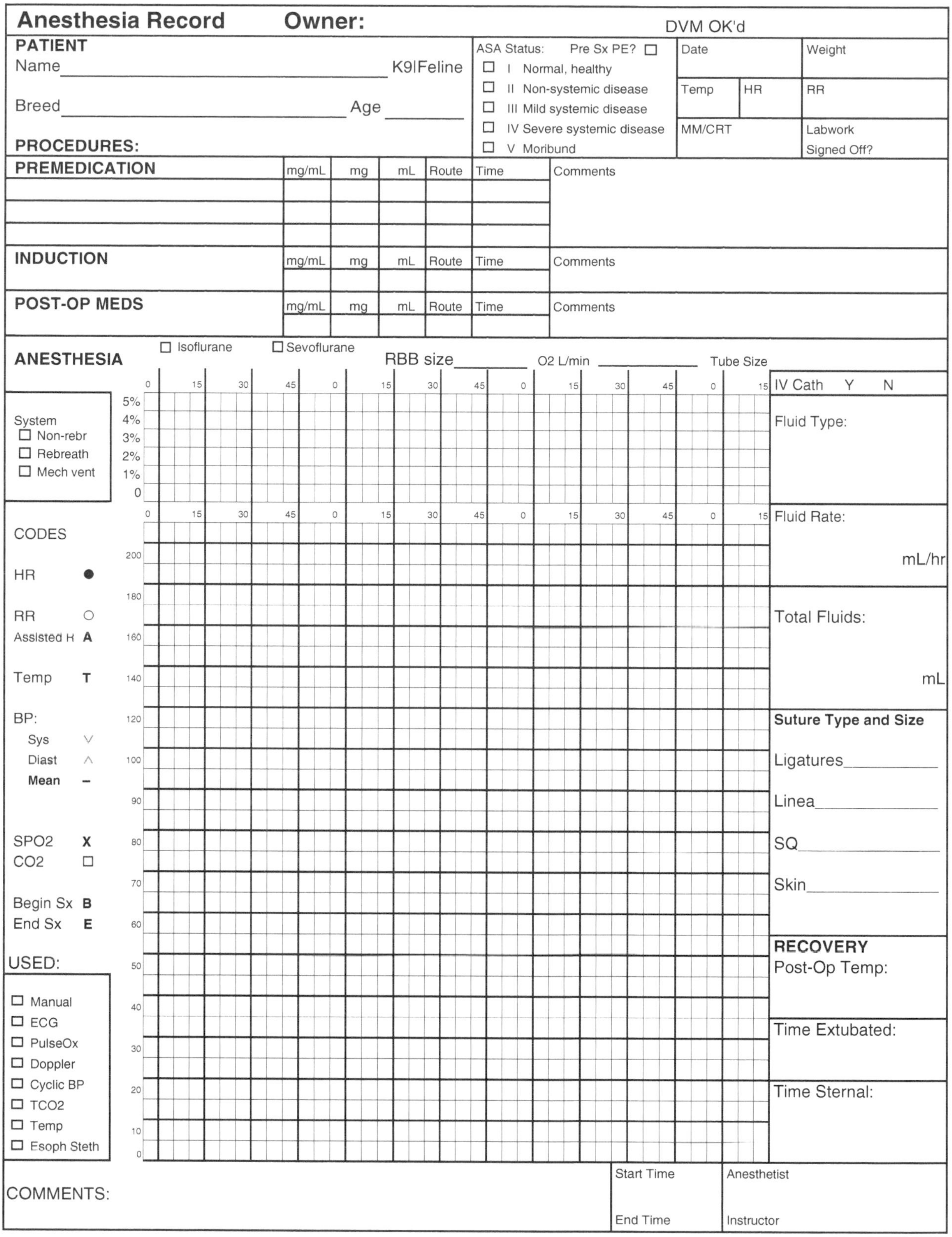

Anesthesia Record **Owner:** DVM OK'd

PATIENT
Name____________ K9|Feline
Breed____________ Age ______
PROCEDURES:

ASA Status: Pre Sx PE? ☐
☐ I Normal, healthy
☐ II Non-systemic disease
☐ III Mild systemic disease
☐ IV Severe systemic disease
☐ V Moribund

Date		Weight
Temp	HR	RR
MM/CRT		Labwork Signed Off?

PREMEDICATION	mg/mL	mg	mL	Route	Time	Comments

INDUCTION	mg/mL	mg	mL	Route	Time	Comments

POST-OP MEDS	mg/mL	mg	mL	Route	Time	Comments

ANESTHESIA ☐ Isoflurane ☐ Sevoflurane RBB size________ O2 L/min ________ Tube Size

0 15 30 45 0 15 30 45 0 15 30 45 0 15

5% 4% 3% 2% 1% 0

System
☐ Non-rebr
☐ Rebreath
☐ Mech vent

IV Cath Y N
Fluid Type:

0 15 30 45 0 15 30 45 0 15 30 45 0 15

200 180 160 140 120 100 90 80 70 60 50 40 30 20 10 0

CODES
HR ●
RR ○
Assisted R **A**
Temp **T**
BP:
Sys ∨
Diast ∧
Mean –
SPO2 **X**
CO2 ☐
Begin Sx **B**
End Sx **E**

USED:
☐ Manual
☐ ECG
☐ PulseOx
☐ Doppler
☐ Cyclic BP
☐ TCO2
☐ Temp
☐ Esoph Steth

Fluid Rate: mL/hr
Total Fluids: mL
Suture Type and Size
Ligatures__________
Linea__________
SQ__________
Skin__________
RECOVERY
Post-Op Temp:
Time Extubated:
Time Sternal:

COMMENTS:

Start Time	Anesthetist
End Time	Instructor

FIGURE 14.34 Anesthesia monitoring chart.

patient should be warmed. Warm water bottles or hot towels can be wrapped around the legs of the patient or around the IV fluid bag attached to the catheter. Both of these will help warm the patient.

The patient is then placed in a position for shaving and prepping the surgical site. This will vary depending on the surgery. Table 14.2 lists the frequently performed surgical procedures and the position required for preparation of the surgical site and the surgery. If you are asked to shave the hair from the surgical area, find out where the incision will be. Shave out an area of 6-8 inches around the incision. If the patient has a limb fracture, the entire leg is shaved. Vacuum as you go or throw the big clumps of hair into the garbage so as not to plug the vacuum. Once the hair is shaved, vacuum all over again, paying attention to the hair that may have gotten caught under the animal and the hair that is on your lab coat or scrub top. You may have to use a roller tape wand to get it all off or you may need to change scrub tops. It is imperative that hair not fall into the scrubbed area on the patient while scrubbing or while moving the patient to the surgery room.

To reduce the chance of contaminating a surgical field or zone, proper dress in the surgical suite includes clean scrubs free of loose hair. Three-quarter to short sleeves to reduce the chance of dragging them across a sterile field. Caps are worn over the hair with long hair tied back or pinned up to avoid it falling out of the cap and into a sterile field (Figure 14.39). Additional PPE include a mask to capture saliva and potential sneezes or coughs, booties worn over the shoes so that hair, dirt, and debris are not dragged into the super clean surgery room. Men with beards will need a beard mask to cover the facial hair. These need to be in place before the

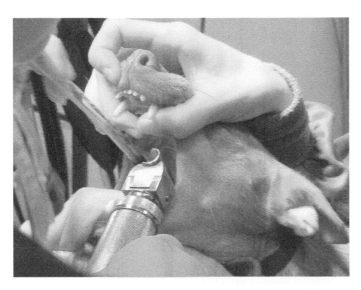

FIGURE 14.35 Insertion of the endotracheal tube.

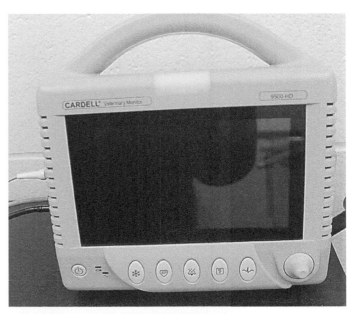

FIGURE 14.37 Multifunctional monitor.

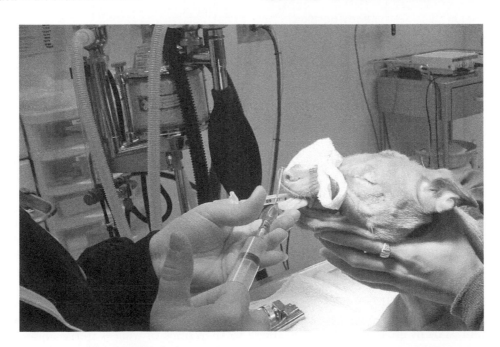

FIGURE 14.36 Secured endotracheal tube and cuff inflation.

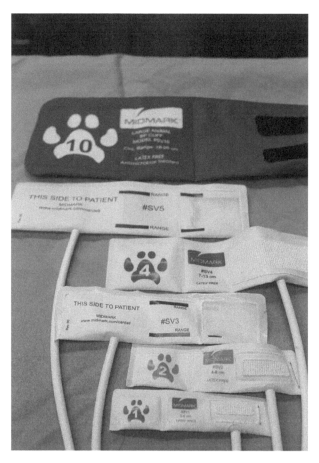

FIGURE 14.38 Blood pressure cuffs.

TABLE 14.2

Frequent Surgical Procedures and Body Position Required for the Procedure

Surgery – with definition	Body position
Ovariohysterectomy – removal of the entire reproductive tract Common name – spay	Ventral – dorsal
Orchidectomy – removal of testicles Common name – neuter or castration	Ventral – dorsal
Pyometra – infection of the uterus Common name – pyo	Ventral – dorsal
Caesarean section – removal of fetuses because of dystocia issues Common name – C-section	Ventral – dorsal
Tail docking – dewclaw removal	Held however it works for surgeon
Onychectomy – removal of distal phalanges Common name – declaw	Lateral recumbency

patient is scrubbed for surgery and before the surgical personnel scrubs for surgery.

To scrub the patient, start by grasping a corner of the gauze sponge soaked in either povidone iodine or in chlorhexidine surgical scrub with index finger and thumb. Bring the other three corners up to the fingers until you have all four between index finger and thumb (Figure 14.40). This will keep your fingers from contacting the patient's skin as you scrub.

Start the scrub over the incision site, scrubbing the gauze over the area in a back and forth pattern for a total of 7–10 times. Then work out overlapping the area scrubbed by a 25–75% ratio: 25% previously scrubbed area with a 75% covering new areas. Most patterns end up being in a rectangle shape especially on the abdomen but not always. Continue to scrub the entire shaved area. This is creating a sterile field and we now have to be careful not to reach across this area or to touch it with anything that is not sterile. Rinse the scrubbed area with either a spray hose set on gentle or with sterile water-soaked gauze sponges working from the incision site outward. Use more than one gauze sponge if you need to in order to remove the surgical scrub from the skin. Repeat this scrub two more times. Then either spray or wipe the surgical area with alcohol.

Peri-Surgical Phase

At this point the patient is moved to the surgery room. Extreme care is taken; to not contaminate the scrubbed surgical site, to keep the patient as level as possible, and not to lose the endotracheal tube! This usually requires two people and if the patient is large the use of a gurney is recommended. The patient is transferred to the surgical table and secured to it with ropes. The ropes are placed upon the limbs using the loop formed by the rope and then a half hitch further down on the leg (see Figure 9.35). The rope is then brought either over the edge or over the end of the table and secured to a cleat (see Figure 9.36) or if there are pinch levers the rope is brought between the rubber stoppers (Figure 14.1d). Once the patient is secured to the table, the surgical site is either sprayed with povidone iodine solution or it is swabbed on with sterile gauze sponges held by a sponge holder.

The surgical lights are turned on and adjusted to shine on the surgical site. The surgical table can be raised or lowered by turning the handle on the base and stepping on the foot pedal (Figure 14.1b). Step and press down to lower, and pump the step to raise the table. Extreme care must be taken not to touch or reach over the surgical site because this is our first sterile field. In the surgical environment, sterile objects must remain sterile and surgical sites and personnel must remain "clean" whereas objects that are no longer or never have been sterile are considered contaminated or "dirty." These two things must not connect in any way. In order to keep track of what is sterile and what is clean, sterile fields and zones are established.

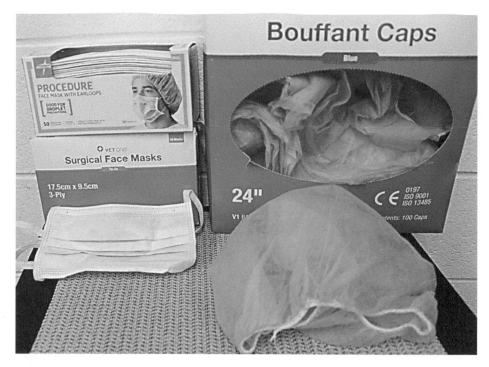

FIGURE 14.39 Surgical caps and masks.

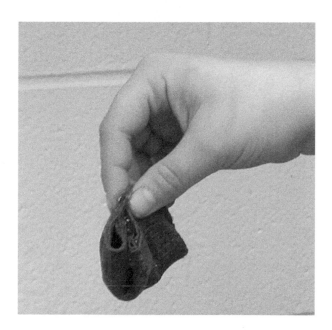

FIGURE 14.40 Holding a gauze sponge for a surgical scrub.

A sterile field is a single area that is prepared aseptically like the surgical prep on a patient and a surgeon's scrubbed hands. We consider these two fields as being "sterile", but they aren't really, because that would actually destroy the tissues, but they are very clean! The sterilized packs, gloves, and suture material are devoid of organic material and so are truly sterile since they were autoclaved. Each of these items are also considered sterile fields. So, we avoid reaching across, brushing against, or touching these fields with bare hands, scrub tops, sleeves, and so on, in order to avoid contaminating

them. Careful movement within the surgery room is vital. Always face any sterile field or zone. Never walk between sterile fields. Keep conversations to a minimum.

When the fields are brought together in the surgical suite, we create sterile zones. For example, when the gloved, gowned, masked surgeon steps up to the prepared patient on the surgery table and proceeds to drape the patient, and pull the surgical pack into reach he/she has created a sterile zone. The sterile zone is even larger than just the physical packs, patient, and surgeon, it extends from the shoulders of the veterinarian down to the draped patient on the surgery table, and the entire length of the draped patient to the open surgery pack. Along with taking care not to touch, reach across, or brush anything in the sterile zone, now we have to be careful not to come between the parts of the sterile zone!

If any sterile field or even a part of a sterile zone is compromised, everything is considered contaminated and must be discarded or re-scrubbed. Even if there is a doubt of contamination it is best to consider it contaminated and switch it out.

The reason for all of this great care is when the integrity of the skin is compromised, which occurs from the incision. This opens a door for contaminants to enter easily. Nosocomial infections occur during surgical procedures because of a break in the sterile fields or zones. These are often staphylococcus or streptococcus bacterial infections that are very difficult to treat and can seriously jeopardize the health and well-being of the patient.

At this point the surgeon is notified there is a patient on the table, and she/he will start their scrub. If there was time, laying out their cap, mask, and booties as well

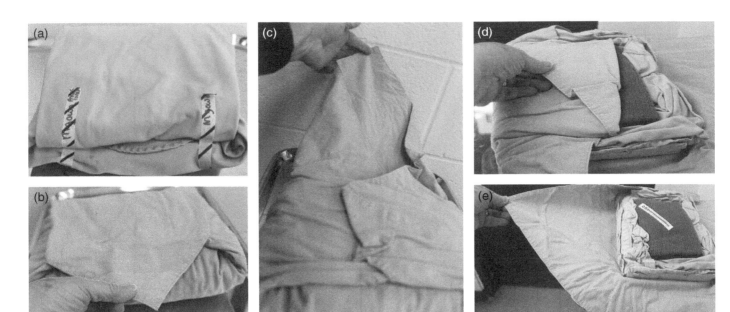

FIGURE 14.41 Opening a surgical pack.

as a sterilized scrub brush will be appreciated. Meanwhile, the surgical packs can be opened. Great care is needed again to not touch or reach across the sterile fields of the open packs. Figure 14.41a–e are the steps to aseptically open surgical packs. Remove the autoclave tape completely from the pack (Figure 14.41a). Either ball it up and put it in your pocket or stick it to your hip, to be thrown away later. If you stick on yourself make sure to do it low enough so that it doesn't fall onto a sterile field. Grasp the cloth tab (Figure 14.41b) on the pack and pull, until it comes completely out of the fold, then swing your arm back to open that fold all the way (Figure 14.41c). Now the reason for making sure the corners of the wraps point out becomes apparent (Figure 14.41d) as they are clearly visible, and your bare hand is as far from the center of the pack as possible. Pinch or pick the corner up on the very point between index finger and thumb and open that fold all the way. Continue until the entire pack has been open. As you can see this was a gown pack, folded neatly with a towel on top but there is a problem with this pack. Can you spot the issue? Should the sterilization indicator be on top of the material (Figure 14.41e)? No, it needs to be in the middle of all that fabric! We don't know if this pack was truly sterile all the way through, so it needs to be changed out for a different one that has the indicator in the correct location. *When in doubt consider an item contaminated!* Open the surgical pack but just the outer most wrap. *Do not* touch or open the inside wrap. That is for the scrubbed, gowned, and gloved surgeon to open. This is to prevent any chance that the instruments used on the inside of the patient are contaminated.

Auxiliary packs are opened upon request of the surgeon (Figure 14.42). This includes gloves, suture

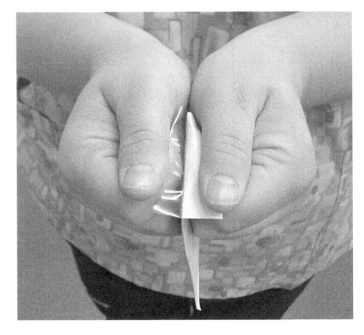

FIGURE 14.42 Opening an auxiliary pack.

material, scalpel blades, and the individually packed instruments in the auxiliary packaging. They are opened by placing both thumbs along the flaps and rolling your hands apart. Don't abruptly tear the flaps apart as the material inside may go flying! Neither should you rip the packaging haphazardly causing a potential for contamination.

Suture packs and scalpel blades are prepackaged and require a bit of skill to determine what it is the surgeon requires. If you know what to look for it is easy enough. In Figure 14.43 there are two kinds of suture material in different sizes and a box of scalpel blades. Note the

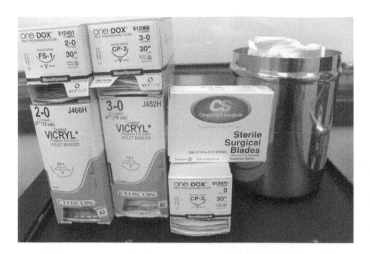

FIGURE 14.43 Suture material and scalpel blades.

names on the suture material: Vicryl™ is the brand name for polyglactin suture and the One-Dox™ is the brand name of polydioxanone suture material. The veterinarian will often ask for them as Vicryl or "Dox" even if the inventory manager ordered the generic suture. So, it's a good idea to ask and then remember which is which! Note too that the size is written in big letters as 2-O or 3-O, the O is pronounced "ought" and the larger the number the smaller in diameter the suture. Note also that each box shows the size and type of suture needle. Most of the time this isn't an issue but every once in a while the surgeon will ask if there are any taper point or cutting-edge needles. In this case there are no taper point suture needles. The box of scalpel blades will indicate the type of blade on the end of the box. Each one of these items is individually packed and are opened on an as needed basis.

During the surgery or the peri-surgical phase, the patient is monitored not only with the multifunctional monitor, but also with manual heart rate and respiratory checks. The heart rate can be taken by slipping a stethoscope under the drapes, taking care not to touch the top of the drape material. The respirations can be taken by watching the non-rebreathing bag or rebreathing bag move in and out (Figure 14.44).

You may also be asked to adjust the flowmeters and the vaporizer during surgery. Find those parts on Figure 14.44. The flowmeter is adjusted if the patient is not getting the right amount of oxygen and the vaporizer is adjust if the patient is not getting the right amount of gas anesthetic.

Another action that may be under taken by the assistant is the application of a drop of surgical glue (Figure 14.45)! This adhesive is specifically engineered to adhere to skin and not cause a reaction. Open the bottle and place a new tip on the top of the container. Many come with multiple tips so the bottle can be used for multiple patients. The surgeon will be holding the tissues he/she wants the glue applied to. Come along

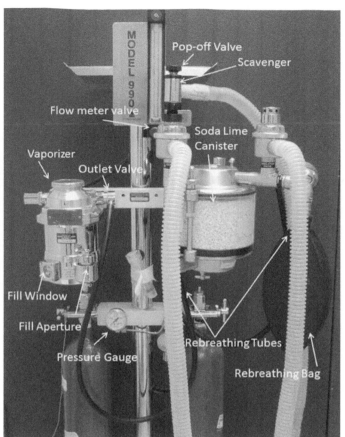

FIGURE 14.44 Gas anesthesia machine.

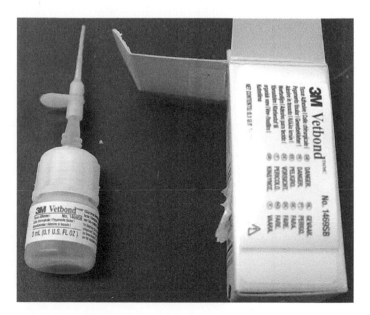

FIGURE 14.45 Tissue adhesive.

side of him/her, but don't touch him/her or the draped patient with any part of your body! Carefully move the tip of the glue close to but not touching the tissue and give a gentle squeeze to dispense a single drop. Then step away from the sterile zone.

Post-Surgical Phase

When the last suture is in place the post-surgical phase is started in the surgery room and finished in the recovery room where the patient wakes up from anesthesia. Veterinary assistants have a vital role in aiding the veterinarian and technician during this phase. The patient is disconnected from the gas anesthesia machine, but the endotracheal tube is left in place. This is to make sure the patient maintains an open airway until fully awake. Pulling a tube too early runs the risk of aspiration pneumonia if the patient should vomit during recovery and inhale the vomitus. The monitoring equipment is usually removed, and the patient is transported to a recovery kennel or run. Make sure to keep the patient's body level as it is transported. This helps to maintain good blood pressure throughout the body.

The kennel and run should have a warming device (see Figure 10.2) and layers of warm blankets either from a towel warmer (Figure 14.46) or from the dryer. Patients lose body heat under anesthesia and if very cold do not recover from anesthesia quickly. Take the body temperature and if the temperature is below 97°F the warm towels are added to the heat blanket and need to be changed out until the patient's temperature is up to 100°F. This can take a long while so if possible get the patient up and moving to help the blood circulate and warm them up.

Someone is required to be with the patient at all times until it swallows, at which point the endotracheal tube can be removed. To remove the tube, deflate the cuff and position the ties that secure the tube to the patient over the incisors. This keeps them from getting hung up on the canine teeth. Watch for a big swallow and then gently pull the tube out. Don't pull the tube out with an inflated cuff as it can cause damage to the trachea! If a tube is left in place and the patient not watched the chances of it chewing the tube apart is great which in turn can cause the patient to suffocate.

The IV catheter is removed once the animal is sternal or standing. A pressure bandage is put over the insertion point for 2–5 minutes and then removed. Then an hourly check on the patient throughout the morning is appropriate. Watch for any vomiting, inability to move or switch positions, and for evidence of pain. Watch for excessive vocalizing, paddling, or thrashing as this is an indication of a rough recovery. Alert the veterinarian or technician if you see this behavior or if you see the patient hunched, whimpering, shivering, or curled in a tight ball. All of these things can indicate the patient is in pain. Follow the orders written for delivery of pain medications and other treatments.

Water is usually offered once the patient is standing. Remember too that IV fluids will filter to the bladder and so a short walk outside to relieve themselves will be appreciated. If the patient can't walk by itself two people may have to carry it outside if it is a bigger patient. If the patient is not to be moved, make sure to provide a raised mat in the kennel or make sure the bed in the run is uphill from the drain. Then point the appropriate body part so the urine can run downhill. If the patient is staying overnight a quarter of the normal volume of food is offered. If accepted and no vomiting occurs after 10–15 minutes the remainder of the food can be offered. Make sure to record all medications and interactions with the patient in the patient's record.

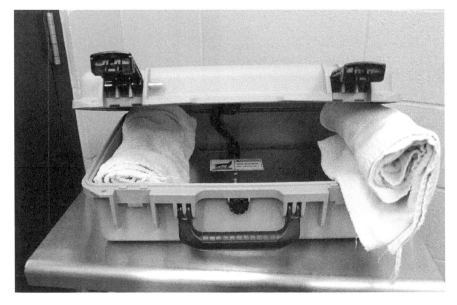

FIGURE 14.46 Towel warmer.

Post-Surgical Emergencies

Good communication with all the team members is essential as you move through the steps it takes to prepare for a surgery.

Anesthetic complications can occur in the recovery phase just as quickly as during the other phases of surgery. Patients can become unable to oxygenate and develop **hypoxemia** when the oxygen is discontinued, or the endotracheal tube is removed, and the airway isn't patent. The mucous membrane color will darken and eventually turn blue if the patient isn't re-intubated and oxygen supplied. Oxygen can come from an ambu bag (see Figure 4.17, upper right corner) or from an oxygen tank. Yell for help as full CPR may be required.

Hypotension is often brought on by a loss of blood causing a drop in blood pressure. This is usually caught while the patient is still in surgery and treated by increasing the volume of IV fluids or administration of blood products. The treatment usually extends into the post-surgical recovery period. Blood pressure cuffs and perfusion parameters like mucous membrane color and capillary refill times are used to monitor the patient.

Cardiac arrhythmia or cardiac arrest can occur and go unnoticed during the recovery period if the heart isn't auscultated regularly. Abnormal heart sounds, arrhythmias, irregular pulse, loss of pulse, and very slow or very fast heart rates must be reported immediately as these can indicate heart failure.

Incision site dehiscence is when the sutures have let go either in the muscle layer or skin layer. This is an extreme emergency and the veterinarian needs to be alerted immediately. Internal bleeding can also occur if a sutured blood vessel leaks. Pale mucous membranes and slow capillary refill are signs of bleeding. Sometimes a large bruise will show around the incision site. Again, alerting the veterinarian if these signs are noted is important.

Once all the surgeries are completed for the day it is time to put the surgery suite in order once more!

Client Communication

Review postoperative patient care with clients. Home care will often determine how well the animal heals. Owners will need complete and understandable instructions in order to help their pet's recovery. Go over the discharge instructions as per the protocols established at your practice. This should be done in a manner that is friendly so as to invite questions and knowledgeably to garner confidence. The highlights of most surgical discharge instructions are pain medications, incision care, exercise restrictions, and when to call the clinic if trouble should arise. A follow-up call the day after discharge will help the patient by catching anything that may be amiss early.

Removing Sutures

The usual incision closure is a buried suture technique using absorbable suture material that does not require removal as the body will absorb it. On occasion, external sutures are placed and the suture material is non-absorbable and must be removed 7–10 days after the surgery. There are two types of suture material used in veterinary medicine: synthetic or natural fibers much like thread or stainless-steel staples. Staples are removed using a special type of removal clip that is slid under the center of the staple and squeezed (Table 14.3). This flares or springs the staples out so they can be "unhooked" from the skin. The "thread-like" suture material can be removed with a small scissors or a specially designed suture removal scissors. One of the scissor blades has a hook that can be slipped under one side of the knot and then closed to cut the suture. Pull on the knot to remove the suture completely. Never cut both sides of the knot as it will leave a half-moon piece of suture inside the patient.

Suture removal appointments are made the day the patient is discharged. The veterinary will evaluate the patient upon arrival and either take the sutures out himself/herself or ask the veterinary technician to do so. The assistant's job at this point is to restrain and distract the patient for the procedure. This is usually painless although some animal may still be a bit sore and it can aggravate the area. Be prepared to keep the patient from biting or scratching.

Some clinics may have these pieces of equipment and other may not. The explanation is included in Table 14.3.

TABLE 14.3

Ancillary Equipment and Instruments

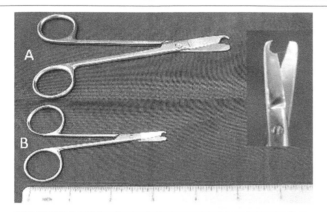

Suture removal scissors
A. Littauer
B. Delicate
The curve in one blade allows it to be slipped under a strand of suture and cut for removal.

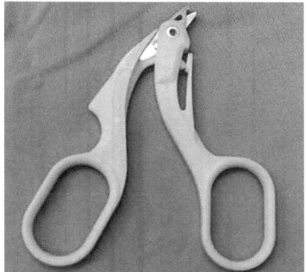

Metal suture removing scissor
One jaw is slipped under the metal suture right in the middle and the handles are squeezed which pries the staple ends apart for easy removal

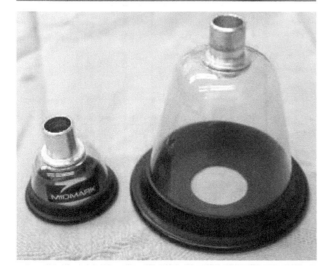

Face masks for "gassing" a patient down or delivering oxygen
On occasion the pre-anesthetics or the induction agent doesn't work on a patient and they need a touch of gas to put them down enough in order to be intubated. PPE for this is a respirator.

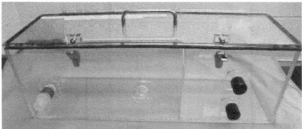

Anesthesia chamber is utilized for "gassing" pocket pets and feral animals down enough in order to be intubated. PPE for this is a respirator

Chapter Reflection

What scares you the most about surgery and anesthesia? How can you take steps to do the best job you can during a surgical procedure?

Reference

Sawyer D. 2016. Best practices for soda lime replacement in veterinary anesthesia machines. https://www.midmark.com/animal-health/resource-library/blog/best-practices-for-soda-lime-replacement-in-veterinary-anesthesia-machines (accessed July 7, 2019).Table 3.3

CHAPTER 15

Dental Skills for the Veterinary Assistant

LEARNING OBJECTIVES

- Provide essential dental education to clients
- Identify and maintain all dental instruments and equipment
- Identify basic tooth anatomy and utilize directional terminology
- Identify each tooth using Triadan or anatomical numbering system
- Assist with dental prophylaxis by charting oral examination
- Identify head types of dogs and cats
- Determine approximate eruption age from dentition
- Recite dental formulas for juvenile and adult dogs and cats, and pocket pets
- Develop and file dental films
- Conduct a thorough dental discharge appointment

Assistant's Role in Veterinary Dentistry

Oral disease is one of the most prevalent diseases in dogs and cats. Eighty percent of adult dogs and 70% of adult cats have some form of oral disease. Dental problems are one of the top three pet concerns among owners, with calculus and gingivitis the most common conditions diagnosed by veterinarians regardless of the age of the animal. The veterinary assistant has a vital role in veterinary dentistry. Dental cleaning, charting, instrument care, and client education falls on the shoulders of the veterinary technician and assistant. Dental care is an important part of patient care.

Dental Anatomy

A basic understanding of dental anatomy is important when assisting with charting, cleaning, and client education. Figure 15.1 shows the exterior and interior of the tooth. The bulk of the mature tooth is composed of dentin. The portion of the tooth above the gumline is covered by enamel and is called the crown. Behind the gum tissue is the neck of the tooth, and below the gumline the dentin is covered by a layer of cementum. Cementum helps to hold the tooth in the socket. In the center of the tooth is the pulp chamber. The pulp chamber contains the blood supply and nerve system for the tooth. The tooth is held in place in the jaw by the periodontium. The periodontium consists of the

Tasks for the Veterinary Assistant, Fourth Edition. Teresa F. Sonsthagen.
© 2020 John Wiley & Sons, Inc. Published 2020 by John Wiley & Sons, Inc.
Companion website: www.wiley.com/go/sonsthagen/tasks

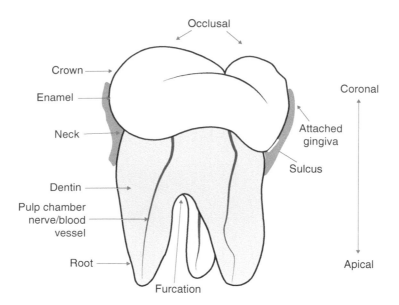

FIGURE 15.1 Tooth anatomy.

gingiva, the periodontal ligament (not shown), and the alveolar bone (not shown).

Teeth have different numbers of roots and it is important to know this when assisting with tooth removal. In dogs, the incisors, canine, first premolar, and the mandibular third molar have one root. The maxillary second and third premolars and the mandibular second, third, fourth premolars, and the first and second molars have two roots. The maxillary fourth premolar, first and second molar have three roots.

The cat has one root on the incisors, canine, maxillary second premolar, and maxillary first molar. The maxillary third premolar and the mandibular third and fourth premolar, and first molar have two roots. The maxillary fourth premolar is the only three rooted teeth in the cat.

Dental Terminology

The following terms are commonly used in veterinary dentistry. A complete list is available at the American Veterinary Dental College website at www.avdc.org:

CEJ – cemento-enamel junction
Coronal – crown
Furcation – area where roots join
Gingiva – gum tissue
Inflammation – swelling, redness, infection
Interproximal – between teeth
Mandible – lower jaw
Maxilla – upper jaw
Occlusion – the way teeth fit together
Recession – loss of gingival tissue
Subgingival – below gingiva
Sulcus – area between free gingiva and tooth
Supragingival – above gingiva.

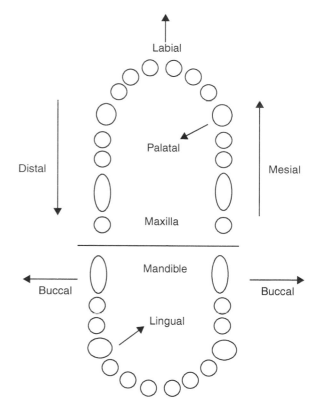

FIGURE 15.2 Directional terms.

Directional Terms

Each surface of the tooth is designated by name. These terms are used for direction and charting of lesions (Figures 15.1 and 15.2):

Apical – toward apex of the root
Buccal – toward the lips
Coronal – toward the crown or top of the tooth

Distal – the surface away from the midline
Gingival – toward the gingiva
Lingual – toward the tongue on the mandible
Mesial – the surface facing the medial incisor, toward the midline
Occlusal – chewing surface
Palatal – toward the tongue on the maxilla.

Dental Formulas

Dental formulas are another means of remembering how many teeth a dog or cat has and in what number. A capital letter is used to designate **I**ncisors, **C**anines, **P**remolars, **M**olars. The numbers separated by a / indicate the number of each type of tooth on the maxilla and mandible, respectively. For example, 2/3M indicates there are two molars in the maxilla and three in the mandible. The 2x refers to the left and right side of the mouth.

Adult dog 2x(3/3I, 1/1C, 4/4P, 2/3M) = 42
Puppies 2x(3/3i, 1/1c, 3/3p,) = 28
Adult cats 2x(3/3I, 1/1C, 3/2P, 1/1M) = 30
Kittens 2x(3/3i, 1/1c, 3/2p) = 26.

Age Approximation Based on Dental Eruption

Age can be estimated by dental eruption. In dogs, the deciduous (primary) canine teeth begin to erupt at 3–4 weeks of age. By 4–6 weeks the deciduous incisors and premolars begin to erupt. By 8 weeks all deciduous teeth are erupted. At 4–5 months the permanent incisors, some premolars, and molars begin erupting. Permanent canines begin to erupt at approximately 5 months. All permanent teeth should be in place by 6 months of age.

In cats, the deciduous incisors begin to come in at 2–4 weeks followed by the deciduous canines at 3–4 weeks. Deciduous premolars begin to erupt in the lower jaw at 4–6 weeks of age. All deciduous teeth are in place by 8 weeks. At 3–4 months the permanent incisors begin coming in. The permanent canines, premolars, and molars begin to erupt at 4–5 months. All permanent teeth should be in by 6 months of age.

Head Type

The head type of each patient should be recorded on the chart as it can affect the number of teeth found. The head type can be indicative of dental problems. Brachycephalic animals have a shortened maxilla and longer mandible. Classic examples are Bulldogs and Persian cats. In mesocephalic animals with medium-length muzzles, both

maxilla and mandible are the same length and will have a scissor bite where the top incisors slide in front of the lower or they have a level bite where the incisors meet crown to crown. Classic examples are Labradors and most breeds of cats. Dichocephalic animals will have very long muzzles with the same bites as the mesocephalic dogs. Classic examples are Dachshunds, Afghan Hounds, and Siamese cats.

Learning Exercise

Produce a dental reference section in your reference book. Utilize a picture of the dental arcades of dogs and cats from the internet. Mark directional terms, dental anatomy, and terminology. Make a note of the dental formulas as well. Select pictures from the internet that depict the various head shapes and add those to your book.

Dental Instruments, Equipment, and Maintenance

Being able to identify and maintain dental instruments and equipment is of great value to the practice. Commonly used hand instruments include a periodontal probe, explorer, scaler, curette, and mirror (Figure 15.3).

From left to right the instruments in the dental kit in Figure 15.3:

- *Mirror* – helps visualize the surfaces of the hard to reach teeth.
- *Periodontal explorer/probe* – the explorer is usually in the shape of a shepherd hook and is used to determine problems on the tooth surface. The explorer is very sharp and should never be used below the gum line. The dental probe end at the top of the instrument is used during the oral examination to measure the sulcus depth of the periodontal tissues surrounding each tooth.
- *Curettes* – the next two instruments in the kit with the yellow and orange colored handles. They have two ends with blunted tips. See Figure 15.4 for a close-up of the curette tip. The curette is designed to remove calculus and debris from under the gingiva. The blunted tip protects the gingival tissues from laceration.
- *Scalers* are the last three instruments; each has two sharp ends and tips that are angled to fit the tooth surfaces. The scaler is used to remove calculus (tartar) from the tooth surface. Due to the sharp tip, the scaler cannot be used below the gum line as it can

cause lacerations. The scaler should always be held with a modified pen grasp and used in a rocking motion from the gum line to the crown of the tooth. See Figure 15.4 for a close-up of the scaler tip.

- *Tartar removal forceps* – used to crack the heavy tartar buildup from the surface of teeth (Figure 15.3, bottom).

Luxators cut or weaken the periodontal ligament that holds the tooth in the alveolar bone. They have a thinner working end and should not be used to leverage a tooth out as they may break (Figure 15.5, upper three instruments). Elevators have a thicker working end and are used to break down the ligament as well as leverage a tooth out of the alveolar bone (Figure 15.5, lower two instruments).

The tooth splitter is the first instrument on the left in Figure 15.6. It is used to help split a tooth if it needs to come out in pieces. Extraction forceps are the other instruments in Figure 15.6 and they are used to remove the tooth from the bone after it is completely elevated.

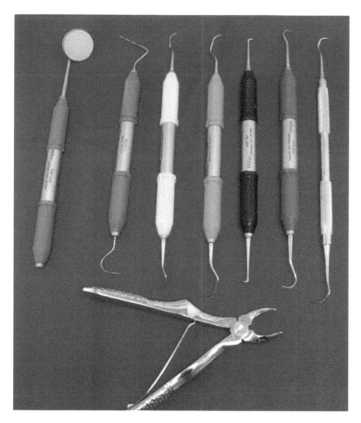

FIGURE 15.3 Dental hand instrument kit.

Learning Exercise

Look carefully at each instrument and notice length, size, curvature of heads, or jaws. What little differences are there to help you learn which instrument is which? Take pictures and perhaps put those in your refence book.

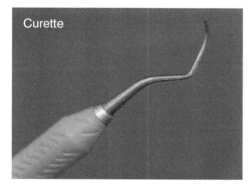
Curette

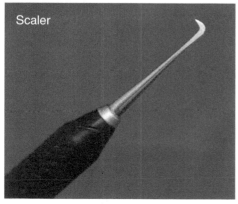
Scaler

FIGURE 15.4 Curette and scaler: close-up of tips.

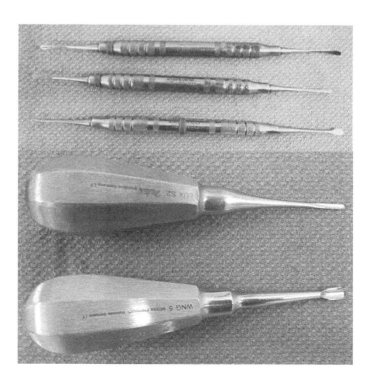

FIGURE 15.5 Luxators and elevators.

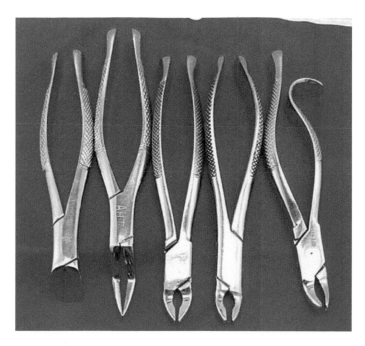

FIGURE 15.6 Tooth splitter and extraction forceps – left to right: incisor/canine, premolar, molar.

Preparation of Dental Instruments

Dental instruments that would be used together can be packaged together in autoclavable pouches or in trays. For example, an oral examination package would include the scaler, curettes, periodontal explorer, probe, tartar removal forceps, and mirror. An extraction package or tray would include the luxator, elevators, and extraction forceps. A periosteal elevator, needle holders, and scissor would be packaged separately as would packets of gauze sponges. These instruments are put into the autoclave with a sterilization indicator and generally, because they are not thick, will sterilize at the minimum setting of 15 psi, 15 minutes at 250°F.

Sharpening Hand Instruments

Sharp instruments can make the dental cleaning more efficient, because they reduce fatigue, improve calculus removal, and save time. A veterinary assistant should learn how to sharpen hand instruments properly. To check an instrument for sharpness, a hard-plastic test stick can be used. A sharp instrument will grab or bite into the test stick while a dull instrument will slide along. These can be purchased where dental instruments are sold. Sharpness can also be determined by visually inspecting the instrument. Hold the instrument under a light and rotate the instrument until the edge is facing the light. A dull cutting edge will reflect light when it has been rounded from use.

The equipment needed to sharpen instruments includes a flat Arkansas stone, conical stone, sharpening oil, cotton tip applicator, gauze sponge, plastic test stick, and a clock. Other helpful equipment includes a magnifying glass. To sharpen an instrument, place a drop of oil on the surface of the stone and gently spread it with a cotton tip applicator in a small circular shape. Grasp the instrument in your non-dominant hand, with your index finger or thumb braced near the shank to counterbalance the pressure caused by the sharpening motion. Hold the stone in your dominant hand, with your thumb on the edge towards you and your fingers on the edge away from you. This grasp will stabilize the stone. It is helpful to use the numbers on a clock to position the instrument correctly and the stone for sharpening. Using the clock as a guide, hold the instrument vertically with the blade to be sharpened at 6 o'clock. Hold the stone initially at 12 o'clock, then angle it to meet the angle of the cutting edge on the instrument. Move your entire arm in an up and down motion when sharpening. One can move either the stone or the instrument to sharpen the edge. When the edge has been sharpened you can take the conical stone and gently remove any metal shards from the cutting surface.

> **TIP BOX 15.1**
>
> There are many helpful dental instrument sharpening videos available. View http://www.youtube.com/watch?v=yUwG0EzyqDY.

> **Reflection**
>
> How do you see yourself learning to sharpen instruments?

Power Scalers

There are two types of powered dental instruments that can be used to clean teeth. Both of these scalers require water during use to prevent thermal damage to the tooth. A properly adjusted water flow will create a fine halo of mist to ensure that the scaling tip is properly cooled. Water must be constantly pumped through the handpiece to not only keep it cool, but to cool the tip as well. Without water the tip can become damaged. Be sure to read the equipment manual for the scaler to ensure proper use and maximize the equipment's life and effectiveness.

The ultrasonic scalers convert high frequency electrical current into mechanical vibrations. It can have either a magnetostrictive insert handpiece that contains tightly stacked metal sheets, or a ferrite rod insert that creates the vibrations. These vibrations knock the tartar off the tooth as the tip of the handpiece is swept along its surface. For both types of handpieces, water must be in the handpiece prior to insertion of the insert. Occasionally hold the magnetostrictive handpiece up to the light; if light is visible between the stacks, it is time to replace the handpiece. Use care with the ferrite rod, if it is dropped it can fracture the rod and render the handpiece unusable (Figure 15.7).

Piezo scalers use crystal technology in the handpiece to provide mechanical vibration. The same care in use should be used with piezo scalers to prevent tooth damage.

Sonic scalers use compressed air to operate thereby producing less heat and reducing the chance of thermal damage to the tooth. Sonic scalers are an excellent choice for the removal of supragingival calculus; however, their inability to descale subgingivally effectively is due to the large elliptical motion of the scaler tip.

Selection of the Correct Handpiece Tip

There are three main types of scaler tips available for power scalers. The tip used to remove gross accumulations of dental calculus or tartar from the crown of the tooth is most commonly called the beaver tail. This tip is broad and effective in rapidly removing debris from the crown (Figure 15.8, first tip on the left). This tip requires a higher power on most units and thus should never be used below the gumline. The periodontal tip is essential to complete a proper dental cleaning (the two tips on the right in Figure 15.8). This tip has a slender end and is designed to be used below the gumline and requires less energy and water to be effective. Using the periodontal tip helps to remove disease-causing dental calculus and plaque found below the gumline. The water flushes out the debris while the vibrations burst the cell

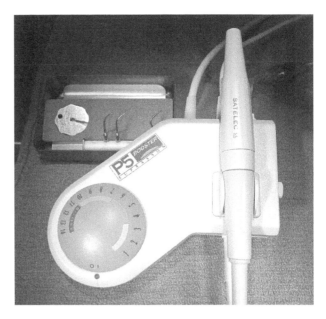

FIGURE 15.8 Ultrasonic dental scaler.

walls of bacteria. It is recommended that each clinic have both the wide or beaver tip and the periodontal tip to perform the most effective dental cleanings. A universal tip can be used both above and below the gumline. However, it is not as effective for cleaning either below or above the gumline.

All tips must be checked regularly using the manufacturers' guides to ensure that they are still effective. They wear down and don't vibrate efficiently. Handpieces and tips will need to be replaced on occasion for the safety of the patients and the effectiveness of the procedures.

Air-Driven Dental Units

Dental units are used by the veterinary dentist that has had training in the removal and periodontal treatment of teeth. There are two types of dental units: one uses compressed gas, usually nitrogen, from a cylinder; the second type uses an air compressor. The pressure in the compressor tank must be released at the end of each day to reduce condensation in the tank. Condensation can lead to ineffectiveness or damage to the tank. Most air-driven compressor systems use oil for lubrication. The oil level must be monitored and changed based on the manufacturer's recommendations. Different types of handpieces can be used on the compressed air systems. Sonic scalers are handpieces often attached to air compressor units. Low speed handpieces use speeds of 5000–20,000 rpm and are used for polishing with prophy angles. High speed handpieces, using speeds of 300,000–500,000 rpm, are used for cutting teeth during extractions and can also be used for creating access

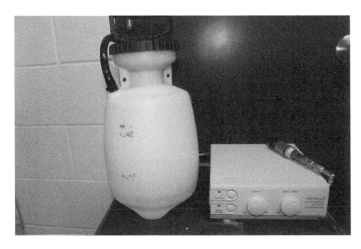

FIGURE 15.7 Dental prophylaxis scaler and polisher.

holes in teeth for root canal therapy. The handpieces may need to be lubricated depending on the manufacturer's recommendations. The dental units also come equipped with a three-way syringe. This syringe has two buttons. One button creates a water spray while the other creates an air stream. The water spray can be used to rinse the mouth to clear debris, excess prophy paste, and irrigate the tissues. The air stream can be used to dry tissues. If both buttons are pressed a mist will be formed.

Reflection

Compare and contrast the differently powered dental machines. What are the advantages and disadvantages of each?

Dental Prophylaxis

The veterinary technician and the assistant will place the patient under general anesthesia and attach the multifunction monitor. Personal protective equipment (PPE) for both are caps, gloves, face masks, and goggles or face shield to protect against the bacteria that is found in the oral cavity of dogs and cats. This is doubly important as the automated scalers aerosolize the bacteria because of the water required to keep the handpieces and tips from overheating.

The technician will often perform the dental prophylaxis. During the procedure the assistant will be monitoring the patient, marking not only the anesthesia monitoring chart but the dental chart as well. As the technician will call out the sulcus depths, lesions found, teeth loose or missing, or fractures or worn teeth. The assistant will be responsible for filling in the dental chart as these pathologies are found. Most charts will have a legend that indicate the marks used to indicate these problems. It will be up to the assistant to make sure the marks are made on the correct teeth.

After using the dental machines, it is recommended that the teeth be gone through once again with the hand instruments. Use the explorer to check for missed calculus by sliding the side of the instrument along the surface of the tooth. Calculus will make the instrument drag or feel bumpy, while on a clean tooth surface the instrument will glide smoothly. If calculus is found it can be quickly removed with the hand-held instruments. Meanwhile, the assistant can help out by changing the handpiece to the polisher and preparing the polishing paste. If the clinic orders the paste in large jars, a portion needs to be taken out with a tongue depressor so as to not contaminate the jar.

Polishing Follows Dental Cleaning

Polishing removes and smooths out the tiny scratches on the tooth surface created during dental scaling. If left unpolished the etching gives the plaque bacteria more surface area to attach to the tooth. Polishing requires a prophy cup filled with a medium to fine grit prophy paste and a prophy tip on a low speed handpiece that moves at approximately 3000–8000 rpm. The prophy paste can be applied with a finger or you can dip the prophy tip into the paste. If that is the method used, make sure to set the prophy tip on the surface of the tooth and then push the foot control to start the rotation. Otherwise you get prophy paste flung everywhere! Disposable prophy tips are available, decrease contamination, and are inexpensive. Each tooth is polished for 1 second or less. The excessive heat from the speed of the handpiece can burn the tooth. For the bigger teeth like the molars polish half the tooth, move to another and then come back and polish the second half.

Charting the Oral Examination

The most effect dental practices implement four-handed dentistry. Four-handed dentistry allows for the veterinarian or veterinary technician to be performing the oral examination while the veterinary assistant records the information onto the dental chart.

A dental chart is a diagrammatic representation of the dentition where information can be entered in a pictorial or notation format. It allows you to keep a record of the patient's oral health, track changes in oral health, and record treatment. The dental chart includes vital information about the patient, history, findings, medications, and, most importantly, a key to interpret the notations used on the format, therefore becoming a legal document.

Triadan Numbering System

There are two systems for identifying teeth, with common abbreviation marks used on both systems. The Triadan system is the most common tooth identification system. It gives each tooth a three-digit number (Figure 15.9). The first digit represents the quadrant of the mouth and the other two numbers represent the tooth based upon its position inside the mouth. The advantages of the Triadan system is that it is quicker and easier to say and can be used with most computers. The disadvantages are that it is not intuitive, it is based upon the canine dental formula and so must be adapted to other species and you

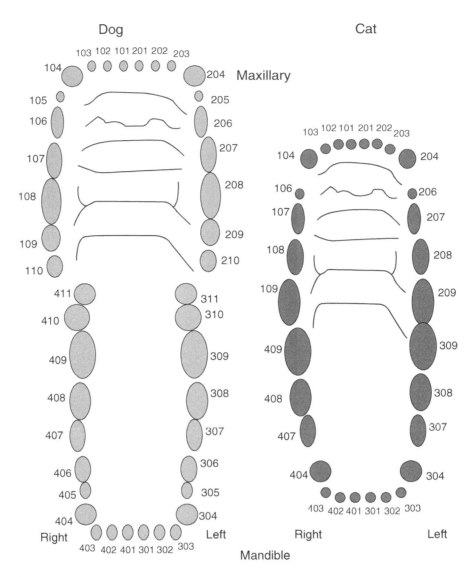

FIGURE 15.9 Triadan numbering system.

must learn the numbering of the individual teeth. If you remember that the four quadrants are numbered 1–4 starting with the upper right quadrant as being 1 and moving counter-clockwise, you'll get the quadrants numbered correctly. They divide the mouth in half with three incisors on each side. Working from the midline out the right quadrant would start 101, 102, 103 for the incisors. The upper right canine tooth is 104. Then in the canine mouth are four premolars numbered 105, 106, 107, and 108. The largest tooth is 108, which is also referred to as the carnassial tooth. The first molar is 109, followed by 110. The upper left quadrant is the same just substitute the 1 for a 2 and you have all the teeth numbered on the top jaw.

The bottom jaw is just as easy, substitute 4 and 3 for right and left, respectively. However, you'll note that the lower jaw has one more molar than the top jaw.

If you remember the "rule of 4 and 9" it will help you adjust the number to other species. As you can see on

Figure 15.9, all four canine teeth are always referred as 04 with the quadrant number in front of the 04. The first molar is always 09. If a species has fewer teeth, identifying the canine tooth is fairly easy as it is the fourth tooth from the midline on both top and bottom jaws. The first molar will always be after the largest tooth in the mouth which is the last premolar or carnassial tooth. Identify the molar then work back toward the canine tooth in species with fewer teeth than a canine. Note the cat chart in Figure 15.9. Find the first molar, as _09, now work toward the canine tooth. You'll notice that there are not as many premolars as there are in the dog.

Anatomical Numbering System

The anatomical system uses the first letter of each tooth type along with a number to identify each tooth (Figure 15.10): I – incisors, C – canine, P – premolars,

M – molars. Capital letters are used for the adult teeth while lowercase letters are used for the **deciduous** (primary) teeth. The teeth are numbered numerically per type of tooth. Look at Figure 15.10 on the dog chart. Note that the teeth left of the midline are identified by placing the number either as a superscript to indicate upper jaw or as a subscript to indicate the lower jaw. So, the upper right teeth starting at the midline and working around the quadrant we have I^1, I^2, I^3, C^1, P^1, P^2, P^3, P^4, M^1 and M^2. The advantage of the anatomical system is that it is easy to remember, and many teeth can be identified at one time. The disadvantages are that is can be more time consuming to identify individual teeth and some computer systems may not be alpha numeric friendly. Note, too, the cat dentition skips numbers when you reach the premolars.

Charting Symbols

During the charting process the technician or veterinarian will call out the abnormal findings as she proceeds through the oral exam. The different lesions are marked with symbols on the dental chart. The following are some of the more common lesions found:

- Sulcus depth is marked with a number on the appropriate surface of the tooth. For example, if the technician says, "105 buccal sulcus 4 mm" you would mark the number 4 next to the first premolar on the cheek side of the tooth.
- Fractured teeth are marked with a wavy line in the direction of the fracture, either transverse or longitudinal.

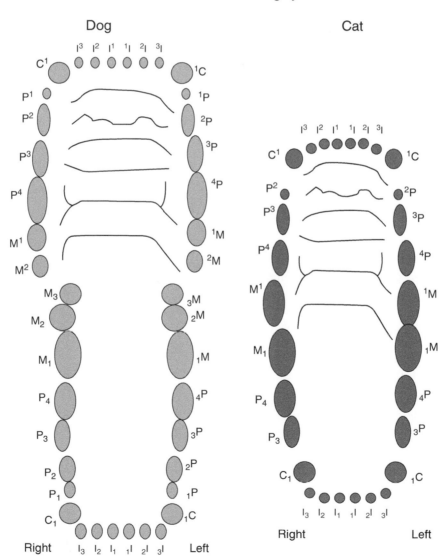

Anatomic numbering system

FIGURE 15.10 Anatomical numbering system.

- Missing teeth are colored in solidly.
- Extracted teeth – if they were taken out by the veterinarian – are marked with an X over the tooth.
- Worn teeth are marked with a straight line at about the level of wear.
- Caries lesions are marked with a filled-in circle on the surface of the tooth.
- Enamel that is missing is drawn in to approximate the missing area on the surface of the tooth.

Learning Exercise

Practice filling out charts, either with a study buddy or by yourself. Print off dental charts and look at a picture of teeth or a skull and imagine the lesion and sulcus depths.

Basics of Pocket Pet Dentistry

Pocket pet dentistry requires special equipment. There are specially designed dental instruments for pocket pets to allow access to the small, long, narrow mouths, assist in retracting cheek pouches, and to cut, file, and extract continuously erupting teeth. A useful set of instruments would include the following:

- Rodent incisor luxator
- Rodent molar/premolar luxator
- Crossley rabbit luxator
- Rodent molar/premolar extraction forceps
- Rodent mouth gag
- Pouch dilators
- Molar/premolar rasp
- Rodent tongue depressor (or use regular wooden tongue depressor split in half lengthwise)
- Low-speed burs to use for crown height reduction
- High speed burs for use in incisor trimming and extraction
- Rodent molar/premolar cutters if no drill available
- Cotton tipped applicators to staunch blood flow from extraction sites or absorb fluid from the mouth.

Oral examination is difficult on an awake pocket pet. The small, long, narrow oral cavity of pocket pets make it very difficult to perform an oral examination, often only being able to examine the anterior portion of the mouth or front teeth. An otoscope may be useful to access the cheek teeth of awake rabbits, chinchillas, and guinea pigs. The canula can be directed back toward the teeth and no fingers get bitten in the process. It is best to give them a light sedation or gas mask them to get a really good look and to fix any issues.

Rabbits and rodents have similar dentition but with some differences. The main dental difference between lagomorphs (rabbits) and rodents (guinea pigs, chinchillas, rats, mice, hamsters) is that lagomorphs have four maxillary incisors – two anterior and two posterior. These posterior incisors are commonly referred to as "peg teeth." The extra incisors of lagomorphs are important in chewing. Rabbits chew in a side-to-side, scissors-like fashion, with the two lower incisors cutting back and forth between the peg teeth and larger, anterior upper incisors.

Rodents have only two maxillary incisors. Another important different between lagomorphs and most rodents (the exceptions being guinea pigs and chinchillas) is that all the teeth grow continuously and must be worn down by chewing or by professional dental treatments. In rodents other than guinea pigs and chinchillas, only the incisors continue to erupt. Also, the incisor teeth of most rodents are normally a yellow–orange in color.

Dental Formula for Pocket Pets

Lagomorphs (rabbits) 2(I2/1:C0/0:PM3/2:M3/3)
Guinea pigs and chinchillas 2(I1/1:C0/0: PM1/1:M3/3)
Rat/mouse/hamster 2(I1/1:C0/0:PM0/0:M3/3).

Ferret Dentition

Ferrets have similar dentition to felines. Because ferrets are carnivores, their dentition appears like the anatomy we commonly see in cats. Their dental formula is 2(I3/3:C1/1:PM3/3:M1/2).

Hedgehog Dentition

As a member of the order Insectivora, the oral anatomy of hedgehogs is very different from other pocket pets. Anatomical characteristics of insectivores include small, long, narrow snouts, and a primitive tooth structure. The incisors are used as forceps for picking up small prey, and the canines often resemble incisors or first premolars. Hedgehogs have 30–46 teeth. A complete oral examination of hedgehogs requires anesthesia or chemical restraint because of their self-protection behavior of rolling into a tight ball when accosted.

Learning Exercise

Make a pocket pet, ferret, and hedgehog section in your reference book. Put in the dental formulas and perhaps a list of the dental instruments used on pocket pets.

Intraoral Radiography

Dental radiographs are an essential part of each and every oral examination. The crown is just the "tip of the iceberg," so to speak. Approximately 42% of dental pathology is found **subgingivally**. Radiographs will help diagnose pathology that is not visible from the surface, confirm suspect pathology, as well as help demonstrate the pathology to the client. Survey radiographs can also increase your clinic's revenue.

Dental radiography is part of the diagnostic workup for dental disease. With the exception of positioning, dental radiography follows the same principles as general radiology, including the use of PPE (see Chapter 16). The dental radiography machine is similar to that used in human dental radiology (Figure 15.11). The major difference is it has a smaller focal area and a much shorter focal film distance than the standard machine. The dental unit is mounted on a moveable arm that is highly positional, which is either wall-mounted over a table or mounted on a wheeled base for portability.

The dental unit can be used to take both traditional film and digital radiographs. Traditional silver halide film is enclosed in a flexible paper cassette, in a full range of sizes 0–4.

1. Size 0 – smallest
   a. Cats or small single tooth

2. Size 2 – small animal
   a. Most common size used

3. Size 3 – cats and dogs
   a. Longer and narrower

4. Size 4 – large dogs
   a. Multiple teeth
   b. Second most common size used.

All intraoral film has a small raised dimple on one corner that always faces the beam. This is a rule every team member working in dental radiology must follow as it orients the veterinarian when reading a dental film.

More and more veterinary clinics are understanding the value of dental radiographs and in an effort to reduce anesthesia time are turning to digital dental radiograph sensors. These sensors allow the radiograph image to appear on a computer monitor within seconds of shooting.

There are two types of digital systems used to produce a dental radiograph. Digital radiography (DL) uses a sensor that is inside a rigid plastic wafer. The wafer is placed inside the patient's mouth and then exposed. The wafer is connected to the computer by a wire or is wireless and transfers the image to the computer. The wafer comes in two sizes and can be damaged if dropped. The other system is a computed radiograph (CR) system. It uses phosphor flexible plates with the same full range of sizes as the dental films and which are positioned and imaged like the silver halide dental films. After exposure, the plate is removed from the patient's mouth, loaded into a laser scanner which projects the digital image and resets the plate for the next image.

The advantage of digital radiography is that it takes less anesthesia time as the images are almost instantaneous. There is no expense for film, chemicals, mounts, envelopes, or storage cabinets for the patient films. Images can be enhanced to change contrast and magnified by adjusting these values on the computer. Finally, images can easily be sent to specialists by email or text.

Patient Positioning for Dental Radiography

There are two intraoral radiograph techniques commonly utilized in veterinary dentistry. The simplest is the parallel technique and, as luck would have it, it can be used for the fewest views. The parallel technique is used for the posterior mandible. This view includes the molars and caudal premolars. The film beam is placed at a 90° angle to the film, which has been placed on the lingual surface of the teeth (see the illustration).

The other technique is the bisecting angle. The bisecting angle is used to minimize distortions of the teeth. The bisecting angle is used for the anterior teeth, maxilla and mandible, and the posterior maxilla teeth. In this technique, the beam is aimed at the imaginary line bisecting the plane of the tooth and the plane of the film.

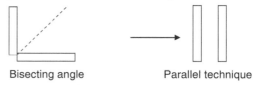

Bisecting angle   Parallel technique

If the beam is not perpendicular to the bisecting angle the tooth will be distorted. If the angle is too low, it

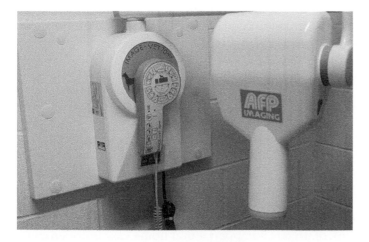

FIGURE 15.11 Digital dental radiography unit.

will cause elongation and too high it will cause foreshortening.

Six to ten intraoral films are needed for a full mouth study in dogs and cats, depending on patient size. Because of this, the patient will need to be in various positions to accomplish these films: right and left lateral, sternal, and dorsal recumbency. Remember when moving an anesthetized patient to keep the body level and take care not to dislodge the endotracheal tube. A mouth speculum is placed in the patient's mouth to keep it open during the radiography procedures. It is often placed on the canine teeth or is moved around to facilitate various views of the dental arcade. There are some dedicated dental positioning devices that can be used intraorally.

Film identification is accomplished during or after the film is exposed and developed. If a separate numbered radiograph log is kept to record dental radiographs, the same number can be placed on a sticky radiopaque label, which is then attached to a corner of the film. A special mount on which patient information and date are written can be purchased to hold the film. These are available from dental product suppliers. An indelible marker can be used on the dry film.

A technique chart just for the dental unit is used to set exposures. The chart is set up based on the size of the animal and for each tooth to be radiographed.

Learning Exercise

If you have access to skulls and dental film or sensors, practice positioning the skull and film with the dental unit.

Manual Developing of Dental Radiographs

Dental films are very easy to develop. Dental film consists of four layers. The outer layer consists of white plastic which protects the film from moisture. The second layer is the lead layer which is silver colored. The third layer is the paper layer which is the black layer. All of these layers surround the film layer, which is gray.

Dental films can be developed in a chairside darkroom. The chairside darkroom contains four cups for rapid film developer, water, rapid fixer, and water, respectively. The cover for the darkroom is a dark red tinted plastic box that allows the developer to see what they are doing without light exposing the film. There are armholes in the chairside darkroom that allows personnel to insert their hands into the side of the unit without allowing light inside. Special clips should be used to hold the film while developing to protect it from fingerprints.

The steps involved in developing dental films are as follows:

1. Ensure that the developer and fixer are fresh
2. Slowly open the film packet, remove the film, and attach the film clip
3. Place in developer – 30 seconds
4. Wash in water – 30 seconds
5. Place in fixer – 10–15 seconds
6. Review the film in 10 seconds
7. If the positioning and exposure are correct, place back in fixer for 10 minutes or until the procedure is completed followed with a thorough rinse for 30–60 minutes.

Dental automatic processors work similarly to regular film processors (see Chapter 16). Follow the manufacturer's directions for use and frequency of cleaning.

Patient Care and Clean-up

The assistant can help out immensely after the dental radiograph. First, take care of the anesthetized patient recovering from anesthesia, extubate as soon as swallowing reflex returns, check body temperature and apply warming devices if necessary. Observe until sternal then return the patient to its housing. Then clean and put away the PPE, endotracheal tube, positioning aids, and gas anesthesia machine. Clean the radiography table and re-cover and store processing chemicals if using the manual technique. Check and complete entries in the dental radiography log, patient's record, and treatment board. Finally, file all the dental radiographs according to the clinic's procedure.

Client Education

Companion animals have become an important part of our lives. Many people consider the pet a part of their family. All members of the veterinary team must be excited and motivated about dental care and project that enthusiasm to the client. As veterinary health professionals it is our job not only to promote dentistry, but to educate our clients about the importance of proper oral health. It is necessary to communicate the importance of dental treatment and oral care in many ways. It should become as routine as vaccinations and heartworm testing in your clinic. This education process starts with clients at the first puppy or kitten visit. Talk with them about the importance of oral care by expressing the fact that the mouth is a mirror to the body. Give handouts explaining the relationship between oral disease and systemic health. Use pictures to give the client an impression of what can happen if oral home care is not given to their pet.

Daily Dental Care

As with many diseases in pets, prevention is the key to good oral health, and demonstrating daily tooth brushing for the client is the first step in preventative care. Tooth brushing is the gold standard of preventive dental care. It is important to not just tell a client to brush their pet's teeth, but to also demonstrate tooth brushing either on their pet, clinic pet, or a model. Demonstrate on one side of the mouth showing the client how to brush the **buccal** and **labial surfaces** of the teeth then observe the client brushing the other side. This allows you an opportunity to make suggestions or give them advice and tips.

Training a pet to accept tooth brushing takes time and patience; it must be done gradually and with plenty of praise. It is best to start with a finger dabbed with pet toothpaste on it. Hold the pet's mouth closed and gently rub the finger over the incisors, canines, and along the molars. As the pet begins to accept the rubbing of the teeth over the course of a few weeks the owner can introduce the toothbrush. Daily brushing is best, especially during the training period. Be sure to tell the client that it is not necessary to brush the **lingual** or **palatal** surfaces of the teeth.

Tooth brushing is the best option for providing quality oral care, but some people are not willing or able to brush their pet's teeth and some pets are not willing to allow their teeth to be brushed. There are options available that can help in the prevention of plaque buildup and the prevention of oral disease. Dental diets are one of the most effective methods of plaque reduction. Good quality chews are also an option. Care should be used when recommending alternative methods of plaque prevention. There are many items that are advertised to prevent plaque or remove tartar; unfortunately, many of these products can actually cause damage to the teeth. Real bones, hard rawhides, cow hooves, bully sticks, and so on, should not be used as they can cause dental fractures. A good rule of thumb is that if you can't easily bend the item in your hands, it is too hard for your pet's teeth.

The pet's jaw is not able to move from side to side like ours so if it bites down on something that is too hard the only option is for the tooth to fracture. The Veterinary Oral Health Council (VOHC) has a seal that is placed on products that have been rigorously tested and have been proven to prevent plaque or calculus accumulations. Products that have the VOHC seal of approval can be found at www.VOHC.org.

Dental Patient Discharge Instructions

Clients need detailed discharge instructions and the use of a dental report card is a great way to help the client understand the treatment that was given to their animal. Include before and after photos and a simplified dental chart on which problem areas can be marked or highlighted. A section for diagnosis, treatment, home care, prescriptions, and follow-up visits should be included on this report card. Keep it simple and use bright, cheerful colors with clipart on the take home sheet.

Learning Exercise

Practice client education with a classmate. Role play with one being the client and the other being the assistant.

Chapter Reflection

What are you most looking forward to when working with a veterinary team on dental procedures?

Suggested Reading

Kesel ML. 2000. *Veterinary Dentistry for the Small Animal Technician.* Ames, IA: Iowa State University Press.

The Why, When, and How of Small Animal Dental Radiology. http://www.dentalvet.com/vets/basicdentistry/whywhenhow_radiology.htm (accessed July 8, 2019)

CHAPTER 16

Diagnostic Imaging and Endoscopy

LEARNING OBJECTIVES

- Practice radiation safety at all times, using PPE and dosimeters
- Maintain a radiology log with every radiograph taken
- Assist with the labeling, positioning, and taking of a diagnostic radiograph
- Differentiate directional terms and abbreviations used in radiology
- Develop films using automatic processing
- Load and unload film from a cassette and cassette maintenance
- File patient films
- Maintain darkroom, automatic processor, and developing chemicals
- Prepare equipment and patient for ultrasonography
- Provide support for endoscopic procedures
- Properly clean and store endoscopic equipment

NAVTA ESSENTIAL SKILLS COVERED IN THIS CHAPTER

VIII. Radiology and Ultrasound Imaging
   A. Follow recommended safety measures
   B. Assist the veterinarian and/or the veterinary technician in the completion of diagnostic radiographs and ultrasound including the restraint, preparation, and positioning of patients
   C. Maintain quality control
   D. Label, file, and store film and/or digital radiographs
   E. Properly care for radiography equipment
   F. Care and maintenance of film cassettes and screens (optional)
   G. Know safety techniques for handling processing chemicals (optional)
   H. Assist in the processing of diagnostic radiographs using:

Tasks for the Veterinary Assistant, Fourth Edition. Teresa F. Sonsthagen.
© 2020 John Wiley & Sons, Inc. Published 2020 by John Wiley & Sons, Inc.
Companion website: www.wiley.com/go/sonsthagen/tasks

1. Manual dipping tank processing, or
2. Automatic processor, or
3. Digital processing
I. Maintain X-ray log

Introduction to Diagnostic Imaging

Diagnostic imaging covers a broad range of tests used to help a veterinarian determine an illness or condition: radiography, ultrasound, computed tomography (CT), magnetic resonance imaging (MRI), and positron emission tomography (PET) scans.

Radiology is the study of how radiographs are produced and used for diagnosing diseases or conditions of the body. A **radiograph** is the "photographic" record or image of a body part on film or in a digital format. Radiograph is preferable to the term X-ray; however, they are used interchangeably. **Radiography** is the act of exposing a film to radiation and a **radiographic study** is a series of radiographs consisting of two or more views with or without contrast media. **Contrast media** is used to show the presence of lesions or items that would normally not show up on a radiograph. A **manual radiograph** utilizes a silver halide film inside a cassette. It is X-ray and light sensitive and placed under a patient, exposed to radiation, and then developed using chemicals to fix the image to the film. **Digital radiography** utilizes radiation, but the image is digitalized and sent to a computer for viewing. More on this later in the chapter.

The specialized equipment used in radiography includes a **view box** which is a box with a light on the inside and a white opaque surface on the outside. The manual radiograph is placed in front of the light source which illuminates the film for clearer viewing. **Cassettes** hold film for manual radiographs or have sensors built in that capture the digital image. **Calipers** are used to measure the body part of a patient; those measurements are then used to set the settings on the radiography machine.

Digital Radiography

Radiation is utilized to produce an image; however, instead of film the image is changed to a digital format. There are two types of digital systems used to produce a digital radiograph. Digital radiography (DR) uses a detector that transforms radiation into an electrical charge which is sent to a unit that processes the image. DR requires specialized equipment that is fairly expensive. The computed radiograph (CR) system utilizes a reusable phosphor plate inside a cassette that is sensitive to radiation but not to light. The plates are positioned and imaged like the silver halide cassettes, using the traditional radiography machine. After exposure the plate is loaded into a laser scanner which projects the digital image to a computer and resets the plate for the next image. The plates are more sensitive than film which allows for a slightly lower radiation dose, reducing radiation exposure to staff and patient.

Both systems project digital images on a computer monitor in about 30–90 seconds. If the radiograph needs to be repeated because of movement or misalignment it can be done immediately. The image can also be altered by increasing or decreasing the contrast and gray scale on the computer, which is called windowing. These radiographs can be sent via the internet to a specialist, which is an example of telemedicine, rather than sending them in the mail. The digital images are stored in the patient's medical record using the practice's management software whereas traditional films are stored in a filing cabinet so they can be retrieved as needed.

Advanced Imaging Technologies

In addition to radiography, there are advanced imaging technologies that provide different visualizations of body structures within a patient: diagnostic ultrasound, CT, MRI, and PET scans. **Ultrasonography** produces sound waves that interact with body tissues. The images produced are echoes converted to electronic signals and processed by a computer. CT scans use X-rays and yield images along a single plane. MRI produces images along three planes using strong magnetic and radio waves that are converted to images by a computer. Both CT and MRI can use intravenous gadolinium-based contrast media that highlights specific structures. Each procedure requires anesthetizing or heavily tranquilizing the patient throughout as the patient must be absolutely still for the duration of the procedure, which can be quite lengthy. PET scans are rarely found in veterinary practices, primarily being used in teaching hospitals or research.

Reflection

Compare and contrast the different diagnostic imaging systems.

Quality Assurance

The usefulness of a radiograph is limited by the quality of the image itself. It is the veterinary technician and the assistant who actually take the radiographs, so their ability to produce quality films is essential. A quality film has subtle shades of white to black contrasts depending on the density of the body parts. For example, a leg bone is mostly white with shades of gray because of its different densities, whereas muscle tissue is a fairly uniform dark shade of gray because it is less dense and fairly uniform in density. This contrast allows the veterinarian to see body structures and determine if there is an injury or condition present. A quality film requires accurate measurement of the body part, correct film exposure settings, accurate patient positioning, and proper developing of the exposed film. With the advent of digital radiography, measurement and proper positioning are still very important but, because the image is digital, the film exposure can be adjusted to be lighter or darker and of course there are no "films" to develop.

Reflection

Discuss the reason for quality assurance and the issues it would cause if films were not diagnostic.

Radiation Safety

The radiation produced by a radiography machine is considered a hazard and regulations regarding use of equipment and personnel safety are governed by the Department of Health at the state level. Radiography machines are registered with a Radiation Safety Board which inspects the equipment to make sure it is operating within parameters.

Radiation is odorless and colorless and it cannot be felt or seen. Radiation causes damage to rapidly dividing cells, such as those found in unborn and immature individuals, bone marrow, skin, and blood-forming tissues. Damage occurs when multiple small doses accumulate over a lifetime or through a single massive dose. This damage may not manifest for years or genetic damage can appear in future generations. Consistently following proper safety measures will prevent harm.

The National Committee on Radiation Protection and Measurements (NCRP) recommends using "as low as reasonably achievable" (ALARA) exposures when taking radiographs. This means that the personnel taking radiographs need to know what they are doing so the image is right the first time. For every radiograph taken there is more exposure to radiation increasing the chance of damage to the personnel over a lifetime. Some states actually prohibit manual restraint of animals during radiographic procedures. Patients are anesthetized and positioning aids are used. This is a sensible guideline even when not required by law. Another option is to rotate staff conducting radiographic procedures, especially in high volume practices.

Major safety measures are used to reduce the amount of radiation exposure to personnel. The following guidelines must be followed to ensure a safe working environment:

1. Each person involved in the radiograph must wear personal protection equipment (PPE) while exposing radiographs. This includes a lead apron that covers the front of the body from the shoulders to mid-thigh, goggles, and a thyroid collar (Figure 16.1).

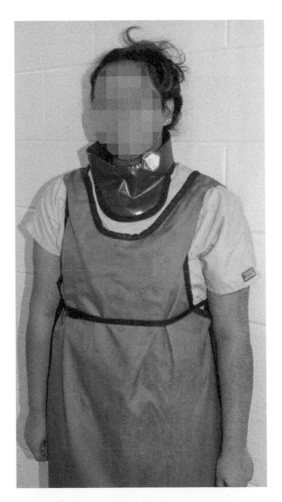

FIGURE 16.1 Lead apron and thyroid collar.

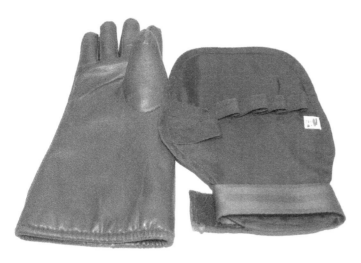

FIGURE 16.2 Lead gloves.

2. Lead gloves are used when a patient has to be held for a radiograph (Figure 16.2). The lead protects the hands from radiation; however, it is never good practice to allow a gloved hand to be within the primary beam.

3. The assistant can facilitate and "enforce" the wearing of PPE. When setting up for a radiograph, locate and lay out all PPE; these are usually stored in the radiology room. Each person will need a lead apron, gloves, thyroid collar, and goggles. The dosimeters are usually stored away from the radiography machine. Gather each person's dosimeter involved in taking the radiograph. Make sure each person attaches their dosimeter on the apron, facing outwards at neck level.

4. A dosimeter is a personal film badge worn facing out at the neck (Figure 16.1) or chest level on the outside of the apron. The dosimeter measures the level of exposure to radiation by the wearer. The standard acceptable exposure is 0.005 sievert/year for occupational and background personnel. An annual report is sent to the practice for each individual badge. A dosimeter should never be placed in direct sunlight or left in the heat of a car as it can give a "false" high radiation reading.

5. Take care of PPE. All lead-containing safety equipment is hung up and never folded. Aprons and thyroid collars have thin sheets of lead in them and folding the lead will quickly cause a break. This break will expose the wearer to radiation. Gloves should be put on a glove rack to ventilate, as they get quite damp from sweat during procedures. Do not allow animals to chew or bite the gloves as the holes will expose the wearer to radiation. All lead-containing equipment should be radiographed at least twice a year to examine for cracks in the shielding. Lay equipment across a cassette and expose; if there are dark spots or lines on the film there are breaks in the lead. Notify the inventory manager so that piece of equipment can be replaced. The assistant can help co-workers by making sure this gets done!

6. Individuals under 18 years of age and pregnant women are never allowed in the room when radiographs are being exposed.

7. Never enter a room denoted by a radiation hazard symbol unless invited or it is known that a radiograph is not being taken at that time. Close and if possible lock the door to the radiation room, or indicate radiographs are being taken by turning on a warning light. This symbol denotes radiation is used in that location ☢

8. Reduce personal exposure by:

   • Staying out of the primary beam which comes from the X-ray tube housing and points down at the table. Never place any human body part within the primary beam as doing so substantially increases exposure to radiation and subsequent damage.

   • Reduce scatter radiation. The radiography machine has an aluminum filter placed between the window of the X-ray tube and the collimator which absorbs soft X-rays referred to as scatter radiation. Scatter radiation is the interaction of the primary beam with objects in its path. As the beam it hits the body part, cassette, and table top it bounces up in an outward projection. Scatter radiation is further decreased by using the collimator to restrict the primary beam from spreading beyond the cassette. Use the smallest cassette size to accommodate the anatomy being radiographed. If restraining a patient, lean as far away from the primary beam as possible.

9. Use only the number of personnel necessary to take the radiograph. Everyone else should evacuate the room or area.

10. Taking exact site measurements using a caliper (Figure 16.3) and subsequent setting of exposure factors are absolutely essential to avoid retakes. Exposure factors are obtained from a technique chart that is prepared especially for that radiography unit.

Position the patient correctly and confirm that the correct body part is being radiographed as per the veterinarian's orders. Tips for accomplishing this are:

   • Anesthetize or sedate the patient if possible, as this reduces struggling with a patient and avoids movements that may require retakes.

   • Use positioning aids: sandbags, foam wedges (Figure 16.4), ropes, and radiopaque "V" troughs to position patients correctly. These will also improve quality by evening out the body.

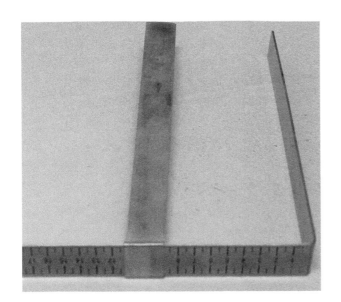

FIGURE 16.3 Calipers.

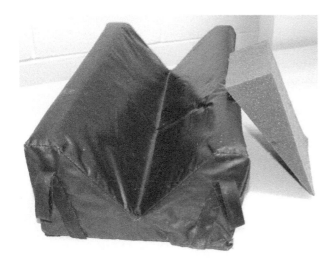

FIGURE 16.4 Positioning devices.

11. Use the correct focal film distance (FFD), usually 36–40 inches from the X-ray generator to the table top or grid under the table top. Most radiography machines have an indicator to show where to place the generator for both tabletop and grid shots.
12. Use the proper film developing techniques if using traditional radiographs.
13. Maintain a "radiology log" of each exposure taken. This can be used to determine if the technique chart is off by comparing settings. It will also help determine if one person is being exposed to too many X-rays. Take care of equipment in the radiography and darkrooms:

- Proper care of PPE equipment, keeping them clean and stored properly.
- Monthly cleaning of traditional cassettes and intensifying screens.
- Proper mixing of processor chemicals and maintenance of automatic processor.
- Annual field service by a qualified representative including machine calibration.

Strict adherence to these recommendations reduces radiation exposure and therefore possible damage. Once the radiation damage occurs, it is not reversible.

Radiography Abbreviations

The American Committee of Veterinary Radiologists and Anatomists (ACVRA) is the source of anatomic and directional terms and abbreviations used in veterinary radiology. Understanding these abbreviations is important because they are used to indicate what body part to radiograph and to fill out the identification label and log. The first letter in an abbreviation represents where the X-ray beam enters the body. The second letter represents where the beam exits the body. Adding these abbreviations to your reference book is a good idea.

The following are some of the most common directional terms and abbreviations:

Left (Lt): a patient's left side or limb
Right (Rt): a patient's right side or limb
Dorsal (D): the upper parts of the body. This includes the top of the head, neck, back, and tail.
Ventral (V): the lower parts of the body. This includes the lower part of the head and neck, chest and abdomen, and tail.
Anterior/posterior (AP): beam directed at the limb from front to back
Palmar (Pa): the forelimb from the carpal joint distally. Used instead of the term caudal.
Plantar (Pl): the hind limb from the tarsal joint distally. Used instead of the term caudal.
Medial (M): the inner surface of a limb or toward the center of the body
Lateral (L): the outer surface of a limb or away from the center of the body
Cranial (Cr): relative to a given point, any point toward the head, also referred to as anterior
Caudal (Cd): relative to a given point, any point toward the tail, also referred to as posterior
Distal (D): relative to a given point, any point on a limb or the tail away from the trunk
Proximal (P): relative to a given point, any point on a limb or the tail toward the trunk
Rostral (R): parts of the head located toward the nostrils
Oblique (O): at a 45° angle, between a horizontal and a perpendicular angle
Recumbent: lying down either on the side (lateral) or sternum (sternal).
An example of the application of this terminology is as follows.

The veterinarian has requested VD and L abdominal radiographs. The positioning of the patient for the VD film is on the patient's back with the front and back legs extended parallel to each other and beyond the patient's head and rear. The beam is centered directly over the caudal aspect of the 13th rib. The second film requires the patient to be lying on its right side to provide better visualization of the kidneys when doing abdominal studies. Again, the beam is centered over the caudal aspect of the 13th rib.

Learning Exercise

Add these abbreviations to your master list.

Radiography Procedure

Although an intimate knowledge of the technicalities of X-ray image creation is not necessary for the assistant, the ability to help during these procedures is essential. Taking a radiograph requires a specific sequence followed every time to ensure a quality image and safety for all involved. The following is that process in a checklist format. Each action is discussed further in the information that follows.

Preparation:

1. Turn on automatic processor if using traditional radiographs (see Developing Radiographs section for these instructions).
2. Enter patient information into the X-ray log. Confirm correct patient positioning and necessary restraint for requested studies.
3. Set out positioning aids if necessary and ready PPE (see Radiation Safety section)
4. Use calipers to measure the thickness of the anatomic site being studied.
5. Set the exposure factors on the X-ray console according to the technique chart.
6. Select the size of film cassette to accommodate the size of the animal.
7. Prepare identification and directional markers.
8. Assist with patient positioning, exposure, and developing of the radiograph.
9. Clean up and restock.

Radiography Log

The radiology log serves three purposes:

1. It is part of the patient's legal record and required by the American Animal Hospital Association (AAHA) to meet the standards for AAHA- accredited hospitals.

2. It facilitates comparison of techniques used on a patient during follow-up studies.
3. It serves as a reference when working toward improved film quality which should be the goal of every team member.

The log is maintained in a binder kept within the radiology area. Entries are made throughout the radiographic process. The format is similar to all logs, being composed of columns and rows. The number of columns will vary but must provide the legal minimum of information. AAHA-approved hospitals will require recording additional details. The log is used whenever a radiograph is taken. *No exceptions. It is the practice's legal means of confirming radiographs were taken and which personnel were involved.*

Maintenance of the log is a job the assistant can take on, thus freeing up other personnel to complete other tasks. The following procedure is followed when making an entry into the X-ray log.

1. Confirm patient identification, using the patient's record for accuracy.
2. Start entry with date, X-ray number, patient/owner identification, breed of animal, sex, age, weight, anatomic location of the radiographs.
3. Record the body measurements and kV, mA, and seconds settings from the technique chart for each radiograph.
4. After the film is developed record film quality, diagnosis (after the veterinarian determines diagnosis), and comments such as whether patient was anesthetized, who took the radiographs (initials will do), and factors impacting film quality (for example, patient panting during thoracic radiographs).
5. Make certain there are enough empty rows to meet the needs of the day or week in the radiography log. Keep a master copy of a blank log page in the binder, under a divider so no one uses it, and make copies as needed. When there is half a page left on the active log sheet, make several copies and place them in the log book. Your co-workers will really appreciate this effort.
6. If the binder is getting full or to prepare a new binder, label and date the spine of the binder with the date of the first and last entries. This facilitates finding a particular entry as binders accumulate. They must be kept as long as the medical records and any other legal documents which varies from state to state.

Measuring the Anatomy with Calipers

The ability of the X-ray beam to penetrate tissue is limited, in part, by the thickness of the tissue so accurate measurements must be taken, and the instrument used is a caliper (Figure 16.3). This instrument is an L-shaped ruler with a moveable bar that slides up and down the vertical axis of the L. The bar is slid up so the body part fits between it and horizontal axis of the L. The vertical axis is marked in both centimeters and inches. Centimeters are used to determine the settings used on the radiograph machine.

Measuring a body part must be done in specific ways to ensure proper settings on the radiograph machine. Place the calipers "around" the thickest portion of the body part to be radiographed. The moveable bar is allowed to settle lightly around the part being measured. For example, the veterinarian orders an AP and ML of the right carpus on a dog. The patient is positioned in sternal recumbency and the right carpus is measured with the caliper. The stationary part of the bar is beneath (or posterior to) the joint, and the moveable bar rests lightly on top (or anterior to) of the joint. The caliper reads 3 cm. Record that measurement under the "cm" area of the log and the direction AP in the "view" section of the same row. Measure the joint again but this time the patient is in right lateral recumbency and the stationary bar is on the lateral side of the joint, and the moveable bar rests on the medial surface of the joint. The reading is 5 cm because the carpus is usually wider than it is thick. Record this measurement and the direction as ML in the log.

There is a temptation, as expertise develops, to "eye-ball" a patient rather than actually using the caliper. This only results in poor quality films and more frequent retakes. Time is actually saved by taking a few moments to measure. When in doubt where to measure, always measure the thickest portion of the area being X-rayed with the animal in the position needed to get the correct radiograph. Correct use of the caliper serves as one of the fundamentals leading to quality films and radiation safety.

Learning Exercise

Practice taking measurements with the calipers on various body parts of a dog or cat.

Setting Exposure Factors Using the Technique Charts

Technique charts are formulated settings for a specific radiography machine based on the thickness of the area to be radiographed, on the type of equipment and techniques being used, and anatomic differences. The constants of the system are predetermined before the technique chart is created; therefore, the assistant should

be aware of them and know how to adjust them if necessary or possible.

The constants of setting up a technique chart are as follows:

1. Because of focal–film distance, a technique chart will be formulated for both tabletop and grid techniques. The grid is used when radiographs of body parts that are 10 cm or more are needed.
2. Intensifying screens on the inside front and back of the cassettes convert the X-rays to visible light to expose the film. The screens are rated high speed, par speed, and slow speed. The high-speed screens reduce the exposure time. Slow-speed screens increase film detail, but blurring is more likely because of patient movement. Usually, a practice will have one type of screen and will formulate the technique chart based on the screens.
3. Radiographic film is rated according to speed and matched to the type of screen. Fast film requires less exposure time but lacks definition. Slower films require greater exposure time and produce films with greater detail. The film–screen system is the combination of the values of the screen and film ratings. The film manufacturers provide tables for their film–screen ratings.

The goal of technique charts is to consistently obtain the greatest detail at the highest speed. Select the chart that corresponds to the body part being radiographed. Charts are set up in rows and columns. The first column lists the thickness in centimeters of the body part to be radiographed. Once the thickness of the study site is located, move across the row to determine the kVp, mA, and exposure time in seconds or milliampere seconds (mAs). The mAs is the mA multiplied by the time in seconds (s).

Based on the constants just discussed and the fact that we have patients that weigh from less than 1 to over 100 lb, the following are recommended charts for a small animal practice. There should be tabletop technique charts and grid technique charts for each of the following areas:

A. Extremities and skull
B. Abdomen
C. Thorax
D. Avian and exotics – usually not grid shots.

While all this may seem confusing, just remember to use the correct chart based on the measurement of the anatomy being radiographed.

Learning Exercise

Look at your programs technique chart. Compare the differences between a small and large animal and the different settings for a bone/skull shot and an abdomen/thorax shot.

Cassette Selection

Cassettes come in three sizes and selection is based on size of animal and area that is to be radiographed. The standard sizes of cassettes are: 8 × 10, 10 × 12, and 14 × 17 inches. Selection is based on making sure the requested body part is on the film with at least an inch above and below the body part. For example, if the radius and ulna are to be X-rayed, the joint above (elbow) and the joint below (carpus) should be included on the film, this ensures the entire radius and ulna are visible. Check your reference book for exact placement of the animal on the cassette.

Film Labeling

Film labeling is very important because radiographs are part of a patient's medical record; as such they are legal documents. Because of this they must be accurately and permanently marked. Basic information required on each radiograph includes the following:

1. Patient/owner's names and/or the medical record number
2. Hospital name this is often on prestamped plates or on "flash" marker tags
3. Date the radiograph is exposed
4. Radiograph number – if used
5. Directional information – left or right – these are lead letters
6. Scout shots and time – for contrast studies.

There are three ways to permanently include the patient information on a radiograph and four other markers that are used to indicate direction and time (Figure 16.5). One type of marker is a holder that allows lead letters and numbers to be slid into a tract (Figure 16.5 A). The holders usually have the clinic's name embossed on them so that information doesn't have to be written each time. A second type is an X-ray label tape (Figure 16.5 B). This consists of a strip of paper that has a graphite bar centered across the strip with adhesive on the back. The information is written on the graphite portion, the back is peeled off to expose the adhesive and then placed on a holder blocker. The holder blocker comes in different thicknesses for tabletop or grid radiographs, most are marked on the back as to when to use for either technique. A third type is a flash marker or flash blocker (Figure 16.5 C). Newer cassettes have a lead blocker shield in one corner preventing exposure of that area. Patient data is written on a card in ink and placed on the flasher plate of the labeler in the darkroom. With the lights, off remove the film from the cassette and place the unexposed corner of the film in the labeler,

press down to expose the information card onto the film. Then process the film as usual.

Directional labeling is very important for the veterinarian to diagnosis an injury or condition. A lead R for right or a lead L for left (Figure 16.5 D) is placed on the cassette adjacent to the corresponding side of the body part being radiographed. For example, if a right limb is being radiographed, the R marker is placed on the right side of the limb. If radiographing the abdomen indicate which side is right or left, or if the patient is recumbent indicate which side is closest to the film.

The Mitchell marker is a gravitational marker used for standing radiographs. A time marker is used to indicate the time since contrast media was administered to a patient.

The markers are usually placed after the patient is positioned to ensure it will not be obscured or it will not obscure the patient. Be certain the markers are placed within the beam, especially if the beam is calibrated to reduce scatter radiation. Once the film is developed, examine the film to confirm that all the required information is visible.

Put labeling equipment away. If using the small lead letters, remove them from the holder and place them back into the proper slots so they can be quickly found for the next label. Remove the X-rite tape from the blocker holder, throw the tape away and store the holder for the next time. Return the directional marker and/or the study markers to their storage place. Make certain there is an adequate supply of blank patient information cards if a flasher block is used. Have a master blank patient information card copy hidden so that it isn't used or in a page protector marked original so more copies can be made.

Learning Exercise

Utilizing the marking devices at your program or clinic, make a label for this patient: Rubi Sonsthagen, today's date, VD/Lat of thorax.

Taking a Radiograph

A minimum of two radiographs for each body structure are taken, usually at right angles to each other. Patient positioning is determined by using a reference text or wall chart providing descriptions of various veterinary patient positioning or the experience of a veterinary technician. Such a reference is customarily kept near the radiology log binder in the radiology area. Any of the following references are highly recommended: Douglas et al. (1987); Morgan (1993); Lavin (2006).

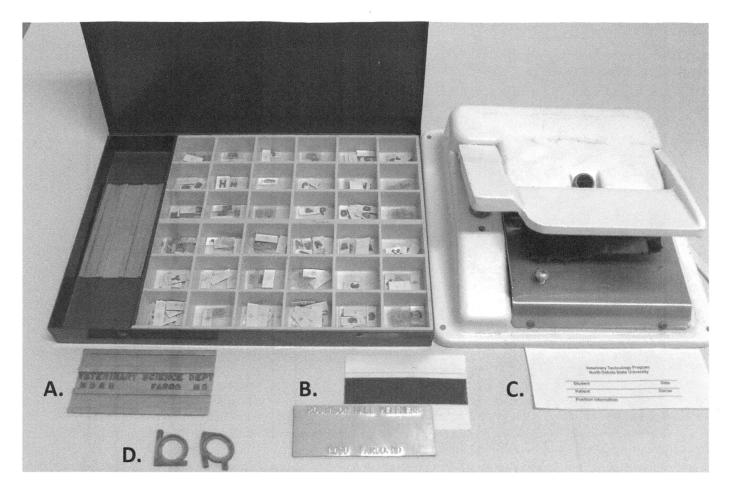

FIGURE 16.5 Labeling and marking devices.

The goal for all radiographs is to maintain as normal an anatomic position as possible while preventing superimposition of extraneous tissues over the study site. This often requires the animal to be placed in often uncomfortable positions. Knowing what is going be radiographed and how it is to be laid on the cassette is important not only for the diagnostic quality, but for the comfort of the animal. Remember to use positioning aids such as sandbags, foam blocks and wedges, ropes, tape, and radiopaque "V" trough if suggested by the reference.

After determining the proper positioning for the patient, it is vital to have everything ready before positioning the animal, so it will only have to be still for less than a second to get the radiograph. Before bringing a patient into radiology, review the sections relevant to positioning for the requested radiographs. Start data entry in the X-ray log, locate positioning aids, determine cassette sizes, prepare identification markers and PPE. Bring the patient into radiology, measure and set the radiography machine. Maneuver the patient into position and take the radiograph by engaging the exposure button. The exposure button can be on the console panel or a foot pedal connected to the console. Either can be pressed to take the exposure. Some machines will have a two-step process to make the exposure, one to start the rotor and the second to trip the exposure. The foot pedal enables someone who is restraining a patient to make the exposure. As the exposure button is pressed a red light will flash on the panel to indicate the emission of X-rays. For patients not requiring manual restraint, the radiologist can simply press the exposure button while standing behind a clear lead shield.

If the radiograph is digital the image should appear immediately on the computer screen. Check to make sure the image is the one ordered by the veterinarian and that it is of diagnostic quality.

Learning Exercise

Using the label you prepared look up the positioning information in the reference book for a VD/Lat Thorax. Describe what you find on how to position a Miniature Dachshund.

Developing Radiographic Film

Manual radiography film is radiation and light sensitive, so it must be handled properly as it can be ruined before, during, or after the radiograph is taken. This requires knowledge about the cassettes that house the film during the radiograph, film handling, and storage and how to use and maintain the processor.

Cassettes are expensive pieces of equipment for both traditional and digital radiography. Traditional film cassettes hold the film flat against the intensifying screens and prevent exposure of daylight to the unexposed film. Cassettes are often dropped by personnel or kicked off tables by the patient. This can cause the screens inside to loosen which in turn will cause film defects. Care must be taken when carrying and using them.

To open a cassette, move to the darkroom and set the cassette with the latches up, onto a dry, clean counter. Lock the darkroom door, turn the overhead lights off, and turn the safety light on. Traditional film cassettes have latches securing the sides tightly together so no light can penetrate. Push or slide the latches to release the sides to access the film inside. Film is handled at the corners only and should not touch anything other than the inside of the cassette. Scratches, static electricity, and water will cause film defects and can be caused by rough handling. Once the film is out of the cassette, place it on the entrance tray to the automatic processor (Figure 16.6). You may have to give it a little push into the machine until the rollers catch it and take it in. While the exposed film is moving through the processor refill the cassette.

Remember radiograph film is light and pressure sensitive. Any work with film must be in the darkroom with the door shut and locked, and the safety light on. Film boxes are stored on edge inside a light-proof safe inside the darkroom. The safe is only opened with the door to the darkroom closed, the overhead light turned off, and the safety light turned on. To open a new box of film, carefully remove the lid by pulling the tear strip and then carefully tearing or cutting the inside wrapper straight across at the very top. Cutting with a scissor is recommended as the paper doesn't tear very well and you are left with ragged edges. This makes it hard to get film out of the box and back inside if too many are removed. Also, the longer wrapper can be folded over and the lid replaced for added protection of the film inside the safe. If the box is already open, carefully try to bring just one piece of film out at a time. Pull the replacement film slowly out of the storage box to prevent static electricity from building up and set it into the cassette without sliding it across the surface. This is all done with just the safety light on, which is a rose-colored light, so you may have to use your fingers to find the corners of the cassette. Set the end of the film into the top edge of the cassette and within the corners, then allow the film to settle into the cassette. Check to make sure it is within the walls and then seal the cassette by pushing the back down until you hear the latches click.

Remove the labeling devices from the outside of the cassette, disinfect and return it to the ready area or pass-through box. A pass-through box is a lead-lined, two-sided cupboard with exposed and unexposed sides. One door opens into the radiography room and the other side opens into the darkroom. The latches for the doors are such that only one side at a time can be opened. This ensures accidental exposure of the film doesn't happen. It is a convenient way to manage cassettes as well. You always know which cassettes are available for use because they are stored on the unexposed side.

By this time the automatic film processor has delivered the developed radiograph and if the film bin and any open cassettes are filled and closed the overhead light may be turned on. Attach the film to a view box and then alert the veterinarian that it is ready for viewing. Record any information in the radiograph log, patient's record, and treatment board. Clean the radiography table off with paper towels and spray disinfectant. Check the automatic processor for enough developer and fixer for subsequent radiographs. Turn the safety light off in the darkroom and leave the door open as you leave.

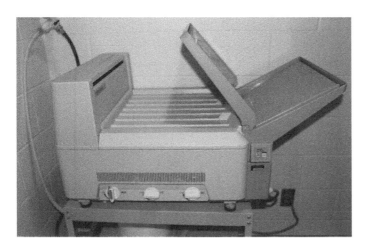

FIGURE 16.6 Automatic processor.

Exploration

Go into the darkroom at your school or clinic. Close the door, turn off the overhead lights, and turn on the safety light. Start counting seconds. How long did it take your eyes to adjust to the red light enough so that you could see your hands?

Cassette Routine Maintenance

Ideally, the exterior is disinfected between patients by spraying with a dilute disinfectant and drying off with paper towels. Monthly they can be wiped off thoroughly using a mild soap and water and then dried thoroughly with towels.

The intensifying screens on the interior of the cassette also requires monthly maintenance. Screen cleaning solutions are used by applying a small amount of solution to a 4 × 4 gauze sponge and wiping the surface of the screens, a second sponge is used to dry the screen. Leave the cassette open to air dry thoroughly, overnight if possible. Clean cassettes at the end of the day so they are not out of commission during business hours. Refill the cassette first thing the next morning. To maintain a record of cleaning, place a small sticker on the back of the cassette with the date cleaned. Replace the sticker after each cleaning. A quick check of the sticker each time the cassette is used will remind personnel it is time to care for the cassette.

Patient Film Filing

Once a film has been read, the diagnosis, film quality, and comments are entered into the radiology log. The assistant can do this from the entry in the patient's record, as the veterinarian will have entered the diagnosis. At this point, the film is ready for filing and storage. The film or films are placed in a large paper envelope specifically designed for radiograph storage. On the exterior of the envelope write the patient's name, owner's name, veterinarian's name, and the dates the radiographs were taken. Some veterinarians also like to put the type of study and the diagnosis after each date.

Radiographs must be filed in such a way that they are easily retrieved. Special storage systems are used to file films as they are too large to file with the patient's paper medical record. The radiograph envelopes are placed in open filing cabinets sized to hold the envelopes in an upright position. There are several methods utilized to file radiographs and they usually follow the same method used to file the patient's medical records. One method is to file them alphabetically under the patient/owner's name. The owner's last name is used first, followed by the first name. This can get a bit confusing with common last names like Smith. Then a middle initial comes into play. If misfiled, these radiographs are difficult and time-consuming to find.

If medical records are filed numerically, the radiograph envelopes are numbered with the patient's file number and filed in numeric order. In either system, all the radiographs for a single patient are filed in one envelope. If the animal is radiographed again, place the new films in front of the old films. The front of the envelope is the side with the writing on it. Hold the envelope so the writing faces you and place the new films in front of the old. Write the information for these new films under the last entry. This will facilitate looking for specific radiographs.

A third system requires filing radiographs using a combination of date and patient name or number. In this circumstance, only the radiographs taken on a specific date for a patient are filed together. The advantage to this system is that location of a specific radiograph is more rapid. The disadvantage is that more envelopes are used, resulting in more cost and more space needed for filing. Likewise, the more items requiring filing increases the chance for misfiling and more personnel time.

The fourth system is filing by date. All films taken on a date are filed together. This requires less filing and fewer envelopes but makes locating all the films of a particular patient for comparison purposes difficult, because they might have been taken on different dates. If many films are taken on a particular date, locating a specific film becomes time-consuming.

Use an out-guide whenever a filed radiograph envelope is removed. This is usually a large card placed in the spot where the radiographs were filed. This makes it easier to return the file or alert personnel that it has been removed.

Accurate filing and quick retrieval are essential! Accurate filing makes radiographs readily available and increases their usefulness. "Lost" or misplaced files require a lot of time to locate the films. Filing radiographs is a daily task for the assistant. Remember these radiographs are legal documents just like the medical record and should be treated with the same care.

Learning Exercise

Find out where and how the radiographs are stored in your school or clinic.

Darkroom Maintenance

The darkroom itself can become a source of poor film quality if it is not properly maintained. Potential darkroom sources for loss of quality include light leaks, improper chemical balance, and artifacts due to chemicals or materials on and in cassettes or on hands. Preparation of a maintenance schedule and strict adherence to it will improve radiographic images.

Checking for Light Leaks

Door seals tend to wear out or get torn loose just from daily wear and tear. To check the darkroom for leaks, close the door, turn off the light, and note the presence of any daylight that might be entering around the door or pass-through box. If there is any light from cracks around the door or any other source, notify the office manager.

Check the safety light as this can deteriorate as the bulb is worn. Close the door, turn off the overhead light, and turn the safety light on. Place an unexposed film on the counter with a metal object such as a paper clip on the film. Let it set for 2 minutes then develop the film. If the object appears on the film, the safety light is not working properly or there is some other source of light in the room.

Check to see if the flasher blocker is working properly. If the light doesn't work, it can be as simple as changing the bulb. Make sure to get the proper wattage bulb, as too bright will cause an artifact on the film and too dim will not show the label very well. Always follow the manufacturer's directions for product maintenance.

Ideally, there are two areas to a darkroom: a wet side and a dry side. The processor side is considered the wet side and the countertops as the dry side. There needs to be sufficient dry counter space for working with cassettes and film boxes. If a flasher block is used for film identification, make sure there is enough room to accommodate the film in the flasher without having to bend the film. Even a slight bend in an unprocessed film can cause an artifact. The cassettes should be able to lie flat on the counter, with the lids open so they don't accidentally fall.

Processor Maintenance

The film processor with the developer and fixer tanks are on the wet side of the room. The processor needs weekly attention. The developer and fixer tanks need to be refreshed or changed as per the quality of the radiographs. The developer and fixer chemicals are pulled from tanks as the film moves through the machine. These tanks usually located on the floor of the darkroom under the processor. When these get too low for the hoses to pump fresh chemicals into the machine or they have reached the expiration date, they need to be refreshed or changed. Follow the instructions on the outside of the developer and fixer chemical concentrates for refreshing or changing. PPE required for this task are goggles, waterproof apron, and gloves. It seems that no matter how careful you are there is always spillage of water or chemicals. These chemicals are not highly toxic but cause skin drying and for some a

headache, so protecting yourself is very important. Film processor rollers are what pulls the radiography film through the processor. These should be wiped off daily to weekly depending on the number of radiographs taken at the clinic. The least often the more they need to be cleaned as the chemicals tend to dry on the rollers causing artifacts on the finished film.

Professional processor maintenance is important to maintain the life of a processor. Read the manufacturer's recommendations and discuss this with the office manager to set up the service.

Floors and counters can become wet. All spills or wet areas need to be cleaned up and dried immediately. Wet spots will make artifacts on the film. Keep paper towels stocked in the room for wiping up spills and cleaning the counter. Mop the floor whenever it becomes wet or at least weekly. Keep a box of examination gloves, an apron, and goggles in the room to be used whenever working with chemicals. Maintain an adequate supply of materials and chemicals in inventory. Note the quantity of each whenever using these items. Add needed items to the want list or notify the inventory manager as supplies become low. Allow for sufficient time for ordering and delivery.

The veterinary assistant can develop daily, weekly, and monthly maintenance charts for the darkroom and materials stored in it. Compose a chart of rows and columns to meet the needs and policies of your practice.

Maintenance tasks include the following.

1. Counters should be wiped down daily with dilute disinfectant. Paper towels are restocked, and the disinfectant is replenished as needed.
2. Developer and fixer chemical levels are checked daily and replenished as needed.
3. Note items that need to be added to a want list or need repair. Next time you are near the want list, copy the information down or pass the note on to the inventory manager if more appropriate.
4. File radiographs daily.
5. Floors are mopped weekly.
6. View boxes are cleaned weekly and bulbs replaced as needed. Any glass-cleaning liquid will do. Dry thoroughly so no streaks are left. View boxes may be

Learning Exercise

Take a look at the automatic processor in your school or clinic if there is one. Lift the covers and look at the rollers. Are they clean? Do they need attention? Are the developer and fixer tanks both sufficiently filled? Is the developer tank dark brown or light brown?

located in the darkroom, each exam room, and even in the surgery and treatment rooms.

7. Clean cassettes monthly inside and out.

Diagnostic Ultrasonography

The use of ultrasonography is increasing as an indirect imaging technique in veterinary medicine (Figure 16.7). The advantages over radiography are the lack of radiation and that the equipment is portable. Ultrasound provides indirect images of organ shape and structure. The principle is based on sound waves. The sound waves are produced by a transducer. As the waves hit tissues within a patient they are "echoed" back to the transducer. The higher the intensity of the returning echo, the brighter (whiter) the image on the screen. It is used for diagnosis of uterine, ovarian, bladder, heart and kidney diseases, confirmation of pregnancy, guided cystocentesis, and tissue biopsies.

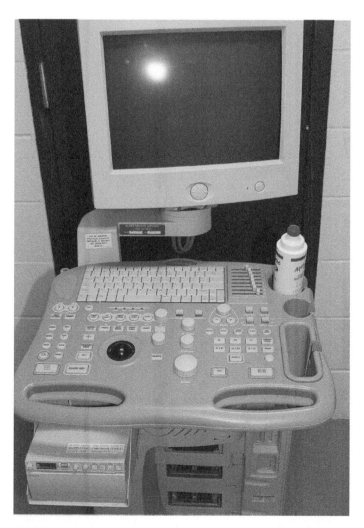

FIGURE 16.7 Ultrasound.

Set-up for Ultrasonography

The role of the assistant in ultrasonography is for equipment set-up, patient preparation, and restraint during the procedure. The ultrasonograph, keyboard, monitor, and acoustic gel are usually kept on a rolling cart making it portable and accessible anywhere in the clinic. Positioning aids can also be stored on the cart. Plug the ultrasound in, turn it on, and place it near the examination table.

The patient is usually to the operator's right with the cart facing the operator. If the operator is left-handed, reverse the arrangement. This allows the operator to hold the transducer in the dominant hand and operate the controls with the other.

Prepare the patient by consulting anatomic charts to learn where to clip a patient for the ultrasound; this will also tell you how to hold the patient for the procedure. The quality of the image is affected by patient preparation. Image quality is decreased by anything that traps air. This can be hair, dirt, or skin scales, which makes skin preparation so important. The study area over which the transducer is placed is clipped with a No. 40 blade to remove the hair completely. The area is gently washed with a surgical soap, rinsed with water, and dried thoroughly. To enhance transducer contact with the skin, a liberal amount of acoustic gel is applied to the skin and allowed to stay in place for 5 minutes before the procedure.

Assist with patient restraint during the procedure. For most studies patients do not need to be anesthetized. After the procedure clean the gel off of the patient with a warm soapy cloth and towel dry. Return the patient to its housing or owner if waiting. Clean the transducer according to the manufacturer's directions and straighten the cart, restock acoustic gel if necessary and put away. File printouts of the images in the patient's record, or if the images are recorded on disk or videotape label in a manner similar to the patient's medical record and store with other patient disks or videotapes.

Reflection

After seeing how images appear on screen during an ultrasound, what did you think of the image? Was it clear? Could you make out the structures? How long will it take looking at these types of images before they become clear to you?

Endoscopy

Oreta M. Samples, RVT, MPH, DHSc

LEARNING OBJECTIVES

- Identify parts of the endoscopic system
- Identify accessory equipment
- List the uses of an endoscope
- Describe the differences between a rigid, semi-rigid, and flexible endoscope
- Gather the needed auxiliary equipment for various endoscopic procedures
- Create a bin filled with materials needed to clean an endoscope
- Correctly clean an endoscope
- Safely transport and store an endoscope
- Restrain and position a patient during the preparation phase of endoscopy
- Effectively assist during the preparation and clean-up phases of an endoscopic procedure

Introduction to Endoscopy

The endoscope is used for diagnostics, but it is also used for surgery and uses highly specialized equipment. It is included with this chapter because it is used for diagnosis by visualizing body structures and can be used for surgical procedures if issues are found. Because patient preparation requires heavy sedation or anesthesia and patient monitoring, refer to those sections in Chapter 14. In instances where entrance to a body cavity is through the skin and musculature, the patient requires a surgical prep (see Chapter 14).

An endoscope is an instrument that allows the veterinarian to have real-time visualization within structures and organs that would otherwise only be visualized indirectly. As the name endoscope implies, the instrument allows the user to see via the end of a complex bundle of glass fibers that allows for the bending of light. These bundles are encased in an insertion tube of varying length and diameter based on the intended location of the instrument's use. The viewer can see through a lens to visualize what is at the other end of the insertion tube or on a video screen.

Parts of an Endoscope

The handpiece is the large end with valves and knobs (Figure 16.8). The valves and knobs are manipulated by the operator to guide the deflection of the tip, control the suction and water valves, and are connected to the umbilical cord, which attaches to the air pump, water bottle for irrigation, and the light source. There may be an eyepiece through which the operator can look, or it may be directly connected to a video screen where the operator can view material directly at the end of the tip.

The tip narrows at the end of the insertion tube and contains the light guide and image lens. The umbilical cord attaches to the handpiece at one end and to various instruments at the distal end or tip. Most important, the light source is attached to the distal end of the umbilical cord. There are connectors for the air pump for insufflation channel for inflating hollow organs with air or gas to increase the visibility of their surface, a connector for a suction channel to remove the irrigation fluid, a connector for the water bottle for irrigation of tissues, and a pressure compensation valve. The last few inches of the insertion tube are known as the "bending section" as this is the portion that is controlled by deflection knobs to bend up and down as well as right and left with remarkable accuracy. This allows the operator to get 360°views within the structures.

Endoscopic findings are documented through video or still pictures (Figure 16.9). Minimally, this requires a camera, light source, and printer. For more sophisticated endoscopic set-ups there is a camera control unit, video recorder, monitor, and keyboard for adding text to the pictures.

All of the equipment is best stored together on a wheeled cart stored out of the way of usual hospital

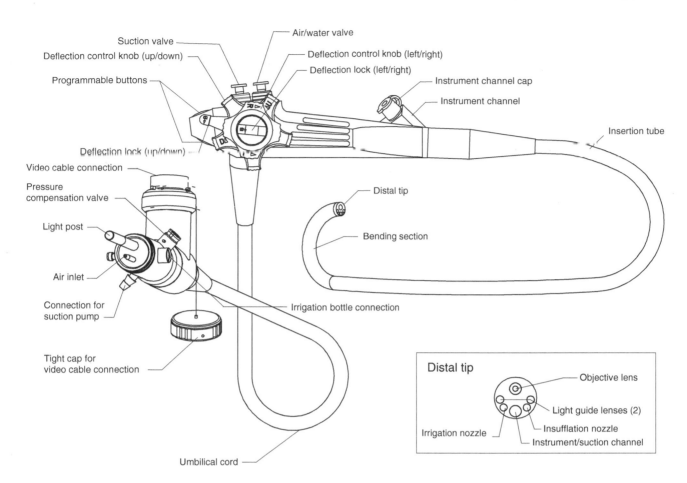

Suction valve
Deflection control knob (up/down)
Programmable buttons
Air/water valve
Deflection control knob (left/right)
Deflection lock (left/right)
Instrument channel cap
Instrument channel
Insertion tube
Deflection lock (up/down)
Video cable connection
Pressure compensation valve
Light post
Air inlet
Connection for suction pump
Distal tip
Bending section
Irrigation bottle connection
Tight cap for video cable connection
Umbilical cord

Distal tip
Objective lens
Light guide lenses (2)
Insufflation nozzle
Irrigation nozzle
Instrument/suction channel

FIGURE 16.8 Labeled parts of an endoscope. Courtesy of Karl Storz Veterinary Endoscopy-America, Inc., Goleta, CA.

traffic near a sink with running water where cleaning functions can be performed immediately after removal of the endoscope from the patient. Ideally, all of this should be in a designated room for endoscopic procedures, as seen in Figure 16.10 showing the special procedures room at the Colorado State University College of Veterinary Medicine.

Unfortunately, many veterinary facilities were built before the advent of endoscopy and lack the additional space dedicated to endoscopic procedures. Endoscopes are usually stored in a special cabinet so they can hang in a vertical position. If a cabinet is not available, endoscopes are most safely stored in the original container in which it arrived from the manufacturer. A possible option is the surgery prep area where instruments are cleaned immediately after surgery or a grated examination table in the treatment area with running water. The cart should have several electrical outlets for plugging in the various machines stored on the cart. The cart itself plugs into a wall outlet providing power for the various outlets on the cart.

Endoscopes are classified as rigid, semi-rigid, or flexible. The earliest endoscopes were little more than a hollow, rigid tube with a light source. The tube was inserted into a patient and the physician looked through the tube to view tissues. Since the advent of fiber optics,

endoscopes have evolved into the highly sophisticated instruments that exist today.

Rigid endoscopes are used for such procedures as ear canal and rectal examinations. These are adaptations of human pediatric endoscopes, and they allow veterinarians to see into structures too small to have been visualized before. These contain fused silica bundles rather than being composed of bundles of very small glass rods that are found in the true fiber optic systems. Semi-rigid scopes are used for such procedures as examination of the urethra, urinary bladder, and the nasal passages.

The flexible endoscopes are larger than the semi-rigid endoscopes, but they have greater flexibility in the bending section, allowing the user to have a wider range of tissue visualization. They are used in a wide range of species and body sites including the gastrointestinal tract.

Endoscopy Preparation

Endoscopy encompasses a variety of procedures, which are named after where in the body the instrument is used. Use is limited only by the length and diameter of the instrument(s) available and the patient size and site of the body into which the instrument is inserted.

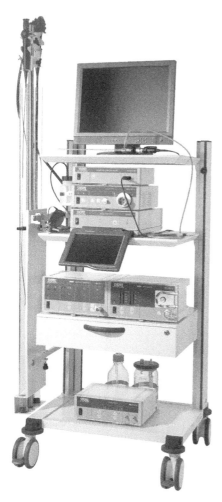

FIGURE 16.9 Basic endoscopy video camera system. Note the endoscope hanging from the hook. Courtesy of Karl Storz Veterinary Endoscopy-America, Inc., Goleta, CA.

Table 16.1 illustrates the more common endoscopic procedures and the location in which the endoscope is used. The assistant can facilitate endoscopy during both the preparation phase and the post-procedural phase of the endoscopic procedure. During the preparation phase, the assistant is helpful by aiding in instrument set-up and patient preparation and restraint. Patients are usually heavily sedated or anesthetized. Refer to Chapter 14 to review the procedure for anesthetizing a patient.

Thoracoscopic and **laparoscopic** procedures require a surgical incision and, to prevent infection, it is important that a surgical scrub be completed whenever the skin and musculature are penetrated to access a body cavity with endoscopic equipment. Patient position depends on the procedure to be performed. Table 16.1 includes the positions required for the various procedures.

Endoscopic procedures require special instruments. Depending upon the procedure you may lay out anticipated equipment:

- Attaching equipment associated with the umbilical cord. Light source, air pump for insufflation, suction pump, and fluid receptacle. Rigid, semi-rigid, or flexible endoscope suitable for procedure and patient.
- Accessory equipment will also depend on the procedure such as cytology brush, coagulating electrodes, dislodger, forceps, biopsy forceps, grasping forceps, needle for injection/aspiration, scissors, trocar, and various snares.
- A basic surgical pack, a towel pack, and surgical drape (see Chapter 14) may also be required together with a bottle filled with sterile normal saline for irrigation. If the procedure is via the oral cavity, an oral speculum of suitable size for the patient will be required. If tissue specimens are to be collected during the procedure, collect appropriate materials (e.g., slides, coverslips, formalin jars, and culture media) labels and laboratory forms, sharpie marker, and ballpoint pen. Label with patient/client name and date.

During the actual procedure, the technician will assist the veterinarian through patient monitoring, helping with instruments and collecting tissue samples, and providing documentation (working the photographic and video equipment). If a licensed or specially training assistant is not available, the assistant might monitor the patient and assist with sample collection and preparation. Special training is usually available through the endoscope manufacturer. Take advantage of it if at all possible.

During gastroscopy, the technician or assistant observes the animal for excessive distention of the stomach with gas or air, which in turn impairs respiratory function.

Endoscopy: Post Procedure

During the post-procedure phase, the technician is busy caring for the patient and the assistant begins cleaning the equipment immediately. That equipment is cleaned immediacy cannot be overemphasized. The endoscope will have mucus and fluids on and around it which will dry and harden very quickly if not removed, making cleaning more difficult. The hollow tubes and valves are so small that foreign materials quickly dry on them making them inoperable.

All of the parts are fragile and very expensive. Do not risk damaging the endoscope by forcibly trying to clear the channel with a small brush or applying too much pressure to work stuck valves. Careful attention to detail in cleaning the accessory instruments is important as the hinges must remain freely movable. The thin wire must never be kinked or bent in any way. Handling requires that the endoscope is never bumped or hit against a hard object or dropped

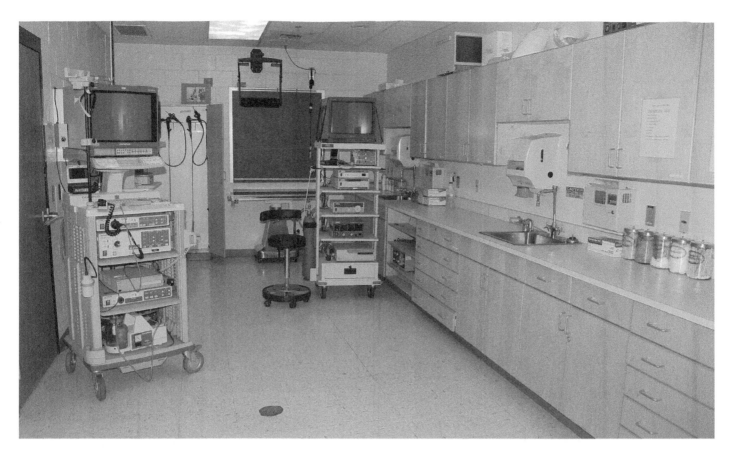

FIGURE 16.10 The endoscopy/special procedures room at the Colorado State University Veterinary Teaching Hospital. Note the cabinet for storage of endoscopes and accessory instruments and a videotape deck and television monitor conveniently located in the work area. Courtesy of David C. Twedt. From Tams, T. *Small Animal Endoscopy*, with permission from Mosby.

Table 16.1

Common Endoscopic Procedures, Locations, and Position

Procedure	Location	Position
Esophagogastroscopy	Esophagus and stomach	Left lateral recumbency
Duodenojejunoscopy	Duodenum and jejunum	Left lateral recumbency
Proctoscopy	Rectum	Any position the endoscopist prefers
Colonoscopy	Rectum and colon	Left lateral recumbency if using a flexible endoscope; right lateral recumbency if using a rigid scope
Thoracoscopy	Thoracic cavity	Dorsal, left, or right lateral recumbency; depends on procedure
Laparoscopy	Abdominal cavity	Dorsal recumbency
Rhinoscopy	Nasal passages	Sternal recumbency with head propped up on a large rolled towel
Bronchoscopy	Larynx and bronchi	Same as above
Cytoscopy	Urethra and urinary bladder	Female: hind legs over the examination table and hips elevated with a large rolled towel Male: lateral recumbency
Arthroscopy[a]	Joints	Depends on the location of the joint; the joint must be uppermost

[a] Requires surgical prep.

(unthinkable!) as the internal glass fibers are easily shattered. This results in black areas in the field of vision when next the endoscope is utilized. No distractions should occur during endoscope cleaning; focus on what you are doing. Be vigilant and thorough in cleaning to avoid cross-contamination with the next patient.

Before a procedure begins, gather all materials that will be needed for cleaning after the procedure is completed. This will allow speedy attention to the fragile equipment. Most clinics only have one endoscope; therefore, it is imperative that it be kept clean and functional. The cleaning of the instrument immediately after a procedure is especially important if multiple endoscopies are scheduled on the same day.

Consult the manufacturer's instructions for cleaning and sanitizing. Failure to follow instructions can cause an existing warranty to be null and void.

Prepare a labeled bin like a household cleaning supplies tote to contain materials for post-procedure instrument cleaning. Place the bin on a lower shelf of the endoscope cart for *immediate* use after procedure conclusion. Materials needed include squirt bottles, with proper secondary container labeling, containing the following:

- Disinfectant soap solution or enzymatic cleanser as recommended by endoscope manufacturer.
- 70% alcohol.
- Hydrogen peroxide. Either cover the secondary container with light and waterproof tape or screw a squirt tip from another bottle onto the original peroxide container as hydrogen peroxide deteriorates in the presence of light.
- Two large dog water dish sized, stainless steel bowls, if there is running water available; if not, have a third bowl for clean tap water.
- Non-sterile cotton-tipped applicator swabs in a large Ziploc bag.
- 4 × 4 inch gauze sponges in a small Ziploc bag.
- Large plastic syringe, 20–35 mL, no needle attached.
- Small bristle brush for cleaning accessory channel and accessory instruments (available from manufacturer of endoscope).
- Roll each of plastic sterilization sleeve and sterilization indicator tape that can be cut to length for enclosing instruments and endoscope if sterilization is used. Indicator tape must be compatible with types of sterilization procedure used. *Or* glutaraldehyde solution or product of the manufacturer's recommendation for cold sterilization *if* the endoscope is submersible.
- PPE: Goggles, gloves, and waterproof apron.

Dissemble each piece of equipment according to the manufacturer's directions. Their recommendations take precedence over any other suggestions.

Put 100–200 mL of cleaning solution (enzymatic cleaner or diluted surgical soap) into one pan. Put diluted disinfectant solution in the second pan. Have tap water available either at a sink or in a third, large bowl.

Clean the working channel first. Using the syringe, draw the cleaning solution through the working channel until the solution exiting the channel is clear. The cleaning brush is passed up and down through the channel. Pass the disinfectant solution through the

channel until it runs clear. Flush with tap water. Flush with alcohol to aid drying *or* use dry air under pressure (large clean, dry syringe).

Clean the air/water valve. Disconnect the water bottle from the umbilical cord. Place one finger on the air/water inlet and one finger on the air/water valve. The light source pump will blow the residual water out of the channel.

Clean the exterior of the insertion tube. Wash using a gauze sponge soaked in soapy solution or enzymatic cleaner. Wipe soap off using a gauze sponge soaked in plain water. Wipe surface with a gauze sponge soaked in 70% alcohol.

Clean the handpiece. Use cotton-tipped swabs soaked in alcohol to clean around the valves and knobs thoroughly.

Clean the accessory instruments. Soak the working end of accessory instruments in soapy water or enzymatic cleanser. Use a soft brush to clean serrations and hinges. Soak wires attached to the working end of accessory instruments, being careful not to bend or kink the wire.

Clean the suction bottle. Dump contents down the drain, flushing with copious amounts of water. Fill the bottle with soapy water. Swirl the contents to loosen debris. Pour out. Rinse with tap water until the water runs clear. Fill with disinfectant solution for designated contact time as per the manufacturer's instructions. Rinse with tap water. Turn upside down on a rack to drain until dry.

To sterilize an endoscope system, either of the following procedures may be used depending on the manufacturer's recommendation.

Gas Sterilization

Place the endoscope and accessory instruments in individual plastic pouches. Insert a sterilization indicator strip into each pouch, seal, and label. Place pouches in the gas sterilizer. Use ethylene oxide gas sterilizer only. Follow the manufacturer's directions for use of the gas sterilizer. Never exceed the endoscope manufacturer's temperature and humidity limits. Allow adequate time after gas sterilization for the gas to dissipate: 7 days in a quarantine area at room conditions *or* 12–18 hours in an aerator (failure to do so results in tissue damage when next used).

Cold (Liquid) Sterilization

Glutaraldehyde (2% Cidex) causes tissue irritation so all channels and surfaces must be rinsed thoroughly with sterile water after sterilization. Follow the product manufacturer's guidelines for contact time and dilution.

Never use a steam autoclave or hydrogen peroxide plasma gas on endoscopes.

After the sterilization process, reassemble the parts. To store an endoscope and accessory equipment, use a designated storage cabinet. Hang vertically on a rack. hang the handpiece up and locked onto rack. This allows for continued drying of the endoscope and parts *or* the cases in which they arrived from the manufacturer; however, be advised that continued drying is inhibited when stored in this fashion which may lead to microbial growth.

End of Procedure Cleaning

Collected tissue samples need to be labeled as to patient, source, and collection method. Complete laboratory requisition forms. Arrange for pick-up or delivery of samples.

Label photographs and video footage with patient's and client's names, date and time, endoscopist, location samples were collected, and procedure(s) performed. File with the patient's medical records.

Learning Exercise

If your clinic has an endoscope ask your supervisor for a lesson in its set up, cleaning, and storage.

Chapter Reflection

What did you think of this chapter? What all did you learn about radiography, ultrasound, and endoscopy?

References

Douglas SW, Herrtage ME, Williamson HD. 1987. *Principles of Veterinary Radiography*, 4th edn. Philadelphia: Bailliere Tindall.

Lavin LM. 2006. *Radiology in Veterinary Technology*, 4nd edn. Philadelphia: Elsevier.

Morgan JR. 1993. *Techniques in Veterinary Radiography*, 5th edn. Ames, IA: Iowa State University Press.

Suggested Reading

Han C, Hurd C. 2004. *Practical Diagnostic Imaging for Veterinary Technicians*. Philadelphia: Elsevier.

Olympus America. https://www.olympusamerica.com/msg_section/cds/index.asp (accessed July 14, 2019).

VetVu. How to clean an endoscope. http://www.vetvu.com/index/cleaning.htm (accessed July 10, 2019).

Suffixes, Prefixes, and Anatomic Terms (Roots)

Suffixes

Characteristic of

English form	Meaning	Example
-al	Relating to, characterized by, of	Mental
-ar	Relating to, being, resembling	Dolar
-able, -ible	Able or capable of	Visible
-oid	Form or like	Hemorrhoid
-plasm	Mold or shape	Cytoplasm
-elle	Small	Organelle

Singular and plural forms

English form	Meaning	Example
-a, -ae	-a means one; -ae means many	Alumna, alumnae
-us, -i	-us means one; -i means many	Radius, radii Alumnus, alumni
-um, -a	-um means one; -a means many	Stratum, strata
-is, -es	-is is singular; -es is plural	Diagnosis, diagnoses

Medical condition

English form	Meaning	Example
-osis	Condition	Prognosis
-ia, -emia	Condition	Anemia
-y	Condition of, state of	Enteropathy
-ic	Condition of	Hydrophobic
-ism	Condition of	Alcoholism

Adjectives (modifiers of the root)

English form	Meaning	Example
-al	Relating to, characterized by	Mental
-ar	Resembling, characterized by	Irregular
-ac, -ic, -tic	Pertaining to, relating to	Cardiac, apneic, acoustic
-us, -ous (vs. ur- meaning urine)	Pertaining to	Various

Characteristics

English form	Meaning	Example
-bryo	Swollen	Embryo
-itis	Inflammation of	Dermatitis
-phlic	Like or love	Hydrophilic
-phob, phobia	Dislike, fear	Hydrophobia
-oma	Mass, bulk	Fibroma
-path, path(y), path(o)	Disease	Enteropathy
-plasm	Related to plasma or the substance of the cell	Cytoplasma
-parous	Bearing	Multiparous
-odyn	Pain, distress	Gastrodynia
-pellent	To drive away	Repellent
-iglia (also: glutin-)	Glue	Neuroglia, agglutination
-stringent	Draw tight, compress	Astringent
-oid	Like	Humanoid

Tasks for the Veterinary Assistant, Fourth Edition. Teresa F. Sonsthagen.
© 2020 John Wiley & Sons, Inc. Published 2020 by John Wiley & Sons, Inc.
Companion website: www.wiley.com/go/sonsthagen/tasks

Person

English form	Meaning	Example
-ist	Person specializing in a disease	Oncologist
-ician	Specialist/practitioner	Physician

Medical operations

English form	Meaning	Example
-ectomy	Excision, removal by cutting	Gastrectomy
-otomy	Incision	Laparotomy
-plasty	Repair, reconstruction	Rhinoplasty
-stomy	Making of an artificial opening	Colostomy
-opsy	Examine	Biopsy
-tome	To cut	Microtome
-cente (vs. prefix cent- meaning 100)	To puncture	Cystocentesis

Communication

English form	Meaning	Example
-gram	Recorded data	Electrocardiogram
-graph	Instrument used to record data	Electrocardiograph

Miscellaneous

English form	Meaning	Example
-ology	The study of	Biology
-rrhea, -rrhage	To flow, discharge	Dysmenorrhea
-zyme	Ferment	Enzyme
-coele, -cele (vs. coel- prefix meaning same is the suffix)	Denotes relationship to a cavity	*Coelenterata* sp.

Prefixes

Characteristics

English form	Meaning	Example
Gnos-	Know	Prognostic
Mal-, cac-, dys- (vs. dis- meaning to separate)	Bad	Malady, cacotrophy, dysphagia
Eu-	Good, normal	Eukaryocyte
Pseud-	False	Pseudocyesis
Noci-	Harmful, deleterious	Nociceptor
Amic-	To love, agreeable	Amicable
Mit-	Thread, small	Mitochondria
Lith-, calc- (vs. calc- meaning heel)	Stone, bone, rock	Urolithiasis, calcium
Nom-	Name	Nomenclature

English form	Meaning	Example
Staphyl-	Cluster	*Staphylococcus*
Strepto-	Chain	*Streptococcus*
Malac-	Soft	Osteomalacia
Scler-	Hard	Sclerosis
Dura-	Hard	Durable
Ton-	Tension	Tonometer
Leva-	Raise	Elevate
Alg-	Pain	Neuralgia
Esthes-	Sensation, perception, feeling	Hyperesthesia
Cata-	Down, negative	Catabolism

Time/space

English form	Meaning	Example
Chron-	Time	Chronology
Templo, tempo (vs. tempo- meaning temple)	Time	Template, temporary
Brady-	Slow	Bradycardia
Tachy-	Fast, rapid	Tachycardia
Neo-	New	Neonate
Poie-	To make, produce	Hematopoiesis
Gene-	Origin, beginning	Genome
Telo-	End	Telophase

Miscellaneous

English form	Meaning	Example
Col(l) (glutin-)	Glue	Collagen, glutinous
Therap-	Treatment	Therapy
Laparo-	Flank, abdomen	Laparoscopy
Febr-	Fever	Afebrile
Ly-	Break down, loose	Lysis

Color

English form	Meaning	Example
Chrom-, chromat-	Colored	Chromatography
Rubri-	Red	Rubrospinal
Erythr-	Red	Erythrocyte
Lute-, lut-	Yellow	Corpus luteum
Xanth-, flav-	Yellow	Xanthophyll, riboflavin
Chlor-	Green	Chlorophyll
Cyan-	Blue	Cyanosis
Leuk-	White	Leukocyte
Alb-	White	Albino
Glauc-	Gray	Glaucoma
Melan-, melano-	Black, dark	Melanoma
Luci-	Clear	Radiolucent
Hyal-	Clear	Hyaline

Relationships/directions

English form	Meaning	Example
A-, an-	Negative, without, absence	Ametria, atrophy
A-, ad- (can become af-, vs. ef meaning away from), abs-	Away from	Abnormal, abduct, afferent
Ad-	Toward	Adduct, addiction
Ant-, anti-	Oppose, prevent, inhibit	Antibiotic
Ante-	Before	Antemortum
Ob- (b can change to c)	Against, toward	Obturator, occlude
Im-	Not, negative	Impossible
Contra-	Against	Contrary
Com-, con- (changes to co- before vowels)	With, together	Contraction, cooperate
Pan-	All, universal	Panleukopenia
Omni-	All, universal	Omniverous
Trans-	Through	Transparent
Amphi- (i can change to a), ambi- (ph changed to b)	Both, doubly	Amphibious, ambidextrous
Sym-, syn-	Together, with	Symphysis, synthesis
Juxta-	Near, close	Juxtaposition
Para-	Apart, beside, beyond	Paranormal
Homo-, hom-	Same, alike	Homogenized
Iso-	Same	Isomer
Hetero-	Different, other	Heterogeneous
Ultra-	High, beyond	Ultraviolet
Meta-	After, beyond, accompanying	Metastasis
Epi-	Above, on top	Epidermis
Super-, supra-	Above, beyond, extreme	Supernatant
Hyper-	Above, beyond, extreme	Hypermotility
Sub- (b can change to f or p)	Beneath, below	Sublingual, suppository
Hypo-	Below, underneath	Hypothermia
In- (n can change to l, m, r)	Negative, beneath	Invalid
Infra-	Beneath	Infraorbital
Inter-	Between, among	Interstitial
Peri-	Around	Perinatal
Circum-	Around	Circumcise
Ec-, ect-, ex- (c can change to x)	Out, outside, away from	Ectoderm, excrete
Extra-	Outside, beyond	Extracellular
Epi-	Upon, addition to, after	Epiglottis, epistaxis
En-, endo- (n can change to m, b, p, or ph)	In, on	Endoscopy, endocarditis
Eso-	Inside	Esophagus
Re-, retro- (o can change to a)	Behind, backward	Retrodeviation, retract

Direction

English form	Meaning	Example
Cept-	Receive, take	Intercept
Later- (vs. lat- meaning carry or bear)	Side	Lateral
Medi-	Middle	Mediolateral
Dorso-	Back	Dorsum
Ventro-	Below	Ventral
Post-	After, behind	Postoperative
Vert-	Turn	Diverticulum
Trop-	Turn	Tropism
Levo-	To the left	Levotorsion
Sinistr-	Left	Sinistrad
Dextr-	To the right, two	Dextrocardia, ambidextrous

Size, number

English form	Meaning	Example
Arith-	Number	Logarithm
Nan-	Dwarf	Nanotechnology
Micr-	Small	Microcyte
Mega-, megal- (can also be a suffix)	Large, great, attached to	Megalothymus, splenomegaly
Semi-	Half	Semiconscious
Hol-	Whole	Hologram
Brachy-	Short	Brachycephalic
Doli-	Long	Doliocephalic
Olig-	Few, small	Oligouria
Poly-	Many	Polydactyl
Multi-	Many, much	Multitude
Uni-	One	Uniform
Mon-	Only, sole	Monochromatic
Di- (vs. dia- meaning through, apart), bi-	Two, twice	Dimorphic, bisexual
Tri-	Three	Triplets
Quad-, quadra, tetra-	Four	Quadrangle, tetradactyly
Pent- (vs. pen- meaning lack or need, pet- meaning seek, toward, and pex- meaning fix or make fast), quin-, qui-	Five	Pentapeptide, quintuplets

English form	Meaning	Example
Sex- (vs. meaning differentiation of gametes produced), hex-	Six	Sexigravida, hexameter
Sept- (vs. sept- meaning wall of, sep- meaning rot, decay, ser- meaning serum)	Seven	Septipara
Octo-	Eight	Octave, octane
Nov- (vs. nod meaning knot, nom- meaning deal out, distribute, nos- meaning disease)	Nine	Novobiocin
Deci-	Ten (metric measure)	Decimal
Centi- (vs. cen- meaning common, cente- meaning puncture, centr- meaning point or center)	Hundred (metric measure)	Centimeter
Kilo-	Thousand (metric measure)	Kilogram

Miscellaneous

English form	Meaning	Example
Commis-	United	Commissure
Tens-	Stretched	Tension
Tetan-	Rigid, tense	Tetanus
Decide-	Falling of	Deciduous
Ortho-	Straight	Orthopedics
Ankyl-	Crooked	Ankyloglossia
Arch- (vs. arachn meaning spider, archo- old term meaning rectum/anus)	Beginning, origin, first	Archiblast
Cusp-	Pointed, a tapering projection	Tricuspid
Delta-	Triangular	Deltoid
Laten- (vs. lat- meaning to the side)	Hidden	Latent
Crypt-	Hidden	Cryptorchid
Actin-	Ray shaped	Actinomycosis
Strat-	Layer, layers	Stratified
Stria-	Furrow, groove	Striation
Fasci- (vs. tear. faci- meaning face, -facient a suffix meaning make)	Band	Fascia
Squam-	Flat	Squamous
Sten-	Narrow, constricted	Stenosis

Visc- (vs. vesic- meaning bladder)	Sticky	Viscous
Append-	To hang, appendage	Appendectomy
Desm-	Band, ligament	Desmosis
Duct-	Lead or draw	Ductile
Bio-	Life	Biology
Vitro-	In a test tube or artificial environment	In vitro
Vivo-	The living body	In vivo

Anatomical terms: roots

English form	Meaning	Example
Abdomi	Abdomen	Abdominal
Acr	Extremities	Acromegaly
Aden	Gland	Adenosarcoma
Adip	Fat	Adiposis
Adren	Adrenal glands	Adrenalism
Angi	Vessel	Angiogram
Aort	Aorta	Aortorrhaphy
Arteri	Artery	Arterial
Arthr	Joint	Arthritis
Bronchi, bronch	Bronchus	Bronchiectasis
Cardi	Heart	Electrocardiogram
Cephal	Head	Cephalocaudal
Cerebr	Brain	Cerebrum
Chondro	Cartilage	Osteochondritis
Col, colon	Colon	Colonoscopy
Cost	Ribs	Costochondral
Crai	Skull	Craniotomy
Cutane	Skin	Cutaneous
Cyst	Bladder	Cystitis
Cyt	Cell	Cytoplasm
Dent	Teeth	Dentist
Derm	Skin	Dermatology
Encephal	Brain	Encephalomalacia
Enter	Intestine	Enteritis
Esophag	Esophagus	Esophagodynia
Gastro	Stomach	Esophagogastric
Gingiv	Gum	Gingivitis
Gloss	Tongue	Glossectomy
Heme	Blood	Hemorrhage
Hepat	Liver	Hepatitis
Hist	Tissue	Histology
Lapar	Abdominal	Laparotomy
Laryng	Larynx	Laryngitis
Lingu	Tongue	Lingual
Lip	Fat	Lipid

English form	Meaning	Example
Lumb	Lower back	Lumbosacral
Myel	Spinal cord, bone marrow	Myeloma
My	Muscle	Myositis
Nas	Nose	Nasopharynx
Nephr	Kidneys	Nephron
Neur	Nerve	Neuropathy
Odon	Teeth	Orthodontia
Ophthal, ocul, opt	Eye	Ophthalmic, oculomotor, optic
Or, Stomat	Mouth	Stomatitis, oral
Oste	Bone	Osteomyelitis
Ot	Ear	Otic

Pelv	Pelvis	Hemipelvectomy
Phalang	Bones of toes	Phalanx, phalanges
Pharyng	Pharynx	Pharyngitis
Phleb	Vein	Phlebitis
Pleur	Pleura	Pleuritis
Pneum	Lung	Pneumonia
Rhin	Nose	Rhinitis
Scler	White of eye, also means hardening	Sclerotomy, Sclerosis
Tend	Tendon	Tendolysis
Thorax	Chest	Thoracotomy
Trache	Trachea	Tracheitis
Vascul	Blood vessel	Vasculitis

GLOSSARY

Abducted   Movement of a limb away from the midline of the body

Abomasum   Fourth ruminant stomach compartment most like the monogastric stomach

Abscess   An accumulation of pus under the skin

Acerbate   Irritate, to make harsh or worse

Acute renal failure   Sudden onset of kidney failure from toxic overload or poisoning

Addison's   See **Hypoadrenocorticism**

Adduction   Movement of a limb toward the midline of the body

Adipose   Body tissue used for the storage of fat

Adrenal gland   Located on top of the kidney, controls inflammation, provides stress hormones

Aerobic organism   Requires oxygen to make energy and to survive

Agonal breathing   Related to the process of dying, patients seem as if they are gasping for breath but in reality it is a muscle spasm

"Ain't doing right" (ADR)   Description of a patient that isn't acting normally

Alcohol (isopropyl or ethyl)   Substance used to disinfect objects or as an antiseptic on skin

Alimentary canal   Entire digestive tract from mouth to anus

Alkalines (lye)   Strong alkaline solutions capable of neutralizing acids. Commonly used for washing or cleansings products

Allele   One of two genes found at the same place on a chromosome

Alopecia   Partial or complete loss of hair

Alveoli   Plural form of the word alveolus, which is an air sac in the lungs or a honeycomb pit in the wall of the stomach

American Animal Hospital Association (AAHA)   Sets standards for veterinary hospitals

American Kennel Club (AKC)   Organization that sets the standard for and registers purebred dogs in the USA

American Veterinary Medical Association (AVMA)   A national organization representing the individual veterinarian

Anaerobic organism   An organism that does not require oxygen for life or growth, oxygen can inhibit or cause death of the organism

Anaphylaxis   An unusual or exaggerated allergic reaction by an animal to foreign protein or other substances

Anogenital distance   An area between the vulva and anus on animals

Anorexia   Lack of appetite or desire for food

Antibodies   Plural for antibody, which is a protein that acts to destroy antigens as an immune response

Anticoagulant   A substance that prevents the process of coagulation or clotting of blood

Antigen   An invader that is foreign to a body and evokes an immune response

Antiseptic   Substance that reduces the spread or growth of microorganisms on living tissue

Apical   Directional term meaning toward apex or the root of a tooth

Apneic   The suspension of breathing or absence of breath

Appendicular skeleton   The bones of the limbs and their means of attachment

Arrhythmia   An irregular heartbeat

Arteriole   Small artery that terminates as capillaries

Arthritis   The inflammation of joints caused by infections, metabolic or developmental causes

Aseptically   Using methods to prevent or protect against the introduction of pathogenic microorganisms

Aspiration   The act of inhaling or of withdrawing of air or fluid from body tissues and medication bottles

Asthma   Respiratory condition marked by a wheezing sound when the animal breathes, often caused by airway obstruction

Astringent   An agent that causes the skin cells to contract

Ataxia   Difficulty coordinating movement, staggering

Atria   The two upper chambers of the heart

Atrial fibrillation   A rapid fluttering beat of the atria of the heart

Aural   In reference to the ear, as in aural medications

Auscultate   To listen to internal organs with a stethoscope

Autoclaving   Common technique using high temperatures, pressure, and steam to sterilize surgical equipment and instruments

Autoimmune   Immune system is attacking the body or organism that is producing the antibodies

Tasks for the Veterinary Assistant, Fourth Edition. Teresa F. Sonsthagen.
© 2020 John Wiley & Sons, Inc. Published 2020 by John Wiley & Sons, Inc.
Companion website: www.wiley.com/go/sonsthagen/tasks

Autolysis   Destruction of cells or tissues by their own enzymes

Autonomous nervous system (ANS)   Nervous system division that responds in times of stress

Axillary   Armpit or space between the underarm and chest wall

Bactericidal   Chemical substance that destroys bacteria

Bacteriostatic   Substance that inhibits growth of bacteria

Basic energy requirement (BER)   The amount of energy from foods required to sustain life or body functions

Beats per minute (bpm)   The number of times the heart contracts and relaxes in one minute

Bight   A sharp bend in the rope

Body conditioning score (BCS)   A subjective evaluation of the body in regards to muscle to fat ratio

Borborygmi   Rumbling or gurgling noise made by the passage of fluid and gas in the intestines

Brachycephalic   Foreshortening of the upper jaw creating a flat face

Bradycardia   Slower than normal heart rate

Break-through pain   Severe pain that occurs in spite of being on pain medications

Bright, alert, and responsive (BAR)   A subjective evaluation of the mental condition of a dog or cat

Bronchiole   Branch of the bronchus in the lungs

Buccal   Refers to the inside of the cheek, a directional term for toward the lips

Calculus   The hardened form of plaque caused by precipitation of minerals from saliva and gingival crevicular fluid

Calorie   A unit of energy defined as the heat required to raise one kilogram of water one degree

Capillaries   The plural form of capillary, tiny blood vessels that are one cell in thickness and are the terminal ends of arterioles; item with wicking action that will lift fluids into it, i.e., "capillary tube"

Cardiac output   The amount of blood pumped by the heart per minute

Carnivore   An animal that feeds on flesh

Catalyst   A substance that increases the rate of a chemical reaction without undergoing any permanent chemical change

Caudal   Refers to moving toward the tail from a current location or being a tail

Cecum   A pouch connected to the junction of the small and large intestine

Cemento-enamel junction (CEJ)   The anatomic border where the enamel and the cementum meet on a tooth

Cementum   A specialized calcified substance covering the root of a tooth

Central nervous system (CNS)   Brain and spinal cord

Cesarean section   Surgical operation for delivering offspring via an incision into the abdomen and uterus

Chattel   Tangible and mobile personal property

Chlorhexidine   Antibacterial compound that is available in three forms: hydrochloride, gluconate, or acetate, used as an antiseptic or disinfectant for both inanimate objects and living tissue

Chlorine   Common substance used in cleaning and disinfecting solutions

Chloroxylenol   Common antiseptic solution, a chlorine derivative

Chromosome   Thread-like structure of nucleic acid that carries the genetic information in the form of genes

Chronic heart failure (CHF)   When the heart does not pump well enough to distribute blood around the body, a progressive state of failure

Chronic renal failure   Ongoing progressive failure of the kidneys to properly filter the blood

Chucks   Absorbent pads to protect against moisture

Cladistics   Method of classifying animals and plants according to the proportion of measurable characteristics they have in common

Clinical pathology   A division within pathology concerned with the evaluation of body fluids and tissues, includes urine, serum, plasma, and tissues

Coenzyme   Non-protein compound that is necessary for the function of an enzyme

Colon   Large intestine

Commissure   The corner of the mouth where the upper and lower lips meet

Congenital   Existing abnormalities at birth, acquired during development inside the uterus

Connective tissue   Category of tissues that includes bones, ligaments, tendons, and fat

Conscious proprioception   Sense of body position, knowing where the appendages are

Contact time   The amount of time required for a disinfectant or antiseptic to destroy pathogens on a surface

Contaminant   Organism or debris that can potentially cause an infection

Contraindication   A condition or symptom that renders a treatment to be inadvisable

Contrast media   Mediums used to improve radiographic contrast often used to distinguish normal from abnormal organs

Controlled drug   Prescription drug with the potential for addiction or abuse, also referred to as controlled substance (CS), regulated by DEA

Coplin jar   Wide-mouth glass or plastic jars with vertically grooved interior walls, used for staining or storage of microscope slides

Coronal   Directional term meaning toward the crown of a tooth

Costochondral junction   Where a rib and the costal cartilage join

Cranial   Refers to moving toward the skull from the current location or relating to the skull

Crepuscular   Animal that is active during twilight

Crown   The uppermost part of the tooth, covered by enamel

Cud   Solid portion of chewed food that is burped up for further chewing

Cushing's   See **Hyperadrenocorticism**

Cyanotic Bluish or grayish color of the skin and mucous membranes

Cystitis An infection of the urinary bladder

Cystocentesis Insertion of a needle and syringe through the wall of the abdomen and urinary bladder in order to collect a sterile urine sample

Cytology Study of cells

Debrided Removal of damaged or dead tissue from a wound

Deciduous tooth A young or "baby" tooth that is shed as the animal matures

Decubitus ulcer Bedsore or ulcer formed from local interference with circulation; pressure sores occurring over a bony prominence such as a hip or elbow

Defecation The act of expelling feces from the anus

Degenerative myopathy Condition or disorder that causes weakness in the affected muscles

Dehydrated Significant loss of body fluid

Dehydration A condition of being dehydrated from loss of fluid

Dentin Material that makes up the bulk of a tooth's structure

Deoxyribonucleic acid (DNA) The carrier of genetic information, the main constituent of chromosomes

Dermatitis Inflammation of the skin

Dermis Vascular layer of skin

Devitalized Weaken or dying

Diabetes mellitus A disease of having too much sugar in the blood, caused by a malfunction of the pancreas

Diarrhea Abnormally watery stool

Diastolic The pressure in the arteries when the heart rests between beats

Dichocephalic Very long head shape, i.e., greyhound

Dilated cardiomyopathy Enlargement of the heart

Dipping The application of a medicine to treat skin infections or parasites

Disinfectant Chemical agent that destroys infectious organisms

Disinfection Reducing the spread of growth of microorganisms on inanimate objects

Distal Locations on appendages that are far from the point of attachment or origin

Distemper Viral disease leading to seizures and tremors

Dolichocephalic A relatively long skull

Dominant gene The effect of one allele of one gene masking the contribution of the second allele

Dorsal Relating to an animal upper surface, moving toward or on the back

Double haircoat A hair coat consisting of two layers, a dense, thick layer of hair called an undercoat, with long guard hairs growing through and protruding above the undercoat

Dram Unit of apothecary weight used commonly in pharmacology that is equal to an eighth of an ounce or 60 grains

Drug Enforcement Agency (DEA) US government agency responsible for enforcing controlled substance laws, specific rules for ordering, storing, and dispensing medications

DUDE normal Acronym for defecating, urinating, drinking, and eating normally

Duodenum First part of the small intestine

Dysplasia Poorly developed or abnormally growing structure

Dystocia Difficult or slow delivery of offspring

Ecological niche How an organism or population responds to the distribution of resources and competitors

Ectoparasite External parasite living on the surface of the host's body

Electrocardiogram (ECG) Graphic record or tracing produced by an electrocardiograph

Electrocardiograph Any instrument that records changes of the electric potential during heartbeats, used to diagnose heart disease

Enamel Thin outer covering of the crown of the tooth, hardest substance in the body

Encephalomyelitis Literally means an inflammation of the brain and spinal cord

End The end of a rope that can be freely moved and be manipulated to tie a knot or hitch

Endocarditis Inflammation of the inside layer of the heart

Endoparasite A parasite that inhabits the internal organs and tissues of a host

Endoscope Fiber optic instrument used for examination of areas of the body not easily seen or accessed. There are three main types of endoscopes: flexible, semi-rigid, and rigid

Endoscopy Visual examination of the interior structures of the body with an endoscope

Endosteum Vascular lining of the inner cavity of a bone

Enervate To cut or drain of energy, used to describe cutting a nerve

Enzyme A substance produced by glands to act as a catalyst to bring about a biochemical reaction

Epidermis Outermost layer of skin

Epithelial Tissues that comprise the linings and coverings of the body and its organs

Ethics Rules or principles that govern right conduct; the values and guidelines that govern veterinary practice

Ethylene oxide Gas fumigant used for sterilizing or disinfecting agent of surgical equipment, has a broad spectrum of activity

Euthanasia A painless death or killing of a patient with an incurable disease or condition

Fascia The outer covering of muscles that cover or bundle them

Fat-soluble vitamin A, D, E, and K are vitamins stored in the adipose tissues in the body

Feces Waste product of food; all living beings expel digested wastes

Fenestration A square, rectangular, or round opening, in this case on a surgical drape

Feral Untamed, term is often used in reference to an animal having escaped from domesticity and running wild

Fight and flight response Physiologic reaction in response to perceived or actual threat, if patient cannot flee it will fight for survival

Flocking instinct A group survival technique of one following the one in front, makes it harder for predators to select an individual

Fomite Inanimate object capable of transmitting microorganisms that can cause disease

Formaldehyde Chemical that is used as a preservative agent for tissues

Fungicidal An chemical compound that destroys parasitic fungi and their spores

Furcation Where the roots of the teeth join

Gastric dilatation and volvulus (GDV) Dilation, expansion, and twisting of the stomach, also known as bloat

Gastric dilatation Dilation and expansion of the stomach

Gastritis Inflammation of the stomach

Gastroscopy Inspection of the interior of the stomach with a gastroscope

Genotype Genetic makeup of an individual

Gestation The time from conception to delivery of offspring

Gingiva Gum tissue in the mouth

Gingival Concerns the gum tissue, directional term toward the gingiva

Glutaraldehyde A disinfectant used in aqueous solution for sterilization of non-heat-resistant equipment

Gonads Gender neutral term for sex organs

Gravid Pregnant, carrying eggs or young

Gross contaminant Contamination visible to the naked eye

Guard hair The long hair that protects the animal from rain and snow

Heart murmur Atypical sound of the heart usually indicating a malfunction or structural defect

Heaves Asthma or emphysema in horses

Hematology Study of the physiology of blood

Hematoma Unclotted mass of blood from a damaged blood vessel under the skin

Hemoglobin Protein responsible for transporting oxygen

Hemolyzed Damaged red blood cells that have released hemoglobin

Hemorrhage Bleeding or abnormal flow of blood

Heparinized saline A mixture of heparin, an anticoagulant, and normal saline used to prevent clotting of IV catheters

Hepatic lipidosis Accumulation of fat in the liver and hypertryglyceridemia that may develop in persistently anorexic obese cats

Herbivore Animal that feeds on plants

Heterozygous Two different alleles of a particular gene or genes

Hip dysplasia Poorly formed hips

Histology The study of body tissues

Hitch The intertwining of loops arranged so the standing part pushes against the end, securing the rope to an animal or object

Homozygous Two identical alleles of a particular gene or genes

Horizontal ear canal A portion of the dog and cat ear canal just in front of the tympanic membrane

Hot spot Common name for pyotraumatic dermatitis, patches of inflamed, painful, moist skin with a secondary bacterial infection

Human–animal bond The emotional bond that exists between humans and their animals

Hydrogen peroxide Mild antiseptic and bleaching agent

Hyperadrenocorticism (Cushing's) Excessive production of adrenocorticotropic hormone (ACTH) by the pituitary gland

Hypertension Abnormally high blood pressure

Hyperthermia Abnormally high body temperature

Hyperthyroidism Excessive functioning of the thyroid gland, results in increased metabolism, heart rate, and high blood pressure

Hypertrophic cardiomyopathy Heart walls enlarge or increase in bulk

Hypoadrenocorticism (Addison's) Insufficient adrenocortical secretion, results in weakness, weight loss, low blood pressure, and gastrointestinal disturbances

Hypodermis Beneath the dermis

Hypotension Abnormally low blood pressure

Hypothyroidism Deficient thyroid activity, low metabolic rate

Hypovolemia Decreased volume of circulating blood

Hypoxemia Low level of oxygen in the blood

Iatrogenic injury Condition not necessarily caused by medical personnel, treatment, or procedure

Idiopathic Disease or condition that arises spontaneously for unknown reason

Ileum Distal portion of the small intestine

Ileus Painful distension of the abdomen, failure of peristalsis resulting in the inability of the intestine to contract normally

Inanimate Not alive or have power of motion

Incontinence The inability to hold urine or feces

Induced ovulator Copulation has to take place in order for ovulation to occur

Inflammation The body's way of protecting itself from infection, illness, or injury; symptoms include swelling, redness, and heat

Inguinal The groin or in the area of the inguinal rings

Institutional Animal Care and Use Committee (IACUC) Sets policies and procedures for the care and treatment of animals at research or educational institutions

Insufflation Blow an agent into the nose, i.e., oxygen

Integument The skin, hair, and nails

Interproximal Directional term meaning between teeth

Intramuscular (IM) Administration of substance into a muscle

Intravenous (IV) Administration of a substance into a vein

Intubation The placement of a tube into the trachea to maintain an open airway or to act as a conduit for medication

Intussusception The slippage of a section of intestine within an adjacent portion of intestine, similar to a "spy glass"

Irritable bowel disease (IBD) Overly sensitive intestines to food or stress

Jejunum Middle part of the small intestine

Knot The intertwining of parts of a rope or two ropes together

Labial Relating to the lips

Laparoscopic Examination of the peritoneal cavity utilizing a laparoscope

Laryngeal paralysis (LP) Folds in the larynx in the throat don't move properly and block the airway

Larynx Upper part of the respiratory passage, contains the voice box

Lateral Away from the middle of the body or limb

Lavage The flushing or washing out of a body cavity or wound

Ligament Strong band of connective tissue that connects bones to other bones or keep organs in place

Lingual Relating to or resembling the tongue, directional term meaning toward the tongue on the mandible

Loop A complete circle made to start a knot or hitch

Lumen The cavity inside a tube

Lymphadenopathy Swelling of the lymph node

Lymphocyte White blood cell that provides an immune response

Lymphoma Cancer of the lymph system

Mandible Lower jaw

Material safety data sheets (MSDS) Sources of information on the hazards of each material found within the hospital

Maxilla Upper jaw

Medial canthus Inside corner of the eye where the eyelids meet

Medial Toward the middle of the body or limb

Meniscus A crescent or crescent shape

Mesial Directional term meaning toward the midline, on the incisors

Mesocephalic A head of "normal" proportions

Metabolism Chemical processes that occur within a living organism in order to maintain life

Microbe Organism not seen with the naked eye, often associated with bacteria

Micturition Urination

Monogastric Digestive system with one stomach compartment

Muscle Tissues that contract to provide movement

Myopathy General term for muscle disease

Nares Opening of the nasal cavity

Nasogastric tube Soft rubber or plastic tube that is inserted through a nostril and into the stomach

Nasopharynx The part of the throat behind the nose

National Association of Veterinary Technicians of America (NAVTA) Professional organization representing veterinary technicians

Necrosis Localized death of tissue

Necrotic Localized tissue death

Negligence Failure to take care to prevent harm to others

Neoplasm New growth, lump, tumor, or growth

Nephron The filtering unit of the kidney

Nerve The tissues that conduct messages by impulses

Neuron Functional cell of the nervous system

Neurotransmitter The chemical messenger that carries messages along the nervous system

Nits The eggs of lice, an ectoparasite

Nocturnal To be active during night-time hours

Nosocomial Infections or diseases that are acquired during a hospital stay

"Not doing right" (NDR) Subjective analysis of a patient that is not acting "normally"

Nucleus Part of the cell that controls the activity of the cell

Nystagmus Rapid flicking motion of the eyes

Occlusal Chewing surface of teeth

Occlusion The way teeth fit together

Occupational Safety and Health Administration (OSHA) US government agency regulating safety in the workplace

Omasum Third of the ruminant stomach compartments

Omnivore Animal that eats both plants and meats

Oocyst A cyst containing a zygote formed by a parasitic protozoan

Operculum A structure that closes or covers an aperture, the end in which parasitic larva break out of egg

Ophthalmic Pertaining to or relating to the eye

Oral Pertaining to relating to the mouth cavity

Orchiectomy Surgical excision of the testicles

Organelle Organs within a cell

Organs Units of specific function within the body

Oropharynx Part of the throat below the soft palate, above the epiglottis, and continuous with the mouth

Orthopneic Position in which an animal stands to breathe easier

Osteosarcoma Bone cancer

Otitis Inflammation of the middle ear

Ova Eggs, female sex cell

Ovary Female reproductive organ that produces eggs and the hormones estrogen and progesterone

Overhand knot Quick and easy way to secure the end of a rope from fraying or to produce a loop to make a fixed bight

Over-the-counter (OTC) drug Non-prescription drug that anyone can purchase

Ovulation The release of eggs

Palatability Acceptable or agreeable taste

Palatal Directional term, meaning toward the tongue on the maxilla

Palpebral reflex The blink of the eyelid when touching the medial or lateral canthus

Pancreas Dual-role gland that produces digestive enzymes and insulin

Pancreatitis Inflammation of the pancreas

Panosteitis Inflammation of all the bones

Parasitic organism A being that lives on or in a host and gets its food from the host at its expense

Parasitology The study of parasitic organisms

Parasympathetic nervous system Part of the nervous system that does not require conscious control; smooth muscle contraction, secretions, breathing, and so on

Parathyroid Glands responsible for calcium regulation

Paresis Partial paralysis

Parturition The act or process of giving birth

Passerine Relating to birds with feet adapted to perching, included all song birds

Patent ductus arteriosus Abnormal persistence of the left sixth aortic arch after birth, leaving an open lumen in the ductus arteriosus, between the descending aorta and the pulmonary artery

Pathogen Microorganism capable of causing disease

Pendulous Hanging skin or in the case of ears cartilage and skin

Penrose drain A tube sutured into a wound cavity to permit body fluids to escape while the wound is healing

Periodontal disease Gum infection that damages the gum tissue and jaw bone

Periodontium The soft tissues and bone that support the teeth

Periosteum Outer covering of a bone

Peripheral field of vision The area of vision to either side of the face

Peripheral nervous system Nerves of the body that correspond with the CNS

Peristaltic wave Involuntary movement of the longitudinal and circular muscles, in the digestive tract

Peritonitis Inflammation of the membrane lining the abdominal wall and covering the abdominal organs

Perivascular Relating to or being the tissues that surround a blood vessel

Personal protective equipment (PPE) Gloves, gowns, masks, and other coverings to protect an individual from infection

Pharyngostomy tube Esophagostomy tube for feeding when the oral cavity must be bypassed following injury or surgery

Phenotype Set of observable characteristics of an individual resulting from the interaction of its genotype

Phlebitis Inflammation of a vein

Pinna The portion of the ear that is formed by cartilage

Pitting edema A resulting pit or depression in tissues that is fluid filled

Pituitary gland Referred to as the "master gland" as it controls other glands

Placenta Life support system for the fetus

Pleural effusion Condition of fluid in the tissues of the lungs

Pneumonia Inflammation and consolidation of the lungs caused by infection

Pneumothorax Air present in the pleural or chest cavity

Polydactyl More toes than normal

Polymyositis Inflammation of many muscles

Popliteal Area of the caudal knee, in reference to finding the popliteal lymph node

Poultice A soft moist mass of material, applied to the body to relieve soreness and inflammation

Predator An animal that naturally preys on or eats other animals

Prehension Taking in food by seizing or grasping

Prescription drug (Rx) Medicines that can be dispensed by a prescription written by a licensed veterinarian

Prey animal An animal that is sought, caught, and eaten by predators

Prion Small infectious protein, self-replicates

Proliferative ileitis Infection of hamsters, characterized by sever diarrhea in weanlings

Protist Member of the kingdom Protista which includes bacteria, algae, slime molds, fungi, and protozoa

Proximal Directional term used for appendages, meaning close to the point of attachment

Pruritus The urge to scratch

Psittacine Relating to birds of the parrot family

Pulmonary artery Takes blood to the lungs from the heart

Pulp chamber The soft area within the center of a tooth that contains the nerve, blood vessels, and connective tissue

Pulse deficit Difference in a minute's time between the number of beats of the heart and the number of beats of the pulse

Punnett square A square diagram used to predict the genotype of a particular cross or breeding

Purulent Containing or flowing with pus

Pustule Elevated or raised spot filled with pus

Quarantine Place or period of detention for animals coming from infected areas; restrictions placed on entering or leaving premises or regions where cases of communicable disease are suspected

Quaternary Bonded to four other atoms, type disinfectant

Quiet, alert, and responsive (QAR) Subjective analysis of a patient's mental state

Radiograph Indirect view of the interior of a patient, produced by gamma rays

Radiology Branch of science dealing with use of X-rays, radioactive substances, and other forms of radiant energy in diagnosis and treatment of disease

Recession Loss of gingival tissue

Recessive gene The second allele that is overshadowed by the first, or dominant gene

Reciprocity Privileges granted to those from another jurisdiction

Reconstitute To restore a product to its liquid state by adding water or other aqueous solution

Recumbant To lay in a prone position, i.e., *laying on its side*

Refractometer Instrument used to determine specific gravity and total protein

Residual activity Compounds that are capable of inhibiting microbial growth that remains active long after being ingested or injected

Respirations per minute (rpm)   The number of breaths per minute

Reticulum   Second part of the ruminant stomach

Ringworm   Highly contagious fungal organism

Rostral   Directional term for locations on the head toward the nose

Rumen   First part of the ruminant stomach

Ruminant   Animal with a four-compartment stomach

Saddle thrombus   Clot that blocks off circulation to the rear of the animal, often manifests as paralysis in hind limbs

Scabies   Infested with sarcoptic mange mites

Sclera   The white part of the eye that surrounds the cornea

Secondary infection   Disease process that occurs after the patient is debilitated from another infection or a weakened immune state

Seizure   Sudden convulsion caused by an abnormal electrical discharge in the brain

Seroma   Swelling from fluid accumulating under the skin

Slough   Devitalized or dead tissue that is splitting away from the body

Species specific   Relating to a parasite that can only continue its life cycle on a specific species of animal

Sperm   Male sex cell

Sphincter   Ring of muscle that can be contracted to control flow from a body opening

Spore   One-cell reproductive unit capable of giving rise to a new individual without sexual reproduction, typically fungi and protozoa

Sporicidal   Disinfectant that destroys spores

Sprain   Overstretching of a ligament

Standing part   The long end of a rope, attached to animal or inanimate object or held still while the end is passed around it to make a knot or hitch

Sterilization   Procedure to make an inanimate object free from living microorganisms

Sternal   Body position where the patient is lying on the sternum

Sternum   Long flat bone located in the central part of the chest, connects to the ribs

Strain   Overstretching, overuse, misuse of muscle

Subcutaneous (SQ or SubQ)   Beneath the skin

Subgingival   Directional term for below gingiva

Submandibular   Beneath the bottom jaw

Sulcus   Area between free gingiva and tooth

Supragingival   Part of the tooth not surrounded by gingiva

Sympathetic nervous system   Responds in times of stress, creating the fight or flight response

Synapse   Space between neurons, where the nerve impulse passes from one nerve to another

Systemic vascular resistance   Resistance of blood flow through the vascular system

Systolic pressure   The pressure on the walls of arteries as the blood is pumped through them from the heart

Tachycardia   Rapid heart rate

Tachypnea   Rapid breathing

Telemedicine   Using technology to practice medicine at a distance

Tendon   Connective tissue that connects muscles to bones

Tertiary   Of third rank, top or third layer of a bandage

Testes   Male reproductive organs

Thorascopic   Use of small equipment to access the interior of the body

Throw   When the end is wrapped around another end or the standing part of the rope being used

Thyroid   Gland that controls the metabolism

Tissue maceration   Occurs when skin is exposed to moisture for a long period of time, skin becomes lighter in color and wrinkly

Trace minerals   Includesodium, potassium, phosphorus, magnesium, sulfur, calcium, iron, chromium, copper, zinc, iodine, manganese, and selenium

Trachea   "Windpipe" that transports air to and from the lungs

Tragi   Fleshy prominence at the front of the external opening of the ear

Transplacental   In reference to an organism or drug that can pass through the placental barrier and into a fetus

Tympanic membrane   A thick membrane that separates the middle ear from the inner ear; it vibrates in response to sound

Ungual process   The modified toe bone of ungulates that ends in a hoof, claw, or nail

Universal precautions   The measures to protect from transmission of infection from a patient or the patient's body fluids to the handler

Urinary tract infection (UTI)   Bacterial infection of the urinary bladder

Urinalysis   Chemical analysis of urine

Urination   Releasing urine

Urolith   Bladder stone

USDA Animal and Plant Health Inspection Service (APHIS)   Regulates the handling of research animals

Vaccination   Injection of microorganisms that have been rendered harmless but will still induce an immune response

Vas deferens   The spermatic vessel

Venipuncture   The act of acquiring a blood sample from a patient

Venipuncturist   The person taking a blood sample from a patient

Ventral   Directional term referring to the belly side of an animal

Ventricle   One of the lower two chambers of the heart

Venule   Small vein

Vertical ear canal   The part of the internal ear canal that runs parallel to the cheek

Vertigo   Sudden internal or external spinning sensation, circling caused by infection of the inner ear

Vestibular disease   Sudden non-progressive disturbance of balance, common in older dogs

Veterinary Practice Act   State laws regulating veterinarians and veterinary hospitals and clinics

Veterinary–client–patient relationship (VCPR)   A legal and medical relationship between the veterinarian, animal, and owner in which the veterinarian has physically examined the animal before providing treatment, surgery, or prescriptions and maintains the relationship through reexamination that occurs at least once yearly

Viricidal   Chemical agent that cause death to viruses

Virustatic   Inhibiting the growth or spread of viruses

Vital signs   Clinical measurements, specifically heart and respiratory rates, blood pressure and temperature indicating state of a patient's body functions

Vitamin   Organic molecule that is an essential micronutrient needed for proper function of metabolism

Volvulus   Twisting of the intestines or stomach

Vomitus   The material that has been vomited

Withholding time   Medication halted to allow for clearance of the drug from the body in animals that are used for meat and milk, or these animals are withheld from the market for a specific period of time after being treated with certain drugs

Zoonosis   Animal disease that is transmissible to humans

Zygote   A diploid cell resulting from the fusion of two haploid gametes; a fertilized ovum

INDEX

Page locators in **bold** indicate tables. Page locators in *italics* indicate figures. This index uses letter-by-letter alphabetization.

AAFCO *see* Association of American Feed Control Officials
AAHA *see* American Animal Hospital Association
AAVSB *see* American Association of Veterinary State Boards
abdominal palpation, restraint of animals   135, *135*
accounts receivable   45
acetaminophen   245
acute renal failure   84
ACVRA *see* American Committee of Veterinary Radiologists and Anatomists
adequacy statement   114–115
adherent bandage material   211, *211*
adhesive tape   211, *212*
adipose tissue   89
admitting patients   39
adrenal glands   88
aerobic organisms   53
age approximation   285
aggressive behaviour   124–127, *125, 126*
Ain't Doing Right (ADR)   174
air-driven dental units   288–289
AKC *see* American Kennel Club
ALARA guideline   299
alert behavior   145, *145*
alkalis   54–55
American Animal Hospital Association (AAHA)   23, 26, 302
American Association of Veterinary State Boards (AAVSB)   2, 22, 23
American Committee of Veterinary Radiologists and Anatomists (ACVRA)   301–302
American Kennel Club (AKC)   96
American Veterinary Medical Association (AVMA)   2, 3, 13, 22, 23, 26
amoxicillin   245–246, 249
ampicillin   245–246, 249
anaerobic organisms   53
anal glands   192–193, *193*
anatomical numbering system   289, 290–291, *291*
anatomy and physiology   73–89
   body systems   75
   cardiovascular system   78–81, *80*
   concepts and definitions   73–75
   dental skills   283–284, *284*
   digestive system   82–84, *83*, **83**
   endocrine system   88–89
   epithelial cells   75, *75*
   immune system   81–82
   integumentary system   88–89, *88*
   muscular system   78, *79*
   nervous system   86–88, *86–87*
   reproductive system   85–86, *85*, **86**
   respiratory system   81, *81*
   terms   74
   skeletal system   75–78, *76–77*
   urinary system   84–85, *84*
ancillary instrument packaging   267–268, *268*
anesthesia
   maintaining and operating gas anethesia machine   255–256, *255–257*
   dental skills   289
   surgery skills and maintaining an aseptic environment   270–271, *272, 277, 277, 280*
Animal and Plant Health Inspection Service (APHIS)   22, 23
Animal Welfare Act (AWA)   22–23
annoyed behavior   126–127, *127, 128*
anorexia   114, 118
ANS *see* autonomic nervous system
anthroponosis   51
antibiotic sensitivity testing   238, 240
anticoagulants   229
antiseptics   54–55, 195
anxiety   169–171, 185
APHIS *see* Animal and Plant Health Inspection Service
appendicular skeleton   75–76, *76*
appointment scheduling   35–37, **35**
Approved Veterinary Assistant (AVA)   3
areolar connective tissue   89
arrhythmias   81
arrivals   38–39
arteries   80
arthritis   78
aseptic environment   270–279
   peri-surgical phase   274–277, *276–277*
   post-surgical emergencies   279
   post-surgical phase   278–279, *278*
   pre-surgical phase   270–274, *270–275*, **274**
aspiration   118, 278
Association of American Feed Control Officials (AAFCO)   113–115
asthma   81
astringent   197
ataxia   88
atrial fibrillation   81
auscultation   176–177, *176*
autoclaves
   ancillary instrument packaging   267–268, *268*
   autoclave operation and indicator strips   258, 268–269, *269*

Tasks for the Veterinary Assistant, Fourth Edition. Teresa F. Sonsthagen.
© 2020 John Wiley & Sons, Inc. Published 2020 by John Wiley & Sons, Inc.
Companion website: www.wiley.com/go/sonsthagen/tasks

autoclaves (*cont'd*)
  cleaning for disease control   67, *67*
  dental skills   287
  folding a cloth drape   265–267, *267–268*
  folding and wrapping a gown for autoclaving   264–265, *264–265*
  instrument packs   258–264, **259–262**, *262–264*
autoclave tape   258, 264, *264*
autoimmune conditions   82
automatic dosing syringes   71, *71*, 202, *202*
automatic processors
  developing radiographic film   306, *306*
  processor maintenance   68–69, 308–309
autonomic nervous system (ANS)   78, 87
AVA *see* Approved Veterinary Assistant
AVMA *see* American Veterinary Medical Association
AWA *see* Animal Welfare Act
axial skeleton   76, *77*

bandaging *see* wound care and bandaging
basic energy requirements (BER)   115–119
bathing animals   172, 181–182, *181*
BCS *see* body conditioning score
beef cattle *see* livestock and poultry
benzalkonium chloride   54
BER *see* basic energy requirements
binocular microscopes   220–221, *220*
biologic hazards   56, 69, 234
birds
  clipping birds' wings   191–192, *192*
  hospitalized patients   169, 174
  oral medications   199
  restraint of animals   123, *123*, 143–144
bladder   78, 84
bleach   54, 59, 62
blood collection and handling   229–240
  antibiotic sensitivity testing   240
  blood chemistry and electrolyte determinations   234–235
  cleaning blood analyzers/blood chemistry machines   69, *69*
  collection of plasma and serum   229–230
  complete blood count   230–234
  equipment set-up   229–230, *229*
  packed cell volume   232–234, *233–234*
  plasma protein   234
  preparing the blood smear   231–232, *231–232*
  restraint of animals for blood sample   229
  sample collection/handling   230–234, 238–240
  serologic test kits   234
  staining protocol   219
  urine collection and urinalysis   235–238, *236–237*
blood pressure cuffs   271, *274*
boarding   170–171, *171*
body conditioning score (BCS)   178, *178*
body language
  professional conduct and foundation skills   10, *11*
  restraint of animals   124–127, *125–129*, 145–146, *145*
body systems   75
borborygmi   177
bowline   160–161, *161*
bowline on a bight   161–162, *161–162*
brain   77, *86*, 87
breeds of animals
  cat breeds   101–103, *102–103*

dog breeds   96–101, *96–101*
  pocket pets   104–107, *104–108*
Bright, Alert and Responsive   174
business managers   3

calculus   289
calipers   295, 300, *301*, 302–303
calorie requirements   112, 115–119
cannulas   66, *66*
capillary refill time (CRT)   177–178
capnography   271, *273*
caps   273–274, *275*
capture poles   139, *140*
carbohydrates   112
cardiac arrest   279
cardiac arrhythmia   279
cardiac muscle   78
cardiovascular system   78–81, *80*
carnivore   112
carriers   127, *130*, 131–132, *132*
cat breeds   101–103, *102–103*
Cat Fanciers Association   96
catheterization   206, 208–210, *208–209*, 236
CBC *see* complete blood count
CNS *see* central nervous system
cecums   112
Center for Veterinary Medicine (CVM)   22
central nervous system (CNS)   87–88, *87*
centrifuges
  blood collection and handling   233, *233*
  cleaning for disease control   69, *70*
  equipment maintenance   221–222
  parasitology   226–227
  urine collection and urinalysis   237, *237*
certificates   43–44
cervical vertebrae   76, *77*, 78
cesarean section   86
charting the oral examination   289–292
  anatomical numbering system   290–291, *291*
  charting symbols   291–292
  Triadan numbering system   289–290, *290*
chemical hazards   56
chemical test strip containers   237, *237*
CHF *see* chronic heart failure
chinchilla breeds   105–106, *108*
chlorhexidine   274
chloroxylenol   55
chronic heart failure (CHF)   81
chronic renal failure   84
chronological order format   42
cladistics   91–92, **92**, *93*
classification systems   91–110
  breeds of animals   96–106
  cat breeds   101–103, *102–103*
  cladistics   91–92, **92**, *93*
  dog breeds   96–101, *96–101*
  genetics   94–95, **94–95**
  phenotypes   92, 94
  pocket pets   104–107, *104–108*
  scientific classification of animals   91–94, **92**, *93*, **93**
  sex determination   107–109, *109–110*
  signalment terms for males, females, and offspring   **93**

cleaning for disease control   51–71
  agents   53
  antiseptics   53, 55
  ancillary instrument packaging   267–268, *268*
  assembling surgical packs   257–269
  autoclave operation and indicator strips   268–269, *269*
  autoclaves   67, *67*
  automatic dosing syringes   71, *71*
  basic cleanliness and orderliness   51–54
  blood analyzers and blood chemistry machines   69, *69*
  centrifuges   69, *70*
  cleaning   54
  cold sterilization   269–270, 314–315
  contact time   53
  crash cart   68, *68*
  disinfecting   54–55
  equipment maintenance   62–71
  facility maintenance   60–62
  folding a cloth drape   265–267, *267–268*
  folding and wrapping a gown for autoclaving   264–265, *264–265*
  gas anesthesia machine   255–256, *255–257*
  hair clippers   62–65, *62–66*
  halters, ropes, leashes, and harnesses   *70*, 71
  hazardous and non-hazardous waste   55–57, *56*
  hospital laundry   61–62
  instrument packs   258–264, **259–262**, *262–264*
  microscopes   69, *70*
  mobile veterinary units   70–71
  order of cleaning   57–60
  otoscope   66, *66*
  radiograph processors   68–69, *68*
  surgical instruments   256–257, *257–262*
  surgical room skills   252–270
  surgical table/tray   252–253, *252–253*
  techniques when caring for hospitalized animals   57–60, *58, 59*
  toenail clippers   65–66, *66*
  vacuums   66–67
cleaning staff   3
cleats   162–163
client communication   10, 279
client education   294–295
clinical techniques   189–215
  administration of medications   193–200
  clipping birds' wings   191–192, *192*
  ear cleaning and medicating   194–196, *194–196*
  emergency support   213–215, *215*
  expressing anal glands   192–193, *193*
  gastric tube   199
  injections   205–208, *205–208*
  IV fluid administration   208–210
  ophthalmic medications   200, *200–201*
  oral medications   197–200, *197–199*
  preparing vaccines   204–205, *205*
  solution bottle preparation   204, *204*
  syringes and needles   201–208, *201–208*
  toenail trimming   190–191, *190–191*
  topical medications   196–197, *197*
  wound care and bandaging   210–213
clipping birds' wings   191–192, *192*
clipping hair or fur   179–180, *180, 197*
cloth drapes   265–267, *267–268*
cloth gown   264–265

cloth wraps   258, *263*
clove hitch   164–165, *164*
cloven foot   77, *77*
cold (liquid) sterilization   269–270, 314–315
combing and brushing   179
commitment   7
communication skills
  client interactions at the facility   38–40, *38*
  day's end protocols   45
  front office skills   34, 36–37
  professional conduct and foundation skills   10–11
  surgical room   279
complete blood count (CBC)   230–234
computed radiography (CR)   298
computed tomography (CT)   298
computer skills   11–12, 40
cone muzzles   140–141, *141*
confidentiality   11–12
conjunctivitis   19
connective tissue   75, 89
conscious proprioception   88
consent forms   25, 43
constipation   172–173, *173*
constructive criticism   7–8
contact time   53
contagious patients   173
    see also quarantine
controlled drugs   244–245
cooperation   4–5
Coplin jars   219, 239
cranium   76
CR *see* computed radiography
crash cart
  cleaning for disease control   68, *68*
  clinical techniques   214–215, *215*
credible web sources   12
cross-training   3
CRT *see* capillary refill time
CT *see* computed tomography
cuff inflation   271, *273*
curettes   285, *286*
customer satisfaction   8
CVM *see* Center for Veterinary Medicine
cyanotic   81
cystocentesis   236

daily dental care   295
daily inventory control   47–48
darkroom maintenance   307–308
day's end protocols   45–46
DEA *see* Drug Enforcement Administration
debriding   210
decubitus ulcers   181–182
defecation   82
degenerative myopathy   78
dental skills   283–295
  age approximation based on dental eruption   285
  air-driven dental units   288–289
  anatomy and physiology   283–284, *284*
  assistant's role in veterinary dentistry   283
  charting the oral examination   289–292, *290–291*
  client education   294–295

dental skills (*cont'd*)
  daily dental care 295
  dental prophylaxis 289
  directional terms 284–285, *284*
  discharge 39, 295
  formulas 83, 285
  head types 285
  instruments, equipment, and maintenance 285–286, *286–287*
  intraoral radiography 293–294, *293*
  patient care and clean-up 294
  patient positioning for dental radiography 293–294
depression 170–171
dermis 88
diabetes mellitus 88
diagnostic imaging and endoscopy 297–315
  advanced imaging technologies 298–299
  cassette routine maintenance 307
  cassette selection 304
  cleaning for disease control 68–69, *68*
  cold (liquid) sterilization 314–315
  concepts and definitions 297, 310
  darkroom maintenance 307–308
  developing radiographic film 306, *306*
  digital radiography 298
  end of procedure cleaning 315
  endoscopy 310–315
  film labeling 304, *305*
  gas sterilization 314
  intraoral radiography 293–294, *293*
  measuring the anatomy with calipers 302–303
  parts of an endoscope/associated equipment 310–311, *311–313*
  patient film filing 307
  post-endoscopic procedure 312–314
  preparation for endoscopy 311–312, **313**
  processor maintenance 308–309
  quality assurance 299
  radiation safety 299–301, *299–301*
  radiography abbreviations 301–302
  radiography log 302
  radiography procedure 302
  setting exposure factors using technique charts 303
  taking a radiograph 304–305
  ultrasonography 298, 309, *309*
diarrhea 172
diet *see* feeds and feeding
digestive system 82–84, *83*, **83**
digital radiography (DR) 293, *293*, 298
dilated cardiomyopathy 81
dilutions 16–18, *17*, **17**
dipping 182
directional terms 74
discharging patients
  dental skills 295
  hospitalized patients 184
  veterinary business protocols 39–40
disinfection 53, 54–55, 252–257
distemper 88
distraction techniques 130, *130*, 148
Doctor of Veterinary Medicine (DVM) 2
dog breeds 96–101
  herding group 96, *97*
  hound group 96–97, *98*

non-sporting group 97, *98*
  sporting group 97–99, *99*
  terrier group 99–100, *100*
  toy group 101, *101*
  working group 100–101, *100*
dorsal recumbency 138, *138*
double leash technique 131, *131*
DR *see* digital radiography
drug calculation 18–19
Drug Enforcement Administration (DEA) 23, 244, 246–247
dry matter basis 115, **115**
DUDE normal 174
DVM *see* Doctor of Veterinary Medicine
dysplasia 78

ear cleaning and medicating 194–196, *194–196*
ear examination 134–135
ear protection 30, *30*
ecological niche 112
ectoparasites
  anatomy and physiology 89
  hospitalized patients 174, 180–181, *180–181*
  sampling/identification of 223–225, *223–225*
electrolyte determinations 234–235
elevators 286, *286*
elimination 168–169, 171–172, 182–183, *183*
Elizabethan collars 141–142, *142*
embryo 85
emergency stations/support 214–215, *215*, 279
encephalomyelitis 19
endocrine system 88
endoparasites
  hospitalized patients 174
  sampling/identification of 225–228, *226–228*
endoscopy 310–315
  cold (liquid) sterilization 314–315
  concepts and definitions 310
  end of procedure cleaning 315
  gas sterilization 314
  parts of an endoscope/associated equipment 310–311, *311–313*
  positioning 313
  post procedure 312–314
  preparation 311–312, **313**
endotracheal tubes
  cleaning and maintaining the surgery suite 254–255, *254–255*
  surgery skills and maintaining an aseptic environment 271, *273*, 279
enemas 172–173, *173*
enervation 88
environmental adaptations 169–171, *171*
Environmental Protection Agency (EPA) 22
epidermis 88
epithelial cells 75, *75*, 88
equipment maintenance
  autoclaves 67, *67*
  automatic dosing syringes 71, *71*
  blood analyzers and blood chemistry machines 69, *69*
  centrifuges 69, *70*, 221–222
  cold sterilization 269–270
  crash cart 68, *68*
  dental skills 285–287, *286–287*

diagnostic imaging and endoscopy   301, 307–308
endotracheal tubes   254
gas anesthesia machine   255–256, *255–257*
hair clippers   62–65, *62–66*
halters, ropes, leashes, and harnesses   *70*, 71
kennels   57–60
laryngoscopes   254
laundry   61–62
microscopes   69, *70*, 220–221
mobile veterinary units   70–71
otoscope   66, *66*
prep sink   253–254
radiograph processors   68–69, *68*
refractometers   222, *222*
sharpening hand instruments   287
stain sets   218–219
surgical instruments   256–257, *257–258*
surgical table/tray   252–253, *252–253*
toenail clippers   65–66, *66*
vacuums   66–67
essential nutrients   112
estimating   16
ethics   13
ethyl alcohol   55
euthanasia   184–186
exercise   170
expressing anal glands   192–193, *193*
eye examination   134–135, *135*

facility logs   44, **44**
facility maintenance   60–62
FARAD *see* Food Animal Residue Avoidance Databank
fats   113
FDA *see* Food and Drug Administration
fear-free techniques   122, 123–124, 126, 129–131, *129–130*
fearful behavior   123, 125–127, *125, 128*
fecal float technique   226
fecal loop   225–226, *226*
fecal matting   171–172
fecal samples   182–183, *183*
feeds and feeding   111–120
    adequacy statement   114–115
    application of basic nutrition   115–116
    calorie requirements   115–119
    concepts and definitions   112
    dry matter basis   115, **115**
    essential nutrients   112–113, **114**
    feeding guidelines   115
    hospitalized patients   117–119, 168–169, 172
    how much to feed   116–117, *116*
    learning to read labels   113, *116, 117*
    list of ingredients   114
    livestock and poultry   119–120
    pocket pets   120
    prescription diets   117, *117*
    surgical room skills   278
    understanding pet food labels   113
    water availability and consumption   112, 119
feline leukemia virus (FeLV)   51
feline lower urinary tract disease (FLUTD)   84
feline restraint bags   *70*, 71, 142, *142*
FeLV *see* feline leukemia virus

female reproductive tract   85–86, *85*
feral domestic animals   173–174
ferrets
    breeds   104, *104*
    dentition   292
    restraint of animals   *122*, 127, 131–132, 143
fetus   85
field of vision   123–124, *124, 144*
fight/flight response   *124*, 124–126
filing systems   41–42, *41*, 307
fleas   180, *180*, 223, *223*
flexibility   4–5
flies   224
fluids   206–207, *207*, 208–210, *208–209*
flukes   227, *228*
fluorescein strips   200, *201*
FLUTD *see* feline lower urinary tract disease
folding a cloth drape   265–267, *267–268*
folding and wrapping a gown for autoclaving   264–265, *264–265*
following directions   5–6
follow-up calls   45
fomites   225
Food and Drug Administration (FDA)
    feeds and feeding   113–115
    laws, regulations, policies, and standards   22
    pharmacy skills   244, 246–247
Food Animal Residue Avoidance Databank (FARAD)   22, 23
foot/hoof inspection   148–149, *149*
footwear   30, *30*
forage   119–120
force feeding   118
forceps   *259–261*, 286, *287*
formaldehyde   54–55
friendly behavior   124, *125*
front office skills   34–37
    handling non-client calls   37
    scheduling appointments   35–37, **35**
    telephone skills   34, 36–37

gallbladder   83–84, *83*
gas anesthesia machine   255–256, *255–257*, 277, *277*
gas sterilization   269, 314
gastric dilation volvulus (GDV)   84
gastric tubes   199, *199*
gastritis   84
gauntlets   142–143, *143*
gauze   211, *212*
gauze sponges   *263*, 274, *275*
GDV *see* gastric dilation volvulus
genetics   94–95, **94–95**
genotypes   94
gerbils   104–105, *106*, 143
gestation period   86, **86**
gloves   27–29, *29*
    cleaning for disease control   53
    diagnostic imaging and endoscopy   300, *300*
    restraint of animals   142–143, *143*
glutaraldehyde   55
goats *see* livestock and poultry
goggles   29, *29*
gowns   264–265, *264–265*

gram stain   218–219, 238–239
grief process   14, 186
grooming
    bathing and dipping   181–182, *181*
    clipping hair or fur   179–180, *180*
    combing and brushing   179
    hospitalized patients   179–182
    identifying ectoparasites   180–181, *180–181*
groove directors   *262*
Guaranteed Analysis   113
guinea pigs   105, *107*, 143

hair clippers   62–65, *62–66*
half hitch   163–164, *163–164*
halters, ropes, leashes, and harnesses   70, 71, 147, *147*
    see also knots and ropes
halter tie   157–158, *157–158*
hamsters   105, *106*, 143
handling shipments   48
handwashing   28–29
hanking   156, *156–157*
Hazard Communication Coordinator (HCC)   26–27
hazardous waste   55–57, *56*
HCC *see* Hazard Communication Coordinator
head types   285
health and safety *see* workplace safety
heart   78–81, *80*
heart rate   175–177, *176*
hedgehogs   292
hematocrit *see* packed cell volume
hematomas   196
heparinized saline   210
hepatic lipidosis   118
herbivore   112
herding group   96, *97*
heterozygosity   94–95
histology   75
hitches   157, 163–165, *163–164*
homozygosity   94–95
honesty   6
hookworms   227, *228*
horses
    oral medications   199
    restraint of animals   144–151, *144*, *145*, *147–149*
hospice care   184–185
hospitalized patients   167–187
    boarding   170–171, *171*
    cleaning for disease control   57–60, *58*, *59*
    collection of fecal and urine samples   182–183, *183*
    concepts and definitions   168
    constipated patients/enemas   172–173, *173*
    contagious patients   173
    discharging patients   184
    environmental considerations   169
    euthanasia   184–186
    feeds and feeding   117–119
    housing requirements/kennel set-up   168
    in-hospital grooming   179–182, *180–181*
    medical records   174
    pain evaluation and monitoring   183–184
    patient care based on reason for being there   170–176
    pocket pets and birds   174
    post mortem protocols   186
    quarantine   173–174
    recumbent patient care   171–172
    socialization and exercise   170
    surgical patients   171, *172*
    treatment plan protocols   175–179, *175–179*
    treatments and procedures   174–179
    understanding the disease process   174–175
    veterinary hospice care   184–185
    vital signs   175–178
    water and food consumption/elimination   168–169
    weight and BCS   178
hospital laundry   61–62
hot spots   89
hound group   96–97, *98*
human–animal bond   13
hurdles   *145*
hydration
    feeds and feeding   112, 119
    hospitalized patients   168–169
    intravenous fluid administration   208–210
    subcutaneous fluid administration   206–207, *207*
    surgical room skills   278
hydrogen peroxide   54, 55
hyperadrenocorticism   88
hyperthyroidism   88
hypertrophic cardiomyopathy   81
hypoadrenocorticism   88
hypodermic needles   202–203, *203*
hypodermis   88–89
hypotension   279
hypothyroidism   88
hypoxemia   279
hysterectomy   19

IACUC *see* Institutional Animal Care and Use Committee
iatrogenic injury   134
IBD *see* irritable bowel disease
idiopathic   84
ileus   84
immune system   81–82
incision site dehiscence   279
incontinence   84, 166, 172
independent working   5–6
infections
    cleaning for disease control   51–55
    clinical techniques   197
    direct/indirect transmission   51
    secondary   52
    surgical room skills   275
infusion pumps   208, *209*
inguinal lymph node   82
injections
    clinical techniques   205–208
    intramuscular injections   207–208, *207*
    intranasal infusion   208, *208*
    proper technique to hold a syringe   205, *205*
    subcutaneous fluid administration   206–207, *207*
    subcutaneous injections   206, *206*
inoculation of media   239–240, *240*
Institutional Animal Care and Use Committee (IACUC)   23
instrument packs   258–264, **259–262**, *262–264*

integumentary system   88–89, *88*
intracardial   19
intramuscular injections   207–208, *207*
intranasal infusion   208, *208*
intraoral radiography   293–294, *293*
   manual developing of dental radiographs   294
   patient positioning   293–294
intravenous fluids   208
inventory control   46–49, **46**, **47**
   daily inventory control   47–48
   handling shipments and invoices   48
   ordering supplies   48
   receiving shipments   48
   restocking shelves   48–49
invoices   48
irritable bowel disease (IBD)   84
isopropyl alcohol   55
ivermectin   246

jugular venipuncture   135, *135*

kennels/cages/runs
   cleaning for disease control   57–60, *58*, *59*
   hospitalized patients   168
   restraint of animals   132–133, *133*, *134*
kidneys   84
knots and ropes   153–165
   bowline   160–161, *161*
   bowline on a bight   161–162, *161–162*
   clove hitch   164–165, *164*
   half hitch   163–164, *163–164*
   hanking   156, *156–157*
   knot tying terminology   153–154, *154*
   overhand knot   154, *154*, 162–163, *162–163*
   preventing fraying   154–155, *155–156*
   reefer's knot   159–160, *159–160*
   sheet bend knot   160, *160*
   square knot   158–159, *158–159*
   types of hitches   157, 163–165
   types of knots   157–163
   types of ropes   154, *155*
   whipping   155, *155–156*

labels
   diagnostic imaging and endoscopy   304, *305*
   feeds and feeding   113, *116*, *117*
   pharmacy skills   245–247
   workplace safety   27, *27*, **28**
laboratory skills   217–242
   antibiotic sensitivity testing   240
   blood chemistry and electrolyte determinations   234–235
   blood collection and handling   229–240
   centrifuge technique   226–227
   complete blood count   230–231
   concepts and definitions   217
   equipment set-up   229–230, *229*
   fecal float technique   226
   inoculation of media   239–240, *240*
   log books   219–220
   maintenance of common laboratory equipment   220–222, *220*, *222*
   maintenance of stain sets   218–219
   microbiology   238–240, *240*

necropsy   240–242
   packed cell volume   232–234, *233–234*
   parasitology   223–229, *223–228*
   plasma protein   234
   preparing samples for shipment to reference laboratory   241–242
   preparing the blood smear   231–232, *231–232*
   restraint of animals   229, 235–236, *236*
   sample collection/handling   222–223, 230–234, 238–240
   sampling/identification of ectoparasites   223–225, *223–225*
   sampling/identification of endoparasites   225–228, *226–228*
   serologic test kits   235
   staining protocol   219, 237–239
   urine collection and urinalysis   235–238, *236–237*
   vaginal cytology collection   242, *242*
laryngoscopes   254, *254*
lateral recumbency   136–138, *137–138*
laundry   61–62
lavage   210
laws, regulations, policies, and standards   21–31
   agencies and their responsibilities   **22**
   common or case law   24–25, *25*
   federal laws   21–23
   guidelines of practice from veterinary organizations   26
   labeling   27, *27*, **28**
   laws and regulations for veterinary practices   21–26, **22**
   lawsuits   24, 43, 171
   local ordnances   25–26
   personal protective equipment   26, 27–31, *29–30*
   policy violations   7–8
   practice act rules and regulations   23–24
   state laws   23–24
   workplace safety   26–31
lead apron   299, *299*
lead gloves   300, *300*
lice   180–181, *180*, 224, *224*
licensing   2, 25
lifetime learning   8
ligaments   76
light–dark cycles   169
list of ingredients   114
liver   83–84, *83*
livestock and poultry
   feeds and feeding   119–120
   oral medications   199–200
   restraint of animals   144–151, *144–150*, 145, *146*, 149, *149*, 150, *150*
log books   47, 219–220
loyalty   7
luxators   286, *286*
lymphadenopathy   82
lymph nodes   82
lymphoma   82

magnetic resonance imaging (MRI)   298
malpractice   24–25, 43, 134, 246
mandible   77
masks   29, *29*, 273–274, *275*
Material Safety Data Sheets (MSDS)   26, 54, 56
maternal behavior   128, 146, *146*
math competence   14–20
maxilla   77
mechanical hazards   56, *56*

medical records
   hospitalized patients 174
   veterinary business protocols 40–45, *41*, **44**
medical terminology 19–20, **20**
medications 243–250
   classification of medications **249**, 250
   concepts and definitions 243
   controlled drugs 243–244
   explaining prescriptions to the owner 248–250
   labeling a prescription container 246–247
   prescription packaging 248
   reading a prescription 245–246
   safe handling of dispensed drugs 247–248, *248*
metabolism 112
mice breeds 104, *105*
microbiology 238–240, *240*
   antibiotic sensitivity testing 240
   inoculation of media 239–240
   stain protocol 237–239
microscopes 69, *70*, 220–221, *220*
micturition 84
minerals 113, **114**
mirrors 285
mites 225, *225*
mobile veterinary units 70–71
Model Veterinary Practice Act 2
molds 120
monitoring charts 271, *272*
monogastric stomach 82–83, *83*
mosquitoes 225
MRI *see* magnetic resonance imaging
MSDS *see* Material Safety Data Sheets
mucose membrane (MM) 177
multifunctional monitors 271–272, *273*
multiple dose syringes 202, *202*
muscle tissue 75, 78
muscular system 78, *79*
muzzles 71, 140–141, *141*
myopathy 78

nasogastric tubes 118, 199
National Association of Veterinary Technicians in America (NAVTA)
   clinical techniques 190
   laws, regulations, policies, and standards 23, 26
   professional conduct and foundation skills 2–3, 13
National Committee on Radiation Protection and Measurements (NCRP) 299
National Institutes of Health (NIH) 22
NAVTA *see* National Association of Veterinary Technicians in America
NCRP *see* National Committee on Radiation Protection and Measurements
necropsy 240–242
necrosis 84
needle holders *260*
nephrons 84
nervous behavior 125–127, *125*, *128*
nervous system 86–88, *86–87*
nervous tissue 75, 86
neurons *87*, 88
no-bite neck brace 142, *142*
noise 169
non-adherent bandage material 211, *211*

non-client calls 37
non-hazardous waste 55–57
non-sporting group 97, *98*
non-verbal communication 10, *11*
Not Doing Right (NDR) 174
nutrition *see* feeds and feeding
nystagmus 88

Occupational Safety and Health Administration (OSHA) 22, 26–31
OD *see* osteochondritis dissecans
odors 169
office personnel 3
Office of Laboratory Animal Welfare (OLAW) 22
ointments 248
omnivore 122
ophthalmic medications 200, *200–201*
ophthalmoscopes *194*
oral dosing needles 199, *199*
oral examination 134–135, *135*, 285, 287, 289–293
oral medications 197–200, *197–199*
ordering supplies 48
OSHA *see* Occupational Safety and Health Administration
osteoarthritis 78
osteochondritis 78
osteochondritis dissecans (OD) 78
osteosarcoma 78
otoscopes 66, *66*, *194*
outer coverings 29, *30*
ovariectomy hook *262*
ovaries 85
ovulation 85
overhand knot 154, *154*, 162, *163*
oxygen pressure gauge 270, *271*
oxygen tanks 270, *270*

packed cell volume (PCV) 219, 232–234, *233–234*
pain 127, 183–184
palatability 118
palpebral reflex 271
pancreas 83–84, *83*, 88
pancreatitis 84
panosteitis 78
paper filing systems 41–42, *41*
paper patient record assembly 41
parasitology
   anatomy and physiology 84
   laboratory skills 223–229, *223–228*
   sampling/identification of ectoparasites 223–225, *223–225*
   sampling/identification of endoparasites 225–228, *226–228*
parasympathetic nervous system 87
parathyroid gland 88
parturition 86
parvovirus 84
pathogens 52
pathologists 75
patient records 40–43
patient positioning 293–294, 311, **313**
Patients' Rights 192–193, 245
PCV *see* packed cell volume
penis 85
Penrose drains 210–211, *210*
perches 170–171, *171*

periodontal explorer/probe 285
peripheral nervous system 88
peristaltic waves 82
personal grooming 8–9, *9*
personal protective equipment (PPE)
   cleaning for disease control 53, 61–62
   clinical techniques 194
   dental skills 289, 293
   diagnostic imaging and endoscopy 299–300, *299–300*
   ear protection 30, *30*
   footwear 30, *30*
   gloves 27–29, *29*, 53
   goggles/safety glasses 29, *29*
   hospitalized patients 173, 181, *181*
   laws, regulations, policies, and standards 26, 27–31, *29–30*
   masks 29, *29*
   microbiology 238
   necropsy 241
   outer coverings 29, *30*
   parasitology 228
   respirators *30*, 31
   sample collection 223, 238
   surgical room skills 255, 273–274, *275*
PET *see* positron emission tomography
pet food labels 113, *116*, *117*
pharmacy skills 243–250
   classification of medications **249**, 250
   concepts and definitions 243
   controlled drugs 243–244, 245
   explaining prescriptions to the owner 248–250
   labeling a prescription container 246–247
   prescription packaging 248
   reading a prescription 245–246
   safe handling of dispensed drugs 247–248, *248*
pharyngostomy tube 118
phenols 55
phenotypes 92, 94
pheromone spray 129, *129*, 170
phlebitis 209
physiology *see* anatomy and physiology
piezo scalers 288
pigs *see* livestock and poultry
pill counting trays 247–248, *248*
pill guns 198, *198*
pill splitters 247–248, *248*
pitting edema 209
pituitary gland 88
plasma protein 234
play 170–171
plural effusion 81
pneumonia 81
pocket pets 104–107
   chinchillas 105–106, *108*
   dental skills 292
   feeds and feeding 120
   ferrets 104, *104*, *122*, 127, 131–132, 143, 292
   gerbils 104–105, *106*, 143
   guinea pigs 105, *107*, 143
   hamsters 105, *106*, 143
   hospitalized patients 174
   mice 104, *105*
   rabbits 106, *108*, 143, 292

rats 104, *104*
   restraint of animals *122*, 127, 143
policies *see* laws, regulations, policies, and standards
polishing handpieces 289
polymyositis 78
popliteal lymph nodes 82
positioning aids 300, *301*
positron emission tomography (PET) 298
post mortem protocols 186
poultices 197
povidone-iodine 55, 274
power scalers 287–288, *288*
PPE *see* personal protective equipment
practice act 23–24
prep room 253–255, *254–255*
prehension 82
prescription diets 117, *117*
presence 4
problem solving 6–7
product quality 8
professional conduct and foundation skills 1–20
   anticipation of workflow 12–13
   application of veterinary ethics 13
   basic math skills 14–19
   computer competency 11–12
   determining credible web sources 12
   determining role within a practice 1–3
   drug calculation 18–19
   effective communication skills 10–11
   estimating 16
   grief process 14
   human–animal bond 13
   medical terminology 19–20, **20**
   meeting employer expectations 4–8
   professional appearance 8–9, *9*
   use/misuse of social media 12
   volume measurements/dilutions 16–18, *17*, **17**
   weight conversion 14–16
prostate gland 85
protein 112–113
protozoans 228, *228*
pulse 175–176, *175*
punctuality 4
Punnett squares 94–95, **94–95**
pustules 89

quadrant method of streaking 239, *240*
quality assurance 299
quarantine 51, 173–174
quaternary ammonium compounds 54
Quiet, Alert and Responsive (QAR) 174

rabbits
   breeds 106, *108*
   dental skills 292
   restraint of animals 143
radiography
   abbreviations 301–302
   cassette routine maintenance 307
   cassette selection 304
   darkroom maintenance 307–308
   developing radiographic film 306, *306*

radiography (*cont'd*)
    digital and computed radiography 293, *293*, 298
    film labeling 304, *305*
    intraoral radiography 293–294, *293*
    log 301, 302
    manual developing of dental radiographs 294
    measuring the anatomy with calipers 302–303
    patient film filing 307
    patient positioning 293–294
    procedure 302
    processor maintenance 68–69, 308–309
    quality assurance 299
    radiation safety 299–301, *299–301*
    setting exposure factors using technique charts 303
    taking a radiograph 304–305
rat breeds 104, *104*
receipts 45
receiving shipments 48
reconstituting medications 248
record keeping
    chronological order or SOAP file format 42
    computerized versus paper patient records 40
    diagnostic imaging and endoscopy 301, 302, 307
    forms, certificates, and logs 43–45, **44**
    hospitalized patients 174, 175
    laboratory log books 219–220
    medical record keeping procedures 40–45, *41*, **44**
    paper filing systems 41–42, *41*
    professional conduct and foundation skills 11–12
    transferring medical records 42–43
recovery room 253–255, *254–255*
recumbent patient care 171–172
reefer's knot 159–160, *159–160*
reference laboratories 241–242
reference ranges 219
refractometers 222, *222*
regulations *see* laws, regulations, policies, and standards
relaxed behavior 126, *127*
reminder cards 45
removing sutures 279, **280**
renal failure
    acute 84
    chronic 84
reporting 7–8
reproductive system
    anatomy and physiology 85–86, *85*, **86**
    sex determination 107–109, *109–110*
respiration
    anatomy and physiology 81, *81*
    surgical room skills 271, *273*
respirators *30*, 31, *280*
responsiveness 174, 271
restocking shelves 48–49
restraint of animals 121–151
    abdominal palpation 135, *135*
    behavior assessment and safe approach 123–129, 145–146
    birds 123, *123*, 143–144
    blood collection and handling 229
    body language 124–127, *125–129*, 145–146, *145*
    companion animals 122–143
    concepts and definitions 122

    contagious patients 129
    dorsal recumbency 138, *138*
    equipment 139–143, *140–143*
    examinations, medications, and procedures 134–139, *134–140*
    eye, ear, and oral examination 134–135, *135*
    fear and pain 127
    field of vision 124, *124*, 144
    fight/flight response *124*, 124–126
    general techniques for dogs and cats 133
    injections 207
    jugular venipuncture 135, *135*
    knots and ropes 153–165
    lateral recumbency 136–138, *137–138*
    livestock and horses 144–151, *144–150*
    maternal behavior 128, 146, *146*
    patient defenses 122–123, *122–123*
    pocket animals *122*, 127, 143
    restraining and lifting large dogs 139, *139–140*
    safe movement of patients between locations 131–133, *131–134*
    sex drive 128, 146
    sternal recumbency 138–139, *138*
    territorial instincts 127–128, 146
    towel wraps 135–136, *136–137*
    urine collection and urinalysis 235–236, *236*
    utilizing fear free techniques 129–131, *129–130*
ringworm 89, 181, *181*
ropes *see* knots and ropes
roughage 119–120
roundworms 227, *227*
ruminant stomach 82–83, *83*, 112

safety glasses 29, *29*
sample collection/handling 222–223, 230–234, 238–240
sarcoptic mange/scabies *180*, 181
scalers 285–286, *286*
scalpels *261*, 276–277, *277*
scheduling appointments 35–37, **35**
scissors 209–210, *209*, 260–261, *280*
scrubs 274, *275*
secondary absorbent/cushion material 211, *212*
secondary infections 52
secondary prescription packaging 248
sedation 127
seizures 88
self-adhesive bandaging products 211, *212*
serologic test kits 235
sex determination 107–109, *109–110*
sex drive 128, 146
sharpening hand instruments 287
sharps disposal 56, *56*, 202
shaving hair or fur 172, 181, 272–274
sheep *see* livestock and poultry
sheet bend knot 160, *160*
silage 120
skeletal muscles 78
skeletal system 75–78, *76–77*
skull 77, *77*
slip leashes 131–132, *131*, 163
smooth muscles 78
SOAP file format 42, 174–175

socialization   170
social media   12
sodium hypochlorite   54
solution bottle preparation   204, *204*
SOP *see* standard operating procedures
species specific   52
sphincters   82
spore-forming organisms   53
sporting group   97–99, *99*
square knot   158–159, *158–159*
staining protocols   219, 237–239
stain sets   218–219
stanchion head gates   149, *149*
standard operating procedures (SOP)   6
standards *see* laws, regulations, policies, and standards
sterile saline   197, 210
sterilization
   cleaning for disease control   55
   cold sterilization   269–270, 314–315
   gas sterilization   314
   indicators   258
   see also autoclaves
sternal recumbency   138–139, *138*
stethoscopes   176, *176*
stocks   148, *148*
stomach   82–83, *83*
stress   112
subcutaneous fluid administration   206–207, *207*, 208–210, *208–209*
subcutaneous injections   206, *206*
subcutaneous tissue   89
submandibular lymph node   82
submissive behavior   125–126, *125*
sunshine therapy   185
supplements   120
   macrominerals   120
   microminerals   120
   vitamins   120
surgical room skills   251–281
   ancillary instrument packaging   267–268, *268*
   assembling surgical packs   257–269
   autoclave operation and indicator strips   268–269, *269*
   cleaning and maintaining the surgery suite   252–270
   client communication   279
   cold sterilization   269–270
   fields and zones   275
   folding a cloth drape   265–267, *267–268*
   folding and wrapping a gown for autoclaving   264–265, *264–265*
   gas anesthesia machine   255–256, *255–257*, 277, *277*
   hospitalized patients   171, *172*
   instrument packs   258–264, **259–262**, *262–264*
   opening an auxiliary pack   276, *276*
   opening a surgical pack   276, *276*
   peri-surgical phase   274–277, *276–277*
   positioning   274
   post-surgical emergencies   279
   post-surgical phase   278–279
   prep room/recovery room   253–255, *254–255*
   pre-surgical phase   270–274, *270–275*, **274**
   procedures and body position   **274**
   removing sutures   279, **280**
   surgery skills and maintaining an aseptic environment   270–279

surgical instruments   256–257, *257–258*
   surgical table/tray   252–253, *252–253*
surgical tables   252–253, *252*
surgical trays   253, *253*
suture needles   *262*
suture packs   276–277, *277*
suture removal   279, **280**
sympathetic nervous system   87–88
sympathy cards   45
synapses   *87*, 88
syringes and needles
   clinical techniques   198–199, 201–208
   injections   205–208, *205–208*
   multiple dose   202
   oral medications   198–199, *198*
   preparing for use   203–204
   preparing vaccines   204–205, *205*
   solution bottle preparation   204, *204*
   types   201–203, *201–203*

tapeworms   227, *228*
telephone skills   34, 36–37, 45
temperature taking   177, *177*
tendonitis   78
tendons   78
terrier group   99–100, *100*
territorial instincts   127–128, 146
testes   85, *85*
thank you cards   45
thoracic–lumbar junction (TLJ)   78
thumb forceps   *261*
thyroid collar   299, *299*
thyroid gland   88
ticks   180–181, 224, *224*
tissue adhesive   277, *277*
TLJ *see* thoracic–lumbar junction
toenail clippers/trimming   65–66, *66*, 190–191, *190–191*
tonometers   200, *201*
tooth splitters   286, *287*
topical medications   196–197, *197*
towel clamps   *259*
towel warmers   278, *278*
towel wraps   135–136, *136–137*
toy group   101, *101*
trace minerals   113
tranquilizers   127
transferring medical records   42–43
treatment plan protocols
   body conditioning score and weight   178–179, *178–179*
   capillary refill time   177–178
   collecting vital signs   175–177, *175–177*
   hospitalized patients   175–179
Triadan numbering system   289–290, *290*

ultrasonic cleaners   257, *258*
ultrasonic scalers   287–288, *288*
ultrasonography   298, 309, *309*
United States Department of Agriculture (USDA)   22–23, 44, 113
United States Equal Employment Opportunity Commission (EEOC)   22
ureter   84

urethra   85
urinalysis   85
urinary system   84–85, *84*
urinary tract infections (UTI)   84–85, *236*
urine collection and urinalysis
    hospitalized patients   182–183, *183*
    laboratory skills   235–238, *236–237*
    restraint   236
urine scalds   171–172
uroliths   84–85, *84*
USDA *see* United States Department of Agriculture
UTI *see* urinary tract infections

vaccinations
    anatomy and physiology   82
    cleaning for disease control   53
    clinical techniques   204–205, *205*
    laws, regulations, policies, and standards   25
    veterinary business protocols   43–44
vacuums   66–67
vacuum tubes   229–230
vaginal cytology collection   242, *242*
vaginal speculum   242
veins   80–81, *80*
verbal communication   10
vertebral column   77–78, *77*
vestibular disease   88
[State] Veterinary Medical Boards (VMB)   22
Veterinariae Medicinae Doctoris (VMD)   2
veterinary business protocols   33–49
    admissions   39
    arrivals   38–39
    chronological order or SOAP file format   42
    client interactions at the facility   38–40, *38*
    computerized versus paper patient records   40
    daily inventory control   47–48
    day's end protocols   45–46
    discharge   39–40
    forms, certificates, and logs   43–45, **44**
    front office skills   34–37
    handling non-client calls   37
    handling shipments and invoices   48
    inventory control   46–49, **46**, **47**
    medical record keeping procedures   40–45, *41*, **44**
    ordering supplies   48

paper filing systems   41–42, *41*
paper patient record assembly   41
receiving shipments   48
restocking shelves   48–49
scheduling appointments   35–37, **35**
telephone skills   34, 36–37, 45
transferring medical records   42–43
Veterinary Oral Health Council (VOHC)   295
Veterinary Technician National Exam (VTNE)   2, 23
viruses   53
vital signs   175–176, *175–177*
vitamins   113, 120
VMD *see* Veterinariae Medicinae Doctoris
vocalization   126–127
VOHC *see* Veterinary Oral Health Council
volume measurements   16–18, *17*, **17**
VTNE *see* Veterinary Technician National Exam

warming devices   171, *172*
waste disposal   55–57, *56*
water availability and consumption *see* hydration
web sources   12
weighing patients   178–179, *178–179*
weight conversion   14–16
welcome cards   45
wet floor warning signs   24, *25*
whipping   155, *155–156*
workflow   12–13
working group   100–101, *100*
working independently   5–6
workplace safety
    diagnostic imaging and endoscopy   299–301, *299–301*
    labeling   27, *27*, **28**
    laws, regulations, policies, and standards   24, *25*, 26–31, *29–30*
    see also cleaning for disease control; personal protective equipment
wound care and bandaging
    applying a simple bandage   211–214, *211–214*
    bandage failure   214
    clinical techniques   209–214
    preparation and drainage   210–211, *210*
    removal of bandages   209–210, *209*, 214
written communication   11

zoonotic disease   173–174, 181